Psychotherapy
and
Medication

Psychotherapy
and
Medication

A Dynamic Integration

edited by
Meri Schachter, M.D.

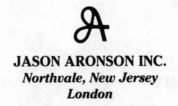

JASON ARONSON INC.
Northvale, New Jersey
London

This book was set in Cheltenham type by Lind Graphics of Upper Saddle River, New Jersey, and printed and bound by Haddon Craftsmen of Scranton, Pennsylvania.

Library of Congress Cataloging-in-Publication Data

Psychotherapy and medication : a dynamic integration / edited by Meri
  Schachter.
     p.   cm.
  Includes bibliographical references and index.
  ISBN 0-87668-296-4 (hard cover)
  1. Mental illness—Chemotherapy.   2. Psychodynamic psychotherapy.
3. Combined modality therapy.   4. Psychoanalytic Therapy—methods.
5. Psychopharmacology—methods.   I. Schachter, Meri.
  [DNLM: 1. Mental Disorders—therapy.   WM 460.6 P974735]
RC483.P7797   1993
616.89′1—dc20
DNLM/DLC
for Library of Congress   92-49162

Manufactured in the United States of America. Jason Aronson Inc. offers books and cassettes. For information and catalog write to Jason Aronson Inc., 230 Livingston Street, Northvale, New Jersey 07647.

This book is dedicated to my teachers,
Sidney S. Furst and Mortimer Ostow

Contents

Acknowledgment

The impetus for this collection of articles came from a study group on Combined Treatment I started with Anna Burton, M.D. (Past President of The New Jersey Psychoanalytic Society), in the fall of 1989. This grew into a course given at Hackensack Medical Center that we called "Introduction to the Combined Approach," which was sponsored by The New Jersey Psychoanalytic Society and The New Jersey Psychiatric Association. The specific speakers in the series were recommended by Steven Roose, M.D. The Valley Hospital Medical Librarian, Mrs. Claudia Allocco, was most helpful in obtaining the reprints. The course and the book could never have been organized without the very able assistance of my secretary, Mrs. Maxine Gottlieb.

My father, Milton Schachter, ran the family furniture manufacturing business. For the rest of us, the family business is psychiatry: my late aunt, Alexandra Schachter Symonds; her husband, Martin Symonds; my uncle, Sherman Schachter; and my brother, David M. Schachter.

Finally, my husband, Lippman Bodoff, has continually encouraged me to pursue this project with his characteristically original suggestions.

Contributors

STEVEN A. ADELMAN, M.D.
Associate Professor of Psychiatry, University of Massachusetts Medical School

ARNOLD COOPER, M.D.
Stephen P. Tobin and Arnold M. Cooper Professorship in Consultation Liaison Psychiatry, Department of Psychiatry, The New York Hospital–Cornell Medical Center.
Supervising and Training Analyst, Columbia University Psychoanalytic Center for Training and Research

PAUL M. GOLDHAMER, M.D.
Staff Psychiatrist, Mount Sinai Hospital, Toronto, Ontario
Assistant Professor, University of Toronto

THOMAS G. GUTHEIL, M.D.
Co-Director, Program in Psychiatry and the Law, Massachusetts Mental Health Center
Professor of Psychiatry, Harvard Medical School

ROBERT S. HAUSNER, M.D.
Assistant Clinical Professor, Department of Psychiatry, University of California School of Medicine, San Francisco, California
Director of Training, Mount Zion Health Systems, Psychiatric Emergency Services–Crisis Center, San Francisco, California
Attending Physician, Department of Psychiatry, Mount Zion Hospital–U.C. Medical Center, San Francisco, California

DAVID A. KAHN, M.D.
Associate Clinical Professor of Psychiatry, Columbia University College of Physicians and Surgeons

SHEPARD J. KANTOR, M.D.
New York Psychoanalytic Institute
Assistant Professor of Clinical Psychiatry, College of Physicians and Surgeons, Columbia University
Gracie Square Hospital, New York City

T. BYRAM KARASU, M.D.
Professor of Psychiatry, Albert Einstein College of Medicine

GERALD A. KLERMAN, M.D.
Professor of Psychiatry, Associate Chairman for Research, Cornell University Medical College

Dr. Klerman died on April 3, 1992.

STEVEN T. LEVY, M.D.
Professor and Chief of Psychiatry, Emory University School of Medicine at Grady Memorial Hospital
Supervising and Training Analyst, Emory University Psychoanalytic Institute

FELIX F. LOEB, JR., M.D.
Clinical Professor of Psychiatry, Oregon Health Sciences University
Member, Oregon Psychoanalytic Study Group

LORETTA R. LOEB, M.D.
Clinical Professor of Psychiatry, Oregon Health Sciences University
Member, Oregon Psychoanalytic Study Group

DONALD B. NEVINS, M.D.
Clinical Professor of Psychiatry, University of California School of Medicine, San Francisco
Faculty, San Francisco Psychoanalytic Institute

MORTIMER OSTOW, M.D.
President, Psychoanalytic Research and Development Fund
Attending Psychiatrist, Montefiore Medical Center

HAROLD W. WYLIE, JR., M.D.
Training and Supervising Analyst, Baltimore–Washington Institute for Psychoanalysis
Clinical Associate Professor of Psychiatry, Georgetown Medical School

MAVIS L. WYLIE, PH.D.
Candidate, Baltimore–Washington Institute of Psychoanalysis
Staff Psychologist, Dominion Hospital, Falls Church, Virginia

Introduction

This book is a collection of papers on the combined approach, medication and psychoanalysis or medication and psychoanalytic psychotherapy. This concept was revolutionary thirty years ago, but even today has not gained very wide acceptance.

For the educated but nonanalytic observer the profound divide between the two approaches has been both puzzling and confusing. They can see no reason for it. In addition, psychiatrists who pronounce themselves eclectic have empirically found their way to the use of medication with psychotherapy. As Klerman says, it is because in practice they have been willing to do "what works" even if it is poorly supported by research data (see Chapter 11).

In recent years the psychiatric residency programs, as if proud to find themselves finally as scientific as the rest of medicine, have been stressing biologic treatments, with the result that it is possible to find many younger psychiatrists with an encyclopedic knowledge of drug treatment who disdain psychoanalysis altogether, convinced that it is ineffective.

Lay analysts, on the other hand, proudly occupy the territory and tradition elucidated by Freud in "The Question of Lay Analysis" (1926). They have joined with Freud in declaring that psychoanalysis is the only process that works in the relief of neurotic misery. It is most interesting to read in that paper, which was an answer to Austria's anti-quackery law that decreed that only medical practitioners might treat the sick, Freud's descriptions of neurotic syndromes:

A patient, then, may be suffering from fluctuations in his moods which he cannot control, or from a sense of despondency by which his energy feels paralysed because he thinks he is incapable of doing anything properly, or from a nervous embarrassment among strangers. . . . He may one day have suffered from a distressing attack—unknown in its origin—of feelings of anxiety, and since then have been unable, without a struggle, to walk along the street alone, or to travel by train; he may perhaps have had to give up both entirely. Or, a very remarkable thing, his thoughts may go their own way and refuse to be directed by his will. . . . And when he has performed simple actions such as posting a letter or turning off a gas-jet, he finds himself a moment later doubting whether he has really done so. . . . But his state becomes intolerable if he suddenly finds he is unable to fend off the idea that he has pushed a child under the wheels of a car. [*Standard Edition*, 20:185]

Today psychopharmacologists would seize upon these patients eagerly as easily recognizable cases of dysthymia, Social Phobia, OCD, and Panic Disorder, with readily available *DSM-III-R* codes. They are satisfied with their approach, despite the fact that it is reported that the most effective drugs work no more than 60 percent of the time in OCD, for example. Here, at least, results are reported. In the intimate, private analytic setting, as Freud describes,

. . . the "analytic situation" allows of the presence of no third person. Moreover the different sessions are of very unequal value. An unauthorized listener who hit upon a chance one of them would as a rule form no useful impression; he would be in danger of not understanding what was passing between the analyst and the patient, or he would be bored. [*Standard Edition* 20:185]

Outcome studies are not done and therefore it is not possible to know what the success rate is.

The underlying assumption for the prohibition of medication in psychoanalysis has been that it would irreparably interfere with the development of the psychoanalytic process. Analysts have been concerned that patients would be so distracted by questions of dosage, side effects, timing of pill-taking, and so on, that they would be unable to concentrate on discovering unconscious processes. Or, an analysis may be brutally thrust off course by the administration of tranquilizers or antidepressants to a patient by his general physician who lacks appreciation for the lengthy struggle that is psychoanalysis.

The passage of time has, inevitably, altered the views of many in the field of psychoanalysis (see Chapter 3). There are the factors of the managed care plans, limited financial resources, and the persistent clinical challenge of patients for whom years of psychoanalytic psychotherapy has been only minimally effective. There has also been medicolegal pressure to demonstrate effectiveness of treatment.[1]

Since psychoanalysis has a long history of resisting popular trends and even villification, these factors may be dismissed by some. But the authors in this volume demonstrate with great care that it is possible to widen the scope of psychoanalysis without destroying it.

In 1940, in *An Outline of Psychoanalysis,* Freud, after 40 years of experience, described the analytic situation as follows:

---

[1]See *Osheroff* v. *Chestnut Lodge, American Journal of Psychiatry,* 1990, volume 147, pp. 409–427.

The position is like that in a civil war which has to be decided by the assistance of an ally from the outside. The analytic physician and the patient's weakened ego, basing themselves on the real external world, have to bond themselves together in a party against the enemies, the instinctual demands of the id and the conscientious demands of the super-ego. [*Standard Edition* 23:173]

Freud goes on to discuss the phenomenon of transference, cautioning the analyst to respect the patient's individuality carefully but acknowledging that a relatively undeveloped patient will require more in the way of influence. In this work, written as he began his exile in England in 1938, Freud is clearly speaking to advanced students, assuming the reader's knowledge of the process of psychoanalysis. To those of us who toil daily in the vineyard of patients' struggles against their illness (and its relief), it is striking in its concise and still current description:

We reach the conclusion that the final outcome of the struggle we have engaged in depends on *quantitative* relations—on the quota of energy we are able to mobilize in the patient to our advantage as compared with the sum of energy of the powers working against us. . . . Here we are concerned with therapy only in so far as it works by psychological means; and for the time being, we have no other. The future may teach us to exercise a direct influence, by means of particular chemical substances, on the amounts of energy and their distribution in the mental apparatus. [*Standard Edition* 23:181]

In December, 1956, Mortimer Ostow and Nathan S. Kline presented a paper at the American Psychoanalytic Association meetings entitled "The Psychic Action of Reserpine and Chlorpromazine." It was not until May 1990 that the subject of combined treatment was again included in the program at the American Psychoanalytic Association although there were discussion groups that met through the years.

The next major publication to appear on the scene, not reprinted here, was Ostow's 1962 landmark *Drugs in Psychoanalysis and Psychotherapy,* which he dedicates

to the psychiatrists of the newer generations, who will understand that a sound psychiatry must be securely based upon a sound psychology, which is the physiology of the mind; but who will not on that account neglect the study of the physiology of the brain, nor disdain to exploit it for the benefit of their patients and their science. [p. v]

As has often been true in the history of science and medicine, the aforementioned new ideas were met with reactions that ranged from indifference and derision to outrage. The implication seemed to be that psychodynamic drug therapy could only be yet another device for destroying the unique purity of analytic treatment. Psychoanalysts and analytically oriented residents in psychiatry staunchly believed as late as the 1970s that they would jeopardize their patients' future analytic success if they relieved any of their suffering chemically. Unfortunately this dictum was often applied to patients who were hospitalized or otherwise in a state of collapse.

In 1975, the Group for the Advancement of Psychiatry prepared a report entitled *Pharmacotherapy and Psychotherapy: Paradoxes, Problems and Progress,* which led to Gerald L. Klerman's paper "Combining Drugs and Psychotherapy in the Treatment of Depression" (see Chapter 11). Here, in tidy, didactic fashion, Klerman organizes the discussion of practical and therapeutic issues, effects of drug therapy on psychodynamic processes, and launches relevant discussions such as the possible positive effects of drug therapy on psychotherapy. He later remarks on a phenomenon that is increasingly important in our era of the "pure" psychopharmacologist: the effects of psychotherapy on pharmacotherapy. Throughout the chapter Klerman lists hypotheses that have been addressed in the Boston New Haven Collaborative Depression Study.

In 1977 two papers examined the pharmacotherapy of schizophrenia from a psychoanalytic perspective. Steven T. Levy, in "Countertransference Aspects of Pharmacotherapy in the Treatment of Schizophrenia" (see Chapter 12) emphasized the largely unconscious aspects of the therapeutic relationship that determine the inappropriate or untimely use of psychotropic drugs. In "Adverse Response to Neuroleptics in Schizophrenia" (see Chapter 4) Donald B. Nevins examined negative therapeutic reactions to neuroleptics in schizophrenic patients through case examples. He described those changes that affect defenses, object relations, and the symbolic significance of medication. In some situations important psychoanalytic issues emerge that may be amenable to transference interpretations.

Ostow's next publication, also not reprinted here but recommended to students of this subject, was *The Psychodynamic Approach to Drug Therapy,* which includes academic discussions of clinical pharmacology, psychoanalytic psychiatry, problems involved in the combination of pharmaceutic agents with psychotherapy or psychoanalysis, observations about a state of mental illness as illuminated by patients' response to pharmaceutic agents, and five cases presented and discussed by a distinguished panel of psychoanalysts. The book's practical orientation is completely relevant today.

Thomas G. Gutheil's 1981 article (see Chapter 1), "The Psychology of Psychopharmacology" discusses what he calls the "mind-brain barrier," which is a tendency on the part of the clinician to shift gears in a marked manner when planning the use of medication in psychotherapy. He recommends a model for the doctor–patient relationship that he calls *the pharmacotherapeutic alliance,* characterized by *participant prescribing.* This is in contrast to the presumed authoritarian attitude of the prescribing physician associated with the compliant, dependent patient's attitude. He discusses the transference implications of prescribing, both positive and negative. He refers to Shader's observations on the treatment of rejection-sensitive patients with Monamine Oxidose Inhibitors and their experience of relief as a narcissistic injury.

With sensitive attention to detail, Gutheil goes on to discuss transference to the medications themselves, including placebo side effects, such as anxiety attacks owing to fear of the medication's effects misinterpreted as an orthostatic hypotensive reaction. He refers to his previous paper about patients' responses to change in so-called drug rituals. This is the sort of material that makes pharmacotherapy so interesting and valid for the analyst. There is also an exploration of important countertransferential issues in prescribing, especially for trainees who inherit patients who are taking medicines prescribed by a departed physician.

In his paper, "Psychotherapy and Pharmacotherapy: Toward an Integrative Model" (see Chapter 2), T. Byram Karasu considers "enlightened eclecticism" to be "a utopian goal for the psychiatrist" (p. 11). He reviews the history of the therapeutic mind–body dichotomy and the resistance to the development of integrated treatment models. He regrets that ". . . when the two modalities are used in clinical practice . . . their concordance is likely to be unsystematic, incompletely understood, and empirically applied to individual cases rather than founded on controlled, preconceived conceptualization and design" (p. 15). In his thorough review of the literature, Karasu further discusses the view each side of the dispute holds of the other, such as the contention of the psychophiles that psychotropic medication is a spurious therapy. He goes on to develop a model of psychopharmacotherapy in which he states categorically that neither form of treatment has a deleterious effect upon the other. He cites studies that demonstrate the differential effects of each modality on each type of patient population. He concludes that ideally, both psychotherapy and pharmacotherapy can be effective in a total therapeutic regimen.

In 1982, Paul M. Goldhamer (see Chapter 13) could still state that the combined approach remained a neglected area of study. He discusses the polarization of the two specialties and the lack of models for psychiatrists in training, leading to "a sense of unease at deviating from orthodox procedure" (p. 217) when combined therapy is employed. Case discussions are well chosen to illustrate the benefits of combining psychotherapy and pharmacotherapy. Here too, countertransferential issues such as therapists prescribing because of a need to be active in treatment, or an inability to tolerate a patient's painful affects are well described.

Felix F. Loeb, Jr. and Loretta R. Loeb in 1983 in "Psychoanalytic Observations on the Effect of Lithium on Manic Attacks" (see Chapter 5) offer with those observations efforts to understand these changes within the context of Freud's structural model. They observed seven patients who were in analysis while being treated for mania with lithium, and report on three of them. They note that the manic episodes could be predicted by a dramatic increase in phallic sexual material. Because this preceded deterioration in ego or superego functioning they hypothesize that the manic symptoms were a response to the inability of the patients' egos to defend against these drives. This is well illustrated by detailed case presentations supported by reports of serum lithium levels. In this chapter the very rewarding possibilities of treating more severely disturbed patients by combining analytic treatment with pharmacotherapy are clearly demonstrated, in that these patients were enabled to be euthymic by the skillful blending of these therapies.

By 1984, Arnold M. Cooper was finally asking "Will Neurobiology Influence Psychoanalysis?" (see Chapter 3). He observes that this question could be phrased another way: "What does it take to change an analyst's theory?"

Cooper points out that despite the claim that psychoanalysis is only interested in the patient's construction of his infancy, nevertheless the results of investigations by Mahler and Bowlby have quietly affected both theory and practice of analysis. He further reminds us that "neurobiologic concepts are built into the core of psychoanalysis" (p. 38) and includes Freud's (1912) comment about the equal importance in etiology of constitutional and accidental factors:

"We shall estimate the share taken by constitution or experience differently in individual cases according to the stage reached by our knowledge; and we shall retain the right to modify our judgment along with changes in our understanding" (*Standard Edition* 12:99) (p. 39).

Cooper attempts to integrate research findings on anxiety with psychoanalytic theory and suggests that "a distinction must be made between psychological coping and adaptive efforts to regulate miscarried brain functions" (p. 41). He shares a clinical vignette of a patient placed on Imipramine for symptom recurrence two years after the successful termination of the analysis. He asserts that "we are alert to the issue of efficacy . . . as physicians, we welcome the most effective treatment" (p. 43) and points out that the "idea of symptom substitution has not been borne out by recent work" (p. 43). Cooper courageously observes that for the patient described earlier, pharmacologic relief might have permitted greater concentration on the conflicts. To fail to appreciate this in analytic work may actually be a cruel misunderstanding of the patient's struggle to understand what he has experienced.

Robert S. Hausner, writing in 1985, decries the lack of attention paid to the use of medication in psychoanalytic psychotherapy and examines the meaning of "Medication and Transitional Phenomena" (see Chapter 6) using Winnicott's concept. Among the illustrations is one of a placebo effect when a patient is initially given antidepressants by a consultant; because the effect was short-lived, the despondency returned and the medication trial was deemed unsuccessful. He cautions that there may be times when the medicine may seem to work to alleviate anxiety, but what may be less clear is the extent to which the effect is pharmacologic and not intrapsychic. Well-detailed cases illustrations are supplied, and countertransferential issues are addressed.

Steven A. Adelman, in "Pills as Transitional Objects" (see Chapter 7), also uses Winnicott's conceptualization of transitional phenomena in his case reports of psychopharmacotherapy with borderline patients. He starts by reviewing the literature, again dismayed by the paucity of material on combined treatment for patients who have personality disorders and affective disorders. Helpful clinical vignettes are included.

In a brief, lucid paper presented in 1986, "An Effect of Pharmacotherapy on the Psychoanalytic Process: Case Report of a Modified Analysis" (see Chapter 17) Harold W. Wylie and Mavis L. Wylie clearly demonstrate how phenelzine permitted a successful analysis in a patient previously unable to engage in the analysis of the transference.

Ostow provides specific and coherent guidance for the psychoanalytic practitioner; in "How Does Psychiatric Drug Therapy Work?" (see Chapter 8) and in his comprehensive and thoughtful "Comments on the Pathogenesis of the Borderline Disorder" (see Chapter 9) he relates the turmoil of these patients to the manic-depressive spectrum, thereby offering the possibility, for some patients, of achieving stability via sophisticated use of psychopharmacology. He also proposes a paradigm of psychic energy with which one can understand the relationship among panic disorder, anxiety, and depression, and therefore understand why antidepressants are so useful in anxiety disorders.

In his well-titled "Transference and the Beta-Adrenergic Receptor: A Case Presentation" (see Chapter 18) Shepard J. Kantor addresses the dynamics and the biology of a patient with more than one illness, and the courage necessary to work with such a patient.

In Chapter 10, "On Beginning with Patients Who Require Medication," Ostow describes how medication is useful to widen the scope of psychoanalysis. This means applying combined treatment not only to patients who are clearly depressed or psychotic, but also to those with masochistic character, anxiety, or even some cases of perversion that we would consider appropriate for classical analysis but who may also respond dramatically to antidepressant drugs. Ostow recommends distinguishing between those patients who will profit from combined treatment and those who should have either treatment alone.

Ostow observes that contrary to his expectations of thirty years ago, he has not seen medication make analysis possible or analysis eliminate the need for medication. Although analytic work does enable patients who need medication to improve their functioning and relationships, in many patients it continues to be contingent upon the control of mood with medication. Ostow takes a strong stand here in urging the analyst to prescribe the medication himself. He recalls the observations of Herman Nunberg in the 1950s that among clinicians, analysts would be the best suited to regulate medications because of their command of psychodynamics and frequent exposure to the patient's mental processes. The author supplies abundant illustrations of the analytic understanding of psychopharmacology, thereby providing guidelines for those who may be just embarking on doing combined treatment.

At the beginning of the '90s, momentum began to gather for openly discussing combined treatment. Often psychoanalysts asked consultants to medicate their patients. This process is well described in papers by Roose and Kahn.

In 1990, Dr. Steven Roose, enlisting his experience as both psychoanalyst and researcher in the pharmacology of affective disorders, considered what was then described as the increasing practice of combining pharmacological treatments with psychoanalytic psychotherapy or psychoanalysis. He refers to the early literature, which reflected a hierarchy in which analytic treatment was felt to be profound and curative and therefore best left undisturbed, whereas medications were to be considered a necessary evil when florid symptoms disrupted the analytic process. As more extensive research was done using double-blind placebo-controlled studies that clearly established the beneficial effects of medications for schizophrenia and affective disorders, in reality the use of combined treatment increased.

Roose refers to comments by Arnold Cooper and Aaron Esman suggesting that the psychoanalytic view of certain conditions might have to be called one-dimensional. He recalls Anna Freud's (Lipton 1985) comments that she was

> surprised at the almost complete rejection of drugs during psychoanalytic treatment. . . . as far as I am concerned I have had great help from medical colleagues used to the administering of modern drugs, with three patients in severe states of depression. In all of these cases the therapeutic use of drugs did not in any way interfere with the progress of the analysis, quite on the contrary it helped the analysis to maintain itself during phases when otherwise the patient might have had to be hospitalized. [p. 1583]

Roose states that the continuing controversies regarding combined treatment still have a strong influence on clinical practice, unfortunately to the detriment of patient care.

In Chapter 14, David A. Kahn reviews the literature on combined treatment, noting the ideological warfare between the opposing camps. He further defines consultation as the triadic therapeutic alliance.

Kantor, in "Depression: When Is Psychotherapy Not Enough?" (see Chapter 16) discusses approaches to a depression that occurs in the course of an ongoing psychoanalysis. He illustrates with an abundance of sharply drawn clinical vignettes the absolute requirement of a psychodynamic understanding of the meaning of medication to the patient, whether the pharmacologist is consulting or the medication is considered a parameter in the otherwise psychoanalytic treatment.

Nevins makes another contribution in "Psychoanalytic Perspectives on the Use of Medication for Mental Illness," (see Chapter 15). He includes extensive discussion of medical countertransference in an effort to explicate the difference in clinicians' readiness to medicate, and describes pharmacotherapy interventions as suggestion, manipulation, and inexact interpretation. A case report of a patient with what might today be called postpartum depression shows illustrative details of both the biological effects of the medications and their management in a dynamic treatment.

In the final chapter Kantor discusses the combined approach: "Analyzing a Rapid Cycler: Will the Transference Keep Up?" In it he describes in awe-inspiring detail his heroic medical-analytic treatment of a bipolar patient. He abundantly illustrates his firm belief that the patient required medication for her biologic disorder and psychoanalysis for her personality disorder. His generous inclusion of process notes serves very well as a guide for learning technique.

Finally, at this moment in history, whether the treatment is called psychoanalysis, psychoanalytic psychotherapy, or psychotherapy, there should no longer remain any rational objection to giving patients whatever treatment they need in whatever combination rather than vowing allegiance to any given modality, thereby sentencing patients to a choice of procrustean beds.

This may mean that it will be necessary to offer courses in psychopharmacology at the psychoanalytic institutes, so that medical and nonmedical candidates alike may be able to learn together what is possible in treatment when the biological and intellectual are integrated. Dedicated clinicians are always most concerned with the well-being of patients.

References

Freud, S. (1958). The dynamics of transference. *Standard Edition* 12:97–109.

_____ (1926). The question of lay analysis. *Standard Edition* 20:179–258.

_____ (1940). An outline of psychoanalysis. *Standard Edition* 23:141–208.

Group for the Advancement of Psychiatry (1975). Pharmacotherapy and psychotherapy: paradoxes, problems and progress, vol. 9, report no. 98, March.

Lipton, M. A. (1985). Editorial: a letter from Anna Freud. *American Journal of Psychiatry* 140:1583–1584, 1983.

Osheroff v. *Chestnut Lodge* (1990). *American Journal of Psychiatry* 147:409–427.

Ostow, M. (1962). *Drugs in Psychoanalysis and Psychotherapy.* New York: Basic Books.

_____ (1979). *The Psychodynamic Approach to Drug Therapy.* Riverdale, NY: The Psychoanalytic Research and Development Fund.

Ostow, M., and Kline, N. S. (1959). The psychic action of reserpine and chlorpromazine. In *Psychopharmacology Frontiers*, pp. 481–513. New York: Basic Books.

Roose, S. (1990). The use of medication in combination with psychoanalytic psychotherapy or psychoanalysis. In *Psychiatry*, ed. R. Michels, vol. 1, pp. 1–8. Philadelphia: Lippincott.

PART I
Analysis of the Resistance to Combined Treatment

1

The Psychology of
Psychopharmacology

THOMAS G. GUTHEIL, M.D.

Despite Freud's appreciation of the biologic role in human experience, there has been a polarization between the psychotherapists and the practitioners of somatic therapies. The author describes the "mind–brain barrier" experienced by clinicians when they prescribe medication and develop an authoritarian attitude. They may develop "the delusion of precision" about the treatment they espouse. The author recommends a pharmacotherapeutic alliance characterized by participant prescribing. This alliance is obviously affected by the transference, positive and negative. One unique aspect is the transference to the medications themselves, such as placebo effects, placebo side effects, and reactions to drug ritual changes. Countertransference issues abound.

In 1960, Menninger and colleagues wrote a seminal article, "The Prescription of Treatment," in which they argued that when prescribing a patient's total treatment, physicians should use medications in conjunction with other forms of treatment, such as pharmacotherapy, psychotherapy, activity therapy, and manipulation of the environment. I agree with their thesis, but I approach the subject from a somewhat different perspective. I believe that psychopharmacology has a psychology of its own, which can be best understood when certain basic principles from psychotherapy are applied.

Freud (1940) struck the keynote to the concept of relating the psychotherapies and the pharmacotherapies when he stated, "The future may teach us to exercise a direct influence, by means of particular chemical substances, on the amounts of energy and their distribution in the mental apparatus. It may be that there are other still undreamt-of possibilities of therapy" (p. 182).

Although Freud entertained no prejudices about the biologic role in human experience and pathology, subsequent generations have failed to share his eclecticism. There has been a polarization between practitioners of the somatic therapies, on the one hand, and of the psychotherapies on the other. Expanding upon this point, The Group for the Advancement of Psychiatry (GAP) Committee on Research (1975) reports that "to a considerable extent, physicians who have been exposed to the theory and practice of psychotherapy and also of pharmacotherapy behave like a split-brain preparation" (p. 272).

I have encountered a similar phenomenon, which I call the "mind–brain barrier"—a tendency on the part of clinicians to "shift gears" in a marked manner when contemplating the use of medications in a psychotherapeutic context. I believe this mind–brain barrier can best be penetrated by exploring the psychotherapeutic aspects of pharmacotherapy and that the best way to accomplish this task is to examine the doctor-patient relationship. According to the GAP report:

> Presumably the prescription of medications promoted an authoritarian attitude on the part of the psychiatrist and enhanced his belief in his biological-medical heritage, while at the same time, the patient would become more dependent, place more reliance on magical thinking, and assume a more passive, compliant role, as is expected in the conventional doctor-patient relationship in fields of medicine other than psychiatry. [pp. 339–340]

One of the temptations toward an authoritarian posture that is inherent in the process of prescribing is to view medication as having the virtues of concreteness, specificity, precision, and straightforwardness—a point of view that I (Gutheil 1977) have termed "the delusion of precision." The same physicians who adopt a receptive, open posture toward their patients' verbal productions may take a rigid, prescriptive stance in relation to drugs, offering direct and specific suggestions, even commands, which they would energetically eschew in the psychotherapeutic interaction.

The physician's authoritarian posture finds its complement in the patient's posture of compliance (the term usually used to refer to the patient's role in pharmacotherapy). I (Gutheil 1978, Gutheil and Havens 1979) have suggested that the appropriate model for the doctor–patient relationship in regard to the prescription of medications is a specialized version of the therapeutic alliance. I referred to this form of alliance as the *pharmacotherapeutic alliance,* characterized by *participant prescribing.* These terms refer to the manner in which active efforts are made by the physician to enlist, recruit, and involve patients in a collaboration with him, a collaboration "involving shared inquiry, shared goals, and mutual participation in both experiencing and observing the process" (Gutheil 1978, p. 219) of using medication. In a discussion of this point, Irwin (1974) notes,

> by making the patient a partner in treatment, the doctor emphasizes and reinforces the patient's strengths as a person instead of his weaknesses in a

dependent, sick role, thus, opening the door for more flexible, appropriate, responsive, and responsible drug therapy. [p. 9]

This desired pharmacotherapeutic alliance, like the treatment process in psychotherapy, is frequently strained and intruded upon by phenomena derived from transference aspects of the relationship. The central point at issue here is the fact that in the process of prescribing, the physician may become the target of transference distortions of his role and intentions, either by prescribing or by not prescribing medication. In either case, the transference may be positive or negative, a point often missed in discussions of this subject. Patients may establish a positive transference with the physician who prescribes medications and see him as giving, responsive, empathetic, and validating. Patients are sensitively attuned to these dimensions, a point captured by the patient who says, "Look, if you really thought I was sick (or really wanted to help me), you would be giving me medication." With this remark, the patient links the prescription of medication to the physician's perceived responsiveness and the seriousness with which he views the patient.

The opposite side of the coin—a negative transference view of the physician who prescribes medication—is less commonly understood. One of my patients expressed his negative transference by saying, "When my previous therapist took out his prescription pad, I knew I could never tell him anything important" (Gutheil 1977). In this connection, Ostow (1979) comments that some patients view the introduction of drug therapy as degrading and interpret it to mean that they are more seriously ill than they want to believe. Also, patients who believe the psychotherapies are somehow the higher or purer forms of the healing arts may view medication as second-rate treatment. For every patient who perceives the prescription of medication as a validation of his distress, there exists another patient who sees the prescription as a dismissal of himself and his suffering. As Blackwell (1973) points out, "Too often a prescription signals the end of an interview rather than the start of an alliance" (p. 252).

Trainees often find it difficult to grasp the paradoxical relationship between the giving of medication by the physician and the feeling of being deprived of valued experiences by the patient. A clear example of this phenomenon is the manic-depressive patient who views the medication (quite correctly, of course) as attacking the mania and, by extension, promoting depression. Similarly, a patient may have negative feelings toward medication if he perceives it as attacking pleasurable, gratifying, or valued symptoms, such as grandiose delusions (Van Putten et al. 1976). Another valued aspect that may be threatened by medication is the patient's "sick role," a role that can result in secondary gain or affect the patient's posture in his family.

Shader[1] notes a peculiar set of circumstances in which "rejection-sensitive patients" experience receiving medications as a narcissistic injury. If such

---

[1]R. I. Shader. Personal communication, 1980.

patients respond well to monoamine oxidase inhibitors, they may discover that they can tolerate rejections that used to cause them considerable dysphoria, distress, and decompensation. Once these patients experience a decrease in symptomatology, they realize that the medication and not the "self" was central to their improvement. That this awareness is experienced as an overwhelming narcissistic injury is supported by observations of what happens to these patients when medication is discontinued.

The physician who does not prescribe medication, either by failing to broach the subject spontaneously or by refusing to prescribe when specifically asked to do so by the patient or by others, may be the subject of positive transference views. The patient can experience his doctor's unwillingness to prescribe medications as a refusal to be distracted from the patient as a person, or as a vote of confidence in the patient and the psychotherapeutic process. Also, a patient may request medication when not really wanting it, merely to see if the physician will make certain emerging issues "go away" before the patient has to experience the conflict of bringing the material into the arena of therapeutic scrutiny.

The failure to prescribe medication may produce negative transference responses as well. In general, patients view the absence of drug prescribing as a type of withholding, with all the attendant overtones, including sadism, lack of caring, and unwillingness to respond or help. Some patients may see the absence of drug prescribing as reflecting negatively on the seriousness and genuineness of their distress, or experience it as a tacit accusation of exaggeration of the degree of illness or outright malingering.

In summary, to prescribe or not to prescribe may evoke in patients positive or negative transference views of the physician. These experiences may relate to the medication's effects but may also be utterly independent of the specific pharmacologic indications, contraindications, or pharmacologic effects of the medication.

In considering the psychology of psychopharmacology, however, an aspect of transference unique to the pharmacotherapies is encountered—transference to the medications themselves. Some people may object to the term *transference* because they believe it is not precisely applicable in this context. However, in using this term, I am incorporating a number of psychic mechanisms, including fantasies, displacements, and symbolizations.

One dimension of the transference to medication that has been extensively described by Shapiro (1966) is the placebo or placebo-related effect—a positive response that is inexplicable either by the actual effects of the medication or by the medication's pharmacokinetics. Placebo effects that act in the desired direction of the medication usually go unchallenged, since questioning them serves no useful purpose. In a drug refusal study, Appelbaum and I (Gutheil 1980) believe we encountered placebo side effects, a much more complex situation. One of the most interesting was an apparent orthostatic hypotensive reaction to a medication known to produce this response as a side effect. Further exploration, however, revealed that the ostensible hypotensive reaction was actually an anxiety attack, based on fear of what the medication's effect would be.

A second dimension of transference to medications relates to drug administration, that is, scheduling, dosage, and the actual form of medication (e.g., pills, capsules). Burgoyne (1976) concludes that patients with schizophrenia are relatively unaffected by changes in what he calls drug rituals, a term describing the concrete parameters of drug administration. However, in a study of drug refusal performed by Appelbaum and myself (Gutheil 1980), we found that a significant number of drug ritual changes had immediate effects on the patients' responses to taking medications. In one case, for example, a patient experienced both decompensation and recompensation around mere discussion of the change in medication, with no actual pharmacologic alteration occurring.

Another case in which a change in the drug ritual had an effect on the patient's response involved a man who suffered from severe chronic schizophrenia. He was given his normal medication, but for the first time, the tablet bore the letters "M.S.D." The patient believed that these letters indicated the medication was analogous to LSD, and he refused to take the suspected hallucinogen. However, he complied readily when his usual brand was reinstituted.

For some patients, medications take on human attributes. This phenomenon is reflected in the case of a male patient with paranoid schizophrenia who began to worry about his homosexual feelings toward his male resident. He complained of somatic sensations, which he attributed to his medication. On exploration, the patient asked, "Why is it that medications are always named after people, like Stella, Thor, and Mo?" The resident inquired about Moban, the medication that the patient was at that time to receive. The patient replied that he felt this was a "male medication," and he believed that "Mo" was inclined to hurt him. He requested a change to "Stella-zine." In this example, the patient's difficulty in the transference to the physician and his paranoid concerns about homosexual attachments were expressed and played out in personifications of the medications.

Another dimension of the patient's transference to the medication rests upon the special form of symbolization alluded to in the last clinical example, that is, personification of the medication. I have indicated elsewhere (Gutheil 1977) that it is possible for the physician to experience the medication as a personified intruder into the therapeutic relationship, "as a rival competitor for control of the patient's positive response, or for efficacy over the patient, as a force acting to take the patient away by making him better" (p. 91). In a similar manner, both patient and physician can use prescribing medication to avoid difficult issues, just as patients may refer to friends as a distraction, or physicians may refer to treatment staff members with a similar intent.

On inpatient services, this phenomenon may be particularly noticeable. For example, when a psychiatrist serves as the medical backup, "the physician may regard . . . [prescribing medication] as the last bastion of authority, the last fortress of uncontested decision making. . . . At worst, physician–staff conflicts may be fought out through the patient's drug regimen" (Vasile and Gutheil 1979, p. 1293).

In the inpatient milieu, the struggles among treatment staff may involve medication. For example, the medical backup may insist on medicating the patient (and occasionally overmedicating the patient) because of unconscious, competitive strivings aimed at devaluing the nonpharmacological psychotherapeutic work of the other members of the treatment team. The reverse situation also applies whereby the nonphysician psychotherapists resist using medication because they fear the invasion of their territory.

Another phenomenon characteristic of inpatient psychiatry occurs because the training program schedule in teaching hospitals results in an annual turnover of resident physicians. In these settings, medication assumes a number of transference-related dimensions by virtue of its specific association with the physician who has his name on both the prescription and the medicine bottle label. The patient is capable of developing an intense attachment to the medication, which he perceives as the embodiment of the departing doctor. This intense relationship may communicate itself to the newly arrived physician, who is now responsible for that same patient's care, and this awareness of these relationships may evoke powerfully rivalrous feelings toward these medications as the "ghost of the departed one." Thus, for some patients, the drug regimen becomes a souvenir—perhaps the only concrete souvenir—of the lost object (Gutheil 1977). Often during the beginning of the training year, the physician and the patient embark upon a struggle about medication. The trainee usually initiates this struggle by discontinuing all the patient's medication. In attempting to rationalize this action, the trainee claims that he needs to "see how the patient does without the medication," or to "evaluate the patient, starting from scratch," or to "reassess whether this patient really needs the medication that he is on." Faced with this planned renovation and distressed at the attempted displacement of the loved object, the patient may energetically resist such "disrespect to the departed" (Gutheil 1977).

In addition, medication and its prescription may enter into countertransference in a variety of ways. The sexual and/or aggressive elements of the patient–physician relationship and the associated conflicts around them may be acted out both in prescribing and nonprescribing actions. The countertransference may express itself not only in gross matters of giving or withholding but in less obvious ways involving the therapist's wish to contain, localize, or disavow the conflicted countertransference issues through medicating the patient (Levy 1977). Struggles around various forms of regressive gratifications of authoritarian control, power, and helplessness may similarly be played out via the medication regimen.

A colleague of mine noted that "telling a doctor his pills aren't working is like telling a mother her baby is ugly." This comment captures the manner in which the doctor may be deeply identified with the medication that he prescribes. One specific area of considerable difficulty, especially for the trainee, is the discussion of sexuality in relation to prescribing medication. For example, many of the phenothiazines, especially the piperidine derivatives, tend to produce retrograde ejaculation, apparently through a reversal of urethral peristalsis. In patients with paranoid trends, the absence of external ejaculate when masturbating can be enormously demoralizing, threatening, and may evoke homosexual panic. All too often patients assume that because this potential side effect is not spelled out by the novice prescriber, any effects that may result are both intentional and expected. While both patient and physician struggle with the same cultural taboos against candor about human sexuality, the fact that the doctor's medication is causing this symptom in the patient makes the entire matter more difficult to discuss from the physician's viewpoint because of conflicts around sadism and castration anxiety. Interestingly enough, an unexpected response to this side effect occurred in the case of a young male with schizo-affective schizophrenia who specifically preferred Mellaril because of its effect of retrograde ejaculation. This patient's personality organization featured powerful obsessive-compulsive trends, and the absence of ejaculate on masturbation suited perfectly the patient's preference for everything to be neat and clean. The absence of "mess" was not threatening but gratifying.

In the supervision process, I recommend that a systematic, routine inquiry be made into the patient's eating, eliminating, sleeping, and sexual functions. The patient should be asked about each of these items, and any changes that the patient reports should be explored. Asking about these issues at regular intervals tends to make both patient and physician more comfortable in discussing these difficult subjects.

An alteration in libido might be a side effect of most of the medications that are used to treat psychosis. This phenomenon is particularly evident in regard to the use of lithium in mania (Fitzgerald 1972). Demers and Davis (1971) point out that in a marriage in which one spouse has manic-depressive illness, their sexual relationship may be predicated on the maintenance of that person's mania. Thus, the normalization of the manic mood swings through the use of lithium produces stress upon the marriage.

Linn (1964) gives two examples of sexual conflict stemming from the successful effects of medication. In one case, the patient believed the relief of anxiety obtained from a minor tranquilizer made him vulnerable to homosexual attack. Another patient with frightening sexual fantasies "compared the effect of the drug to the cutting of the wires to a fire alarm. 'The clamor of the fire alarm is silenced, but the fire goes on unabated and nobody is warning me to fight it' " (p. 141). This example gives new meaning to the concept of "signal anxiety" and the possible undesired consequences of its alleviation.

Another aspect of difficult countertransference manifestations involves money. Havens (1968) points out that "for patients marginally employed, the cost [of medications] may be prohibitive. . . . Many people would rather be sick than poor, or at least they would be willing to be less than healthy if they could remain relatively wealthy—something doctors seldom understand" (p. 44).

Resolutions of difficulties in this area are frequently based on whether the doctor is free to explore conflicted material in a manner that recruits the patient's collaboration. By exploring and discussing with the patient the virtues of generic medications or the rationale for prescribing nongeneric medications, when such may be indicated, the physician demonstrates that he has the patient's interests, broadly speaking, at heart. This attention to the cost to the patient may be remarkably effective in cementing the alliance between the two. Establishing such an alliance, as I have stressed throughout this article, is the key to effective pharmacotherapy.

References

Applebaum, P. S., and Gutheil, T. G. (1980). Drug refusal: the study of psychiatric inpatients. *American Journal of Psychiatry* 137:340–346.

Blackwell, B. (1973). Drug therapy: patient compliance. *New England Journal of Medicine* 289:249–252.

Burgoyne, R. W. (1976). Effect of drug ritual changes on schizophrenic patients. *American Journal of Psychiatry* 133:284–289.

Demers, R. G., and Davis, L. S. (1971). The influence of prophylactic lithium treatment on the marital adjustment of manic-depressives and their spouses. *Comprehensive Psychiatry* 12:348–353.

Freud, S. (1940). An outline of psycho-analysis. *Standard Edition* 23:144–207, 1964.

Fitzgerald, R. G. (1972). Mania as a message: treatment with family therapy and lithium carbonate. *American Journal of Psychotherapy* 26:547–554.

Group for the Advancement of Psychiatry (1975). *Pharmacotherapy and Psychotherapy: Paradoxes, Problems and Progress.* Vol. 9, Rep. No. 93. New York: Group for the Advancement of Psychiatry.

Gutheil, T. G. (1977). Improving patient compliance: psychodynamics in drug prescribing. *Drug Therapy* 7:82–83, 87, 89–91, 95.

―――― (1978). Drug therapy: alliance and compliance. *Psychosomatics* 19:219–225.

Gutheil, T. G., and Havens, L. L. (1979). The therapeutic alliance: contemporary meanings and confusions. *International Review of Psycho-Analysis* 6:467–481.

Havens, L. L. (1968). Some difficulties in giving schizophrenic and borderline patients medication. *Psychiatry* 31:44–50.

Irwin, S. (1974). How to prescribe psychoactive drugs. *Bulletin of the Menninger Clinic* 38:1–13.

Levy, S. T. (1977). Countertransference aspects of pharmacotherapy in the treatment of schizophrenia. *International Journal of Psychoanalytic Psychotherapy* 6:15–30.

Linn, L. (1964). The use of drugs in psychotherapy. *Psychiatric Quarterly* 38:138–148.

Menninger, K., Pruyser, P., Mayman, M., and Houston, M. (1960). The prescription of treatment. *Bulletin of the Menninger Clinic* 24:217–249.

Ostow, M., ed. (1979). *The Psychodynamic Approach to Drug Therapy.* New York: Psychoanalytic Research and Development Fund.

Shapiro, A. K. (1966). Semantics of the placebo. *Psychiatric Quarterly* 42:653–695.

Van Putten, T., Crumpton, E., and Yale, C. (1976). Drug refusal in schizophrenia and the wish to be crazy. *Archives of General Psychiatry* 33:1443–1446.

Vasile, R. G., and Gutheil, T. G. (1979). The psychiatrist as medical backup: ambiguity in the delegation of clinical responsibility. *American Journal of Psychiatry* 136:1292–1296.

2

Toward an Integrative Model

T. BYRAM KARASU, M.D.

The author reviews historical trends, hypotheses, and problems in the application of pharmacotherapy and psychotherapy and uses research findings to develop an integrative model. He portrays a chronology of models over three decades; an "additive" relationship represents the decade of 1970 to 1980. He presents factors that must be considered in determining the effects of pharmacotherapy plus psychotherapy and recommends refinement of these variables in future research.

The rapid proliferation of assorted treatments for mental illness has increasingly enhanced the alternatives for alleviation of man's symptoms and suffering. Meeting the growing need for enlightened eclecticism in psychiatry, however—which means approaching each clinical situation from multiple theoretical perspectives and selecting those which are in closest accord with an individual patient's needs—is as yet a Utopian goal for the psychiatrist (Yager 1977). Rather, the positive potential of various practices and the integration of concurrent treatments are usually undermined by partisan, competitive, and conflicting credos and claims in behalf of one modality over another. This polarization has characterized the internal arena of the psychotherapies (Parloff 1975) as well as the broader spectrum of psychological versus somatic therapies (Van Praag 1972), whether the latter has encompassed physical, biologic, chemical, or neurophysiologic forms of treatment such as electroconvulsive therapy (ECT), psychosurgery, sleep deprivation, biofeedback, or pharmacotherapy. Separatist tendencies and fragmentation of the field have occurred throughout the history of psychiatry and are largely reflective of a complex evolution of disparate belief systems, social trends, and hidden biases about the nature of man, the origin of his psychopathology, and how he can be healed (Ehrenwald 1966, Lazare 1973, Karasu 1977).

The splitting of "pharmacotherapy" and "psychotherapy" in particular has become a chronic (albeit changing) characterization of the field of psychiatry to the present day. This is a product of several forces, including limited vision on the part of pharmacotherapists and psychotherapists (Linn 1964). The resilience and reification of this split may be considered symptomatic of a longstanding legacy in psychiatry—the post-Cartesian mind–body dichotomy that still resides at the core of modern medicine (Miller et al. 1978).

A major manifestation has been the alternating ascent and fall of each of the ostensibly opposing sides of the mind–body hyphen at selected times in psychiatry's history. Thus the field in Freud's day was preoccupied with cerebral pathology and changes in the soma of the brain; it was not until the 1940s and 1950s that there was a dramatic change toward dynamic conceptualizations of etiology and treatment. The primacy of the "mind" was ultimately expressed in the psychoanalytic approach. This trend was partially preempted in the late 1930s and 1940s, when the use of insulin coma, ECT, and, to a lesser extent, psychosurgery provided the first efficacious physical treatments of mental pathology. Subsequently, at the turn of the half-century, the advent of major psychotropic drugs marked the dawn of modern pharmacotherapy; this meant the precipitation anew of an important trend in favor of biological psychiatry, its "second heyday" (Van Praag 1972) since Virchow's cellular pathology.

The 1960s also brought the beginnings of the judicious use of drugs into psychoanalytic circles (Ostow 1962, Sarwer-Foner 1960), which had long been resistant to such practices. However, Freud's own view of the potential of pharmacotherapy was more open and optimistic than that of many of his analytic followers. In 1938 he anticipated, "The future may teach us to exercise a direct influence, by means of particular chemical substances, on the amounts of energy and their distribution in the mental apparatus. It may be that there are other still undreamt-of possibilities of therapy" (Freud 1938). Along with proliferating pharmacologic advances, of simultaneous significance in the 1960s were major hospital reforms, the ascendancy of social and community psychiatry, increased application of outpatient and maintenance treatments, short-term therapies, and experimentation with new methods of psychological, social, and behavioral intervention. These have often served to both balance and confound the "mind-body" score: it is difficult to discern to what extent each set of factors has been responsible for radical changes that have occurred in length of hospital stay and patient improvement. Today the two modalities—psychotherapy and pharmacotherapy—each a hallmark of the decade of the 1970s, coexist in great profusion and diversity as pervasive influences on the mental health field.

The Special Nature of the Problem

Ironically, there has been both tremendous need for and, at the same time, great resistance to the development of integrated treatment models for pharmacotherapy and psychotherapy. The overall paucity of guidelines for their conjoint use (simultaneous, intermittent, or sequential) has been created and compounded by a host of interrelated ideological, administrative, moral, scientific, and clinical factors and their manifestations. These include the following:

1. Deeply rooted conceptual antagonisms inherent in developing a comprehensive psychobiological view, including conflicting organic (e.g., neurochemical) versus psychogenic (e.g., psychodynamic or psychosocial) orientations toward the etiology of mental illness and goals of treatment (Group for the Advancement of Psychiatry 1975, Van Praag 1979).

2. The reinforcement of these concepts by parochialism, rigid cultism, overallegiance to one's own affiliation (Halleck 1978), and deficient training and learning experiences, especially insufficient or biased information implicitly transmitted through selective curriculum and prejudicial faculty attitudes and practices (Grinker 1964, Gottlieb 1978, Klerman 1965).

3. Lack of resources or availability of institutions administratively, economically, or practically able to offer broad exposure or extensive experience with a diversity of modalities (Lesse 1980).

4. Ethical and regulatory barriers to psychopharmacological investigation and treatment. These encompass external factors of societal biases and lack of public and institutional endorsement and internal issues regarding the morality and pragmatics of informed consent, patient participation, and staff support (Cole 1977, Gallant 1978). An antiresearch climate in the last decade and the rising emphasis on patient rights have resulted in social pressures against treatment studies, especially research on drug therapy. Public pressures and concerns about patient coercion, possible misuses of treatment, or irreversible toxic effects, for example, have led recently to the abandonment of several proposed investigations despite the fact that they met all federal and local institutional requirements. Some feel that current Department of Health and Human Services regulations present inherent regulatory difficulties by requiring a "disinterested" institutional review board composed of unpaid citizen members and by constructing a multilevel review process not subject to appeal, which increases the chances of bureaucratic delays and vetoes (Gallant 1978). In addition, medical and psychological treatments are objects of substantial legal constraints, including complex legislation, administrative regulation, and malpractice litigation. Greater sensitivity to ethical precepts and advocacy pursuits has therefore meant an increased need to reconcile and balance the competing interests of civil libertarians and legislators. It has also heightened staff differences between scientists and clinicians when well-designed research comes into basic ethical conflict with individualized treatment and the establishment of the relationship between therapist and patient. Such ethical and regulatory problems are perhaps most manifest in the issue of informed consent, which some feel is a major barrier to psychopharmacological research (Cole 1977, Gallant 1978). Ample evidence suggests that giving complete information to the patient and obtaining his or her full informed consent may not only influence and possibly invalidate study results but seriously threaten the conduct of the entire

investigation (Gallant 1978). Others (Cole 1977) suggest that the very patients who need better therapies the most (e.g., treatment-resistant chronic schizophrenic patients, those with senile dementia, or those with marked behavioral disturbances) are often the least able to give informed consent at all. The appointment of legal guardians for such patients may solve the legal issue, but not necessarily the ethical one, by presumably protecting patients' "rights" but at the same time denying them any chance to benefit from the investigation of new therapies and their combinations.

5. Methodologic, diagnostic, and statistical problems involved in complex research with drug and psychosocial environments (Halleck 1978, Lesse 1978, Marholin 1976, May 1968, May and Goldberg 1978, Overall 1969, Reich 1975, Schooler 1978). These include, first, the special scientific difficulties in arriving at stringent statements about the respective efficacy of either drugs alone (Morris and Beck 1976) or psychotherapy alone (Luborsky et al. 1971, Malan 1973) as necessary prerequisite controls for studies of their combined effects (Klerman 1976). In addition, problems exist in the complexities of multivariate design; criteria of outcome, diagnoses, and definitions; differential attrition; patient noncompliance; and generalizability limitations deriving from the application of data from heterogeneous populations to individual patients, or from research wards to natural clinical settings (Fisher 1976, Gillum 1974, Gunderson 1977, Halleck 1978, May 1968, Schooler 1978). Ultimately, there is a lack of definitive data for establishing interactive effects that combine subjective experiences with objective behaviors or psychodynamic insights with the biochemical actions of drugs (Docherty et al. 1977).

6. Clinical constraints, including characterologic limitations of the therapist's personality and suitability for the practice of combined treatments (Lesse 1980). In addition, therapeutic dangers during treatment, like misinterpreting drug side effects as psychological phenomena or defensively turning to drugs at difficult points in psychotherapy, have been noted (Barondes 1966). Others have pointed out interpersonal misunderstandings of communication between physician and patient specific to joint treatment (Havens 1963), especially the basic problem of "bimodal relatedness" in the physician–patient relationship (Docherty et al. 1977). Here the differing interpersonal modes of pharmacotherapist and psychotherapist, respectively, result in inappropriate emphasis and alternation or substitution between relating to the patient as a diseased organ or object of study (i.e., "subject-object" mode) and as a disturbed person (i.e., "subject–subject" mode). These incompatible modes of functioning place a special strain on the psychopharmacotherapist, who must safeguard and maintain a delicate balance between the two interpersonal approaches in clinical practice, despite the host of extrinsic and intrinsic forces that act to exaggerate one or the other in a setting of combined treatment. In addition to this pressing problem for the therapist, the imbalance of approaches might have a direct antitherapeutic impact on the patients themselves.

When the two modalities are used in clinical practice, therefore, their concordance is likely to be unsystematic, incompletely understood, and empirically applied to individual cases rather than founded on controlled, preconceived conceptualization and design. The gap between the researcher and the clinician has also been compounded by the parallel problem that broadly generalizable results based on large, heterogeneous groups may not be of clinical use with the individual patient (Downing and Rickels 1978). Thus, as clinical considerations have followed along the falsely frozen conceptual lines and unresolved research lines between drug treatment and psychotherapy, additional or alternative therapies to one's own experience and expertise have often become relegated to secondary positions in the total treatment armamentarium. Not only have psychotherapists been resistant to the use of drugs, but drug advocates have been skeptical about the value of verbal, psychodynamic, or psychosocial methods. A major implication of this phenomenon is that adherence to one or another conceptual or clinical frame of reference often fails to be in close concordance with evidence about comparative (or nondifferential) therapeutic efficacy of various treatment approaches (Halleck 1978, Luborsky et al. 1976).

In 1975 the Group for the Advancement of Psychiatry (GAP) addressed these issues in its report of pharmacotherapy and psychotherapy's "paradoxes, problems, and progress" (1975), a comprehensive summary encompassing all major diagnostic entities. This paper, based on my survey of research studies of the decade 1970–1980 (unpublished 1981 manuscript), draws on the GAP material and represents an update of the subject. As such, it especially reflects the most current directions of work in this area—the broadened application (and success) of both treatments, the newest thrust of research on major depression, the greater concentration on outpatient samples and follow-up studies, the enlarged spectrum of therapeutic modalities (e.g., cognitive-behavioral techniques), and, ultimately, the increasing specificity of application of these two major treatment interventions based on refinements in our knowledge of the interactive variables.

Differential Efficacy and Therapeutic Process

A major pivot point on which the ambiguity and ambivalence of combined treatment turn has been the critical issue of psychotherapy's and pharmacotherapy's separate efficacies and the inextricable question of what relative role each modality reciprocally plays in a conjoint treatment regimen. In brief, the evidence for both the prevention of relapse by antipsychotic drugs in schizophrenia and lithium prophylaxis in affective disorders has been considered by some to be unequivocal (Davis 1975, 1976). The efficacy of psychosocial treatments in the 1970s has also been found to be increasingly positive even for major disorders (Mosher and Keith 1979), despite Eysenck's pessimistic report on psychotherapy of three decades ago (Eysenck 1952). However, psychotherapy is still more ambiguous and vulnerable to scientific scrutiny than the pharmacotherapies (Gunderson 1978, Klein 1980). Beyond their separate efficacies, there still remain the dual enigmas of the natural course of some mental diseases and spontaneous remission over time without either, indeed any, treatment (Eysenck 1965, GAP 1975) and, conversely, the very negative outcomes that occur with the best of modern-day treatments (Harrow et al. 1978).

Thus, naturally subject to dispute depending on which side of the therapeutic fence a clinician is on, the pharmacophile often places the psychotherapy function in an elective position, useful essentially as ameliorative treatment. In essence, this particular stance of drug advocacy is said to view psychological intervention as "rehabilitative" but not therapeutically curative (Overall and Tupin 1969). The contention here is that psychotherapies do not operate on fundamental mechanisms residing at the core of the disease process, but they can correct related difficulties in interpersonal relations, self-esteem, and psychological problems secondary to the impact of the symptoms per se. Alternatively, the psychophile may contend that drug treatment can serve to alleviate the major symptoms or mood of the patient without substantially altering his or her underlying clinical state or dynamic status (Ostow 1979). In such instances psychotropic medication may be falsely claimed to be a spurious therapy, a kind of anesthesia that effaces the "true" causes of the psychopathology (Van Praag 1979).

Simultaneously, pharmacotherapists frequently extol the "prophylactic" properties of certain psychotropic drugs because they can prevent relapse, especially in acute or exacerbating states (Davis J. M. 1976a,b). But their critics still raise the knotty problem of whether antipsychotic drugs do or do not prevent recidivism (Tobias and MacDonald 1974). They have also challenged symptom prophylaxis as the unilateral criterion of drug efficacy, viewing it as an insufficient basis for extensive use of drugs in the light of the following:

1. Serious and often irreversible toxic effects or negative symptoms, such as extrapyramidal disorders (predominantly tardive dyskinesia), anhedonia, social isolation, depression, and amotivational syndromes, which may make the pharmacologic cure even worse than the disease (Carpenter et al. 1977, Gardos and Cole 1976);

2. Equivocal hospital readmission rates and/or quality of adjustment of nonrelapsed patients who are taking standard drug doses compared with those taking low doses or placebo (Engelhardt and Freedman 1969, Hogarty et al. 1974);

3. A lack of ample long-term follow-up studies to determine how much pathology is sufficient to justify drug continuance and a lack of clinically useful research evidence on the natural course of the disease without treatment (Carpenter et al. 1977, Davis 1975, 1976a); and even

4. As serendipitously suggested from a 5-year follow-up study, the prolongation of the social dependency of discharged patients who take drugs (Bockoven and Solomon 1975).

Thus, for those involved in the dark dilemma of how to interpret drug efficacy figures (e.g., how to explain the less than 60 percent nonrelapse rate to the over 40 percent relapse rate of patients given drugs), which has been likened to the philosophical question of whether the glass is half-full or half-empty (Gardos and Cole 1978), greater attention to a balanced risk–benefit ratio is urged (Gardos and Cole 1976, Rifkin et al. 1976). It has been suggested that further studies should review both agent and dose strategies so that short- and long-term toxicities can be better known (Rifkin et al. 1976). It is also recommended that social and community measures be added to behavioral and pharmacological ones in the complex problem of drug evaluation (Gardos and Cole 1976, Watt 1975). This means a broadened vision that includes not only the likelihood of patient relapse following drug withdrawal but the total impact of withdrawal on the patient's interpersonal, economic, and familial life. It includes consideration of whether one is at most providing some protection against future recurrences, yet failing to offer a positive therapeutic agent that will continue to enhance improvement. Comparably, incorporation of a risk–benefit ratio for psychotherapy might weight differently in the total psychopharmacotherapy balance—less manifest risk in terms of observable toxicity or danger, but also less tangible or immediate effects. The latter factor is reflected in those findings which took timing (as well as multiple outcomes) into account; they suggested that the results of psychotherapy may not only be of a different order than the effects of pharmacotherapy but emerge at a later time (Grinspoon and Shader 1975, Klerman 1975, Weissman et al. 1974, Weissman et al. 1976). Thus the efficacy question is inextricably bound to issues of outcome criteria and latency, which have yet to be elucidated.

Aside from the question of efficacy, the vicissitudes in the therapeutic process of these two large and complex domains—the psychotherapeutic and the psychopharmacologic—are far from clear. That is, controversy still exists not only with regard to outcome (e.g., if, when, for whom, and to what extent each works) but with regard to mode of action (i.e., how each works) (Davis 1976, Frank 1974). This refers to the degree of specificity versus nonspecificity of their respective therapeutic ingredients, including the symbolic meaning of treatment, the place of positive expectations, the influence of historical, psychological, and social variables, the role of the physician–patient relationship, and the overall so-called placebo effect (Downing and Rickels 1978, Lesse 1964, Uhlenhuth et al. 1970). It has been amply pointed out that even with therapies with known specific effects, there is always some degree of placebo reaction, and it is usually quite difficult to differentiate between the contributions of both in a given therapy. It is even more difficult to evaluate to what degree one type of reaction is present as compared with the other (Lesse 1964). For example, there is still much controversy over "what is psychotherapy" (Lesse 1964, Strupp 1970, 1973, 1974, 1975, Tseng and McDermott 1975). The unique nature of the interpersonal relationship between therapist and patient and its centrality for cure is generally recognized as substantially different from the traditional physician–patient relationship in medicine. In psychotherapy the special relationship established may be the crucial therapeutic agent. Nonetheless, the nature of the psychological influence exerted by the professional therapist may not be intrinsically different from that exerted by others influencing the patient (Strupp 1973). In this regard, data have suggested that the patient–physician relationship may override, even reverse, the expected effects of drugs (Wolf 1965) and that the more intense the relationship, the more obscure the differences between drug and placebo, because the latter effects are enhanced and the former ones are depressed (Rickels and Cattell 1969). According to considerable research, however, the nonspecific influence in drug therapy is not as pervasive as previously thought (Fisher 1970). By contrast, in the light of common elements that can be found to occur across all psychotherapeutic modalities (Frank 1974, Strupp 1974), the reverse may be true for psychotherapy.

Interactive Effects of Psychotherapy and Pharmacotherapy

A variety of positive and negative effects of drugs and psychotherapy on each other have been postulated (GAP 1975, Klerman 1975, 1976, Lehmann 1967, Linn 1964, Rioch 1958, Sarwer-Foner 1957, 1960). Only rarely, however, have broad classificatory models been posed for the results of the two interventions when combined (Klerman 1963, Uhlenhuth et al. 1969).

Negative effects of drugs on psychotherapy have included the possibility that they may have deleterious effects on psychotherapeutic expectations because their introduction often relegates the patient to unsuitability for insight, that their easily accomplished reduction of anxiety or symptoms may become a motive for discontinuing psychotherapy owing to a decreased desire to work toward more difficult characterologic change, that drug treatment merely produces state-dependent learning that is not transferable to nondrug situations, and that there may be negative placebo effects or nonpharmacologic countertherapeutic reactions to the pill-taking experience itself (Klerman 1975). Emphasizing the highly subjective nature of drug response by patients in psychoanalysis, others have warned against sudden anxiety crisis, thought disorder, or increased depression in patients threatened by the passivity resulting from potent tranquilizers and the fact that patients with somatic fears might be thrown into a state of acute panic due to body image alterations resulting from the side effects of psychotropic drugs (Sarwer-Foner 1957, 1960).

An assumption of high potency pervades the above positions. Many feel that because physical therapies can bring about rapid, observable changes that require little or no active participation on the part of the patient, he or she is likely to view them as the sole initiator of change. As a negative consequence, the patient may develop a passive outlook toward therapy in general and be less motivated to engage in nondrug treatments. Others have expressed concerns that the patient receiving drug treatment loses his or her sense of autonomy, that drugs become a crutch leading to the fear of functioning without reliance on external aides, and that the concurrent use of drug therapy attenuates the power and meaning of the individual psychotherapeutic relationship (Halleck 1978). More in line with psychodynamic orthodoxy, still others have suggested that the introduction of drugs to the analytic situation necessarily introduces artifacts that confound the therapeutic transference; that drugs reduce the ability to respond affectively to psychotherapy explorations (Semrad and Klerman 1966); that they unwittingly mask feelings necessary for the resolution of conflicts and undercut the need to "suffer" through the reeliciting of repressed events (Linn 1964); and, alternatively (concordant with the thinking of authors like Laing and Perls), that drugs prevent the patient from participating fully in the psychotic experience itself (May and Goldberg 1978).

Positive effects of pharmacotherapy on psychotherapy include the possible role of drugs as "facilitators" to psychological functioning required for participation in psychotherapy (for example, the inducement of abreactive effects); reduction of discomfort, which may help to promote accessibility and communication; and positive placebo effects from pill-taking per se (Klerman 1975, 1976). Sarwer-Foner (1957, 1960) has suggested in this regard that some patients may perceive drugs as a welcome protection against overwhelming aggressive or sexual impulses. Rioch (1958) observed that drug therapies during psychotherapy serve to facilitate the development of different types of identification (that is, transference) with the therapist, which would enhance or impede treatment depending on the kind of pharmacologic agent.

Postulated effects of psychotherapy on drug action have generally been of less concern. The beliefs here are that psychotherapy's input is irrelevant because drugs alone will serve as "biochemical replacement" for the respective deficiencies or excesses of psychiatric illness; that psychotherapy largely serves an ameliorative function secondary to the effects of drugs; or, more potently (and negatively), that psychotherapy may disrupt pharmacologic relief by uncovering areas of conflict which countertherapeutically serve to increase anxiety and symptoms (Klerman 1975, 1976). It has also been more positively suggested that psychotherapy in conjunction with pharmacotherapy may serve to enhance drug compliance (Schooler 1978). This was evidenced in investigations of Hogarty and his associates (1976), which serendipitously suggested that social therapy could function to reinforce medication taking.

Theoretical Models of Combined Treatment

In light of the range of possibilities of positive and negative interdigitation between the two interventions, it is understandable that few models have been posed for the theoretical effects of psychotherapy and pharmacotherapy when combined (Klerman 1963, Uhlenhuth et al. 1969). Klerman (1963) originally hypothesized five models directly concerned with the interface between the social (hospital) milieu and the influence of psychiatric drug treatment:

1. Drug effects are independent of the milieu (drug effects are similar in all milieus);
2. Drug effects are augmented by the milieu (drug and milieu factors combine additively so that the drug is more effective in the better milieu);
3. Drug and milieu factors bear a reciprocal relationship (in the maximally effective milieu, drug effects are not important, but in the poor milieu they are important);
4. There are negative interactions between drug and milieu factors (drug effects are detrimental to the particular environment); and
5. There are negative interactions between placebo and psychotherapy factors (the mere giving of a pill hinders the patient's psychotherapy progress).

Klerman concluded that evidence was insufficient for making any definitive choice among these five models of drug–milieu interaction.

In another attempt at delineating psychotherapy and pharmacotherapy, Uhlenhuth and associates (1969) proposed four nonindependent models:

1. Addition (the effect of the two interventions combined equals the sum of their individual effects);
2. Potentiation (the effect of the combined interventions is greater than the sum of their individual effects);
3. Inhibition (the combination is less than the sum of the individual effects); and
4. Reciprocation (the combination equals the individual effect of the more potent intervention).

As defined, the order of maximal to minimal effects would be potentiation, addition, reciprocation, inhibition, with the former two reflecting different degrees of positive interaction, the latter two different degrees of negative interaction. Uhlenhuth and associates applied these models to their review of research on combined treatment in the 1950s and 1960s. They concluded that there was minimal or no evidence for either potentiation or inhibition effects, minor evidence for additive effects, and that a reciprocal model (in the sense that one modality could replace the other) was the prototype for the interaction between psychotherapy and pharmacotherapy. That is, the combined effects of pharmacotherapy and psychotherapy were no better than the effects of pharmacotherapy alone. Specifically, out of nineteen relatively well-controlled studies, none was inhibitive, one was potentiating, three were additive, and ten were reciprocal. Interpreted somewhat differently, four showed positive interaction and ten negative interaction. But in a later research review Luborsky and his associates (1976) analyzed comparable findings somewhat differently and less stringently, thus favoring a more positive additive model. Specifically, they found that two treatments were better than one in 69 percent of the comparisons (eighteen out of twenty-six), two treatments were equal to one approximately 25 percent of the time, and one treatment was never better than two treatments.

Although the above proposed models have been globally useful in the quantitative analysis of research results, there are limitations even at this broad level of generalization. The categories are not mutually exclusive, nor do they cover all contingencies, and the two sets of definitions have not been consistent in name or application (e.g., Uhlenhuth's definition of "reciprocal" was narrower and more negative than Klerman's, which suggests more of a "seesaw" effect; although the term "additive" theoretically refers to joint treatment as the sum of both treatments, in practice it has been more loosely applied when joint treatment is simply better than either treatment alone).

Van Praag's later analysis favoring combined treatment (1979) suggested that in principle the therapy of psychiatric disorders can take place through two complementary channels: an attempt can be made to normalize the disturbed brain functions (the cerebral substrate of the psychiatric disorder) with the aid of pills ("tablets"); simultaneously, the pathogenic input from the individual's inner world and his environment may be attenuated, or possibly eliminated, with psychotherapy ("talking"). This notion is based on the thesis that "every disorder of behavior has its neurochemical substrate, which in turn can have been induced by (among others) psychogenic and psychosocial factors" (Van Praag 1979). More specifically, Klerman (1976) analyzed the advantages of combined treatment into two basic forms: (1) "facilitation of psychotherapeutic accessibility" and (2) "two-stage treatment strategy." The former reflected the hypothesis that there is a direct relationship between psychotherapeutic accessibility and symptomatic distress (i.e., when the patient is not sufficiently distressed or, in counterpoint to that, if there is too much anxiety or too many symptoms, he will not be accessible to psychosocial influence). The major function of pharmacotherapy here would be to assist the patient in reaching the ideal level of stress, calibrated toward maximal accessibility of the patient to psychological intervention. Such "facilitation of psychotherapeutic accessibility" is the interactive hypothesis most supported by Klerman's research study (1975). The second combined treatment form reflected the thesis that drugs can be useful initially in treatment to reduce disturbance or excitation in order to assist the patient in the early or acute phase of illness. Psychotherapy would be initiated for maximal effect at a later stage for supportive purposes and establishing a relationship. Aside from their consecutive effectiveness and usefulness at different stages of treatment, each could thereby address different targets or goals—the symptomatic, then the interpersonal.

A Model of Psychopharmacotherapy for the Future

In an attempt to derive a model of psychotherapy and pharmacotherapy, certain consistent trends may be considered as characteristic of the current decade in relation to previous decades (see Table 2–1 and Figure 2–1). First, on the broadest level, a chronological order emerges: different prototypal combined treatment models can be recognized as one traverses the course of treatment over time. In the decade of the 1950s, when the psychoanalytic study of the neuroses prevailed, the swing of the psychotherapy–pharmacotherapy pendulum resided primarily on the psychotherapeutic side. Here a model in favor of psychotherapy may be said to have applied, with drug treatment considered as inhibitory or, at best, superfluous. Subsequently, in the decade of the 1960s, with the advent of psychotropic drugs as a major treatment modality for chronically ill, hospitalized schizophrenic patients—usually combined with group therapy as a psychosocial, supportive intervention—the swing of the psychotherapy–pharmacotherapy pendulum shifted to the pharmacotherapeutic end. Here a reciprocal model (using Uhlenhuth's definition) still applied, but with a bias in favor of drug treatment; psychotherapy was considered inconsequential or, at best, adjunctive. Later still, in the decade of the 1970s, especially in the latter years, with an increasing focus of attention on affective disorders—especially major depression—and on new cognitive-behavioral formats, the swing of the psychotherapy–pharmacotherapy pendulum started to settle toward center. Here an additive model may be said to apply: both modalities are being given relatively equal weight in the treatment process. It is this model which resides on the threshold of the 1980s (see Table 2–1). This additive trend may reflect more flexible thinking as well as a reaction to research evidence. May (1976), for example, whose previous findings have strongly supported the efficacy of pharmacotherapy, has warned that they should not be interpreted as meaning that all schizophrenic patients should receive antipsychotic drugs or that other forms of treatment are unnecessary. He expressly cautioned against doctrinaire attitudes and staunchly advocated thoughtful adjustment of goals and methods to meet the needs of the various individuals and situations involved in treatment.

TABLE 2–1. Major Trends in Psychotherapy and Pharmacotherapy Models and Modalities Over Three Decades

Decade	Prototypal Model	Diagnostic Focus	Type of Drug	Type of Psychotherapy
1950–1959	Reciprocal (bias toward psychotherapy)	Neurosis (anxiety)	Antianxiety	Individual psychoanalytic
1960–1969	Reciprocal (bias toward pharmacotherapy)	Schizophrenia	Antipsychotic	Psychosocial supportive
1970–1979	Additive (psychotherapy and pharmacotherapy)	Depression	Antidepressant	Interpersonal behavioral

Model	Reciprocal	Additive	Reciprocal
Modality	Pharmacotherapy		Psychotherapy
Diagnosis and Subtypes		SCHIZOPHRENIA	
	Acute hospitalized		Chronic outpatient
		AFFECTIVE DISORDERS	
	Major depression (endogenous) Mania		Minor depression Reactive (nonendogenous)
		NEUROSES	
	Panic attacks (agoraphobia) Endogenous anxiety		(Nondepressive) Object phobia (simple) Reactive anxiety
Type of illness	"State" disorders (psychoses, severe depression, and anxiety)		"Trait" disorders (neuroses, character disorders)
Duration	Time-limited		Long-lasting
Origin	Genetic or biological		Social or learned
Severity	Severe or major		Mild or minor
Chronicity	Acute or prophylactic		Chronic
Goal	Symptomatic relief		Interpersonal adjustment
Latency	Early stages of treatment		Later stages of treatment
Process	Facilitation of accessibility		Therapeutic relationship established

FIGURE 2–1. Factors Toward a Model of Pharmacotherapy and Psychotherapy

Second, in elaboration of the above, my findings for the decade 1970–1980 have confirmed earlier findings for the preceding decade (Uhlenhuth et al. 1969), where there were virtually no or minimal inhibitory effects of either treatment on the other. In particular, the fears of the orthodox psychoanalyst that drug treatment would interfere with the vicissitudes of the therapeutic transference or reduce patient motivation remain essentially unfounded. Nor does the introduction of psychotherapy to a drug regimen serve to undermine the effects of the latter. Beyond this, there appears to be less evidence for the reciprocal model with a bias toward pharmacotherapy (which characterized the research results of 1960–1969, and which may have been in part an artifact of the type of populations studied). Concurrently, there is greater evidence in the evolution of combined treatment for additive or potentiating effects: each modality plays a variable, albeit differential role in the total regimen. This is most true for the affective disorders, including both acute and chronic depression, but it may yet apply to other diagnostic subgroups as well.

Third, the establishment of models of psychotherapy and pharmacotherapy is beginning to be formed along certain diagnostic lines (see Figure 2–1). Basic are the prototypal reciprocal model with a bias toward pharmacotherapy for schizophrenia, according to which the efficacy of drugs alone may be equal to (or better than) combined treatment; the reciprocal model with a bias toward psychotherapy for the nondepressive neuroses and character disorders, in which the efficacy of psychotherapy alone may be equal to combined treatment; and the additive model (pharmacotherapy plus psychotherapy) for affective disorders, in which combined treatment is deemed better than either treatment alone. In addition, other related or more specific diagnostic factors have been implicated as guidelines for establishing the model of best fit in the combined treatment of mental disorders. The type of illness, rather than the diagnostic category per se, may be one such variable. In this regard, Extein and Bowers (1979) have suggested that "state" disorders, encompassing all psychoses—schizophrenia, depression, and mania—as well as severe anxiety, are amenable to pharmacotherapy, whereas "trait" disorders, encompassing neuroses and character disorders, are most amenable to psychotherapy. Supporting variables here would be the duration of the illness (time-limited disorders would be most treatable by pharmacotherapy and long-lasting ones by psychotherapeutic modalities) and the origin of the illness (those disorders whose etiology suggests genetic or biological vulnerability are best treated by pharmacologic means and those whose etiology suggests social or learned factors are best treated by psychological means) (White et al. 1977).

Others have posed a clinical continuum for pharmacotherapy and psychotherapy according to severity of illness (Zitrin et al. 1978): severe or major depression would require maximal pharmacotherapy relative to psychotherapy and mild or minor depression would require increasingly less. Comparably, it has been suggested that the chronicity of the illness and, bearing on this, the basic setting in which it is treated influence the therapeutic effectiveness of the modality. For example, Schooler (1978), who organized combined treatment studies of schizophrenia on the basis of "newly hospitalized," "chronic hospitalized," and "chronic outpatient" populations, found that the closer to the latter end of the spectrum the patient was, the better the relative results with psychotherapeutic approaches. Alternatively, inpatient acutely ill populations fared best with drug treatments. Much more specifically, Zitrin and associates (1978), working with phobic neuroses, found significant differences in response to treatments between simple phobic and agoraphobic or mixed phobic diagnostic subtypes.

Apart from diagnostic types and subtypes, other factors with implications for treatment also appear to reside on a pharmacotherapy–psychotherapy continuum. These include consideration of outcome criteria or goals of treatment (Claghorn et al. 1974, DiMascio et al. 1979, Friedman 1975, Grinspoon and Shader 1975, Hogarty and Goldberg 1973, Hogarty et al. 1979, Linn et al. 1979, May 1968, Weissman et al. 1976), the duration or stage of treatment (Davis et al. 1972, DiMascio et al. 1979, Friedman 1975, Grinspoon and Shader 1975, Hogarty and Goldberg 1973, Hogarty et al. 1976, 1979, Karon and Vandenbos 1970, Klerman 1975, Linn et al. 1979, Paul et al. 1972, Podobnikar 1971, Sheehan et al. 1980, Weissman et al. 1976, Zitrin et al. 1976, 1980), and the major therapeutic processes involved (Klerman 1975). For example, a variety of research studies revealed the importance of the particular outcome criteria in favoring one or the other treatment modality. In his now classic study of schizophrenic inpatients, May (1968) found that combined treatment or drugs alone were most effective, especially when time and cost were included in the outcome criteria. When relapse was the primary criterion, drugs alone were favored, and when insight was the goal, psychotherapy was favored. In a similar vein, the work of Weissman and her associates on combined treatment of neurotic depression (1976) suggested that drugs were effective in reducing relapse rates and preventing symptom return, whereas psychotherapy served to improve the social adjustment of patients who did not relapse. More specifically, drugs affected vegetative symptoms like sleep disorders, somatic complaints, and lack of appetite, whereas psychotherapy affected suicidal ideation, work, and interests (DiMascio et al. 1979). In addition, differential duration of effectiveness was reflected in these (and similar) findings that drug effects occurred early in treatment, often within the first week, whereas psychotherapy effects occurred later, at approximately 1 to 2 months (DiMascio et al. 1979).

In brief, one could use research results to form a combined treatment model of pharmacotherapy and psychotherapy based not only on diagnostic groups or subgroups but also on the goals and stages in the treatment process. In the development of such a model, concordant with the "two-stage treatment strategy" (Klerman 1976), one could apply the data that pharmacotherapy fared best for relief and remission of symptoms, whereas psychotherapy appeared to be best when the goals of therapy included interpersonal and social adjustment, family relationships, and work performance. In addition, relief and remission of symptoms tended to occur relatively quickly and were perhaps best accomplished when drugs were administered during acute stages at the onset of the study. The effects of psychotherapy often took longer to emerge. Psychotherapy, therefore, was best instituted, it appeared, during longer term therapy and/or at the latter stages of the treatment regimen. Klerman (1976) suggested that pharmacotherapy might be used to set the stage for the establishment of a therapeutic relationship by facilitating accessibility to the therapist and the therapeutic process. Psychotherapeutic modalities might be best applied after the patient's acute symptoms have abated and a therapeutic relationship between patient and therapist is possible.

In total, the diagnostic considerations in combined treatment could be substantiated by data suggesting that pharmacotherapy and psychotherapy selectively tap different disorders or different subgroups of the same disorder. The goal, length of treatment, and process considerations could be based on data suggesting that pharmacotherapy and psychotherapy, in addition to the above, influence different manifestations of the same disorder and occur at different latencies and durations along the varied course of illness and treatment.

The above-mentioned variables (e.g., diagnosis or subtype of disorder, criteria for outcome, duration or stage of treatment) are only a few of the important factors that may influence the ultimate model of combined treatment with pharmacotherapy and psychotherapy. Research studies have also implicated a variety of drug, psychotherapy, therapist, and patient variables that may also be crucial to the effects of the two modalities and their interaction. According to a review of the research of 1970–1980, these include the following:

1. Drug variables—the type of drug (Grinspoon et al. 1972, Lipman and Covi 1976, Sheehan et al. 1980, and Lesse 1980), dose (Paul et al. 1972), frequency of administration (Podobnikar 1971), route of administration (oral or depot) (Hogarty et al. 1979), and who regulates its intake (doctor or patient) (Chien 1975);

2. Psychotherapy variables—the type of psychotherapy (Davenport et al. 1977, Friedman 1975, Rush et al. 1977, Zitrin et al. 1980) and degree of contact (Covi et al. 1979);

3. Therapist variables—his or her type (A or B) (Grinspoon et al. 1972) and level of experience (Karon and Vandenbos 1970);

4. Patient variables—premorbid adjustment (Goldstein et al. 1978) and gender (Goldstein et al. 1978, Hogarty et al. 1976); and

5. Setting variables—the type of clinic (Lipman and Covi 1976) or day treatment center (Linn et al. 1979).

More specifically, several studies that used different drugs in combination with psychotherapy suggested that combined effects often depended on the particular drug. In a study of combined treatment of affective disorders comparing phenelzine plus group therapy with imipramine plus group therapy (Sheehan 1980), the former combination produced significantly better outcomes. In another combined treatment format using diazepam versus imipramine plus group therapy (Lipman and Covi 1976), the imipramine–group-therapy combination was significantly superior in reducing symptoms and improving interpersonal perceptions, whereas diazepam proved no better than placebo. Similarly, in combined treatment of acute schizophrenia, thioridazine plus individual psychotherapy produced significantly better outcomes than haloperidol plus individual psychotherapy, which was no better than placebo (Grinspoon et al. 1972). In addition, other drug factors of differential dose, frequency of administration, and route of administration proved significant. Patients who received higher or more frequent doses of chlordiazepoxide (Gottlieb et al. 1978), patients who were given long-acting fluphenazine decanoate (Hogarty et al. 1979), and patients who received physician-regulated continuous medication (Chien 1975) did better than patients given lower doses, those given shorter-acting drugs (i.e., oral fluphenazine hydrochloride), and those taking irregular doses (i.e., patient-regulated), respectively. The complexity of the drug variable in combined treatment was additionally highlighted in the study of regular doses versus intermittent doses by the fact that successful patients who regulated their own doses received less than half the dose of successful patients whose doctors regulated their doses (Chien 1975).

The differential effects of the psychotherapy variable emerged first in controlled studies revealing that the particular type of psychotherapy significantly affected outcome (Zitrin et al. 1980) or was attributed by the researchers themselves to be relevant to treatment effects (Davenport et al. 1977, Friedman 1975, Rush et al. 1977). In a study of women with phobic neuroses, patients receiving group exposure in vivo plus drug or placebo showed significantly more improvement than those who received the same drug plus behavioral therapy with imaginal desensitization (at least at the midpoint of treatment) (Zitrin et al. 1980). In a study of outpatients with chronic unipolar depression, Rush and associates (1977) attributed the greater improvement found with psychotherapy than drugs to the special form of psychotherapy offered (i.e., cognitive therapy). In the combined treatment of married manic patients with lithium and couples therapy, the finding of no rehospitalizations, marital failures, or suicides in the combined treatment group (which did not occur with lithium alone or community care alone) was attributed to the marital psychotherapy format (Davenport et al. 1977). Other studies of combined treatment that explored the psychotherapy variable suggested that the factor of greater therapist experience was significant in effecting less hospitalization, better overall functioning, and less thought disorder in a group of newly hospitalized, acutely ill schizophrenic patients (Karon and Vandenbos 1970). The variable of therapist type (type A versus type B) also produced differential outcomes. Patients receiving individual psychotherapy plus drug treatment fared better with type A therapists, whereas those receiving psychotherapy plus placebo did better with type B therapists (Grinspoon et al. 1972).

Patient variables of premorbid adjustment (Goldstein et al. 1978) and gender (Goldstein et al. 1978, Hogarty et al. 1976) have also emerged in combined treatment. Goldstein and his associates' study of first-admission schizophrenic patients (Goldstein et al. 1978) revealed that those with good premorbid adjustment fared best with psychotherapy, those with poor premorbid adjustment did best with drugs, and women fared best with psychotherapy and men with drugs. By contrast, in the treatment of chronically ill schizophrenic patients Hogarty and associates (1976) found that drug effects were significantly greater for women, but there were no differences by sex for placebo users (Goldstein et al. 1978).

Finally, the factor of treatment setting in differentially affecting outcomes was suggested by Linn and associates (1979) in a study of chronic schizophrenia and by Lipman and Covi (1976) in a study of affective disorders. Lipman and Covi highlighted significant outcome differences dependent on the particular day treatment or clinic setting.

These studies suggest that we are gradually attaining greater understanding of the complex interactive factors that must be taken into account in drug-psychotherapy research.

Conclusions

The increasing wealth of scientific data on combined treatment during the decade of the 1970s augurs well for the joint future of pharmacotherapy and psychotherapy. That the gap between the two modalities has been slowly closing is evidenced by the results of much recent research and clinical observation. It is increasingly suggested that in the best of all psychopharmacotherapy worlds, psychotherapy and pharmacotherapy would have a cooperative rather than competitive or inconsequential interaction, an additive or even mutually potentiating relationship. Ideally, then, psychotherapy and pharmacotherapy would work both separately and sequentially in a total therapeutic regimen.

The above would be concordant with the separatist, though potentially *integrative* theses:

1. Each has differential effects or loci of outcome—drugs have their major effects on symptom formation and affective distress, whereas psychotherapy more directly influences interpersonal relations and social adjustment (Claghorn et al. 1974, Frank 1961, Friedman 1975, Grinspoon and Shader 1975, Klerman 1975, 1976, Parloff et al. 1954, Weissman et al. 1974, 1976).

2. Each is activated and sustained on a different time schedule—drugs may take effect sooner, be of shorter duration, and be used prophylactically; psychotherapy results may not reveal themselves until later, but they last longer (Davis 1976a,b, Grinspoon and Shader 1975, Hogarty et al. 1975, Klerman 1975, Weissman et al. 1974, 1976, Zitrin et al. 1976).

3. Each may best relate to different disorders and their subtypes—drugs for time-limited and autonomous "state" disorders, psychotherapy for long-lasting "trait" disorders (Extein and Bowers 1979).

The ideally noncompeting, noninhibiting, positive synergism of the two modalities, then, may occur through both simultaneous and sequential interactions. They would work in mutual enhancement through the complementarity of their interdigitating effects, temporal activities, aims, and sites of action. Thus, for example, in clinical practice, symptom removal or relief, reduction of anxiety and depression, improvement in attention and control, and correction of perceptual disturbances could be addressed with the use of pharmacologic agents; by thus laying the groundwork for the facilitation of interpersonal accessibility, drugs can serve both as a prerequisite and a continuing condition for the establishment of a therapeutic relationship and, thereafter, for ongoing psychotherapeutic interventions.

Future directions will entail increasing refinement of significant variables toward a greater understanding of individual differences in response to pharmacotherapy and psychotherapy. Such refinement will depend on ongoing research, which must take into account specific interventions (rather than "pharmacotherapy" or "psychotherapy" as entities). It must also consider specific disorders or patient subgroups of responders and nonresponders, specific doses, specific durations, and specific combinations and sequences of the two treatments—in short, the ultimate establishment of carefully delineated criteria for titrating the nature and timing of pharmacotherapy and psychotherapy. In the light of the contributions of the 1970s and the gaps in the field that are pressing to be filled, this would be a fitting task for the decade of the 1980s.

References

Barondes, S. H. (1966). General discussion. In *Psychiatric Drugs*, ed. P. Solomon, pp. 118–119. New York: Grune & Stratton.

Bockoven, J. S., and Solomon, H. C. (1975). Comparison of two five-year follow-up studies: 1947 to 1952 and 1967 to 1972. *American Journal of Psychiatry* 132:796–801.

Carpenter, W. T., Jr., McGlashan, T. H., and Strauss, J. S. (1977). The treatment of acute schizophrenia without drugs: an investigation of some current assumptions. *American Journal of Psychiatry* 134:14–20.

Chien, C. (1975). Drugs and rehabilitation in schizophrenia. In *Drugs in Combination with Other Therapies*, ed. M. Greenblatt, pp. 13–34. New York: Grune & Stratton.

Claghorn, J., Johnstone, E., Cook, T., et al. (1974). Group therapy and maintenance treatment of schizophrenics. *Archives of General Psychiatry* 31:361–365.

Cole, J. O. (1977). Research barriers in psychopharmacology. *American Journal of Psychiatry* 134:896–898.

Covi, L., Lipman, R. S., Derogatis L. R., et al. (1974). Drugs and group psychotherapy in neurotic depression. *American Journal of Psychiatry* 131:191–198.

Davenport, Y. B., Ebert, M. H., Adland, M. L., et al. (1977). Couples group therapy as an adjunct to lithium maintenance of the manic patient. *American Journal of Orthopsychiatry* 47:495–502.

Davis, A. E., Dinitz, S., and Pasamanick, B. (1972). The prevention of hospitalization in schizophrenia: five years after an experimental program. *American Journal of Orthopsychiatry* 42:375–388.

Davis, J. M. (1975). Overview: maintenance therapy in psychiatry. 1: schizophrenia. *American Journal of Psychiatry* 132:1237–1245.

_____ (1976a). Overview: maintenance therapy in psychiatry. 2: affective disorders. *American Journal of Psychiatry* 133:1–13.

_____ (1976b). Maintenance antipsychotic drugs do prevent relapse: a reply to Tobias and MacDonald. *Psychological Bulletin* 83:431–447.

DiMascio A., Weissman M., Prusoff, B., et al. (1979). Differential symptom reduction by drugs and psychotherapy in acute depression. *Archives of General Psychiatry* 36:1450–1460.

Docherty, J. P., Marder, S. R., and van Kammen, D. P., et al. (1977). Psychotherapy and pharmacotherapy: conceptual issues. *American Journal of Psychiatry* 134:529–533.

Downing, R. W., and Rickels, K. (1978). Nonspecific factors and their interaction with psychological treatment in pharmacotherapy. In *Psychopharmacology: A Generation of Progress*, ed. M. A. Lipton, pp. 1419–1428. New York: Raven.

Ehrenwald, J. (1966). *Psychotherapy: Myth and Method.* New York: Grune & Stratton.

Engelhardt, D. M., and Freedman, D. (1969). Maintenance drug therapy: the schizophrenic patient in the community. In *Social Psychiatry*, vol. 1, ed. A. Kiev. London: Routledge & Kegan Paul.

Extein, I., Bowers, M. B., Jr. (1979). State and trait in psychiatric practice. *American Journal of Psychiatry* 136:690–693.

Eysenck, H. J. (1952). The effects of psychotherapy: an evaluation. *Journal of Consulting Psychology* 16:319–324.

_____ (1965). The effects of psychotherapy. *International Journal of Psychiatry* 1:97–178.

Fisher, S. (1970). Nonspecific factors as determinants of behavioral response to drugs. In *Clinical Handbook of Psychopharmacology*, ed. A. DiMascio and R. Shader, pp. 17–39. New York: Jason Aronson.

_____ (1976). Discussion: do psychotherapeutic interventions really influence the drug treatment of depression? In *Evaluation of Psychological Therapies*, ed. R. L. Spitzer and D. F. Klein, pp. 219–224. Baltimore, MD: Johns Hopkins University Press.

Frank, J. (1961). *Persuasion and Healing.* Baltimore, MD: Johns Hopkins University Press.

_____ (1974). Common features of psychotherapies and their patients. *Psychotherapy and Psychosomatics* 24:368–371.

Freud, S. (1938). An outline of psychoanalysis. *Standard Edition* 23:144–207.

Friedman, A. (1975). Interaction of drug therapy with marital therapy in depressed patients. *Archives of General Psychiatry* 32:619–637.

Gallant, D. M., and Force, R. (1978). Ethical and regulatory issues in psychopharmacologic research and treatment. In *Psychopharmacology: A Generation of Progress*, ed. M. A. Lipton, A. DiMascio, and K. F. Killam, pp. 1–6. New York: Raven.

Gardos, G., and Cole, J. O. (1976). Maintenance antipsychotic therapy: is the cure worse than the disease? *American Journal of Psychiatry* 133:32–36.

_____ (1978). Maintenance antipsychotic therapy: for whom and how long? In *Psychopharmacology: A Generation of Progress*, ed. M. A. Lipton, A. DiMascio, and K. F. Killam, pp. 1169–1178.

Gillum, R. F., and Barsky, A. J. (1974). Diagnosis and management of patient noncompliance. *Journal of the American Medical Association* 228:1563–1567.

Goldstein, M., Rodnick, E., Evans, J., et al. (1978). Drug and family therapy in the aftercare of acute schizophrenics. *Archives of General Psychiatry* 35:1169–1177.

Gottlieb, R., Nappi, T., and Strain, J. J. (1978). The physician's knowledge of psychotropic drugs: preliminary results. *American Journal of Psychiatry* 135:29–32.

Grinker, R. R., Sr. (1964). A struggle for eclecticism. *American Journal of Psychiatry* 121:451–457.

Grinspoon, L., Ewalt, J., and Shader, R. (1972). A research overview of drug–psychotherapy interactions in acute schizophrenic patients. In *Schizophrenia: Pharmacotherapy and Psychotherapy.* Baltimore, MD: Williams & Wilkins.

Grinspoon, L., and Shader, R. (1975). Psychotherapy and drugs in schizophrenia. In *Drugs in Combination with Other Therapies*, ed. M. Greenblatt, pp. 49–66. New York: Grune & Stratton.

Group for the Advancement of Psychiatry (1975). *Pharmacotherapy and psychotherapy: paradoxes, problems, and progress.* Vol. 9, Rep. No. 93. Group for the Advancement of Psychiatry: New York.

Gunderson, J. G. (1977). Drugs and psychosocial treatment of schizophrenia revisited. *Journal of Continuing Education in Psychiatry* 38:25–40.

———— (1978). The value of psychotherapy in schizophrenia: a Semrad memorial. *McLean Hospital Journal* 3:131–145.

Halleck, S. L. (1978). *The Treatment of Emotional Disorders.* New York: Jason Aronson.

Harrow, M., Grinker, R. R., Sr., and Silverstein, M. L., et al. (1978). Is modern-day schizophrenic outcome still negative? *American Journal of Psychiatry* 135:1156–1162.

Havens, L. L. (1963). Problems with the use of drugs in the psychotherapy of psychotic patients. *Psychiatry* 26:289–296.

Hogarty, G., and Goldberg, S. (1973). Drug and sociotherapy in the aftercare of schizophrenic patients: one-year relapse rates. *Archives of General Psychiatry* 28:54–64.

Hogarty, G., Goldberg, S., and Schooler, N. (1974). Drug and sociotherapy in the aftercare of schizophrenic patients. *Archives of General Psychiatry* 31:609–621.

———— (1975). Drug and sociotherapy in the aftercare of schizophrenia: a review. In *Drugs in Combination with Other Therapies,* ed. M. Greenblatt, pp. 1–12. New York: Grune & Stratton.

Hogarty, G., Schooler, N., and Ulrich, R. (1979). Fluphenazine and social therapy in the aftercare of schizophrenic patients. *Archives of General Psychiatry* 36:1283–1294.

Hogarty, G., Ulrich, R., Goldberg, S., et al. (1976). Sociotherapy and the prevention of relapse among schizophrenic patients: an artifact of drug? In *Evaluation of Psychological Therapies,* ed. R. L. Spitzer and D. F. Klein, pp. 285–293. Baltimore, MD: Johns Hopkins University Press.

Karasu, T. B. (1977). Psychotherapies: an overview. *American Journal of Psychiatry* 134:851–863.

Karon, B., and Vandenbos, G. (1970). Experience, medication, and the effectiveness of psycho-therapy with schizophrenics: a note on Drs. May and Tuma's conclusions. *British Journal of Psychiatry* 116:427–428.

Klein, D. F. (1980). Psychosocial treatment of schizophrenia or psychosocial help for people with schizophrenia? *Schizophrenia Bulletin* 6:122–130.

Klerman, G. L. (1963). Assessing the influence of the hospital milieu upon the effectiveness of psychiatric drug therapy: problems of conceptualization and of research methodology. *Journal of Nervous and Mental Disease* 137:143–154.

———— (1965). The teaching of psychopharmacology in the psychiatric residency. *Comprehensive Psychiatry* 6:255–264.

———— (1975). Combining drugs and psychotherapy in the treatment of depression. In *Drugs in Combination with Other Therapies,* ed. M. Greenblatt, pp. 67–81. New York: Grune & Stratton.

———— (1976). Combining drugs and psychotherapy in the treatment of depression. In *Depression: Biology, Psychodynamics and Treatment,* ed. J. Cole, A. Schatzberg, and S. Frazier, pp. 213–237. New York: Plenum.

Lazare, A. (1973). Hidden conceptual models in clinical psychiatry. *New England Journal of Medicine* 288:345–351.

Lehmann, H. E. (1967). Psychodynamic aspects of psychopharmacology. In *Excerpta Medica International Congress Series 150: Proceedings of the Fourth World Congress of Psychiatry.* New York: Excerpta Medica.

Lesse, S. (1964). Placebo reactions and spontaneous rhythms: their effects on the results of psycho-therapy. *American Journal of Psychotherapy* 18(Suppl.):99–115.

———— (1978). Psychotherapy in combination with antidepressant drugs in severely depressed outpatients: 20-year evaluation. *American Journal of Psychotherapy* 32:48–73.

———— (1980). Psychotherapy on ambulatory patients with severe anxiety. In *Specialized Tech-niques in Individual Psychotherapy,* ed. T. B. Karasu and L. Bellak, pp. 220–235. New York: Brunner/Mazel.

Linn, L. (1964). The use of drugs in psychotherapy. *Psychiatric Quarterly* 38:138–148.

Linn, M. W., Caffey, E. M., Klett, C. J., et al. (1979). Day treatment and psychotropic drugs in the aftercare of schizophrenic patients. *Archives of General Psychiatry* 36:1055–1066.

Lipman, R., and Covi, L. (1976). Outpatient treatment of neurotic depression: medication and group psychotherapy. In *Evaluation of Psychological Therapies*, ed. R. F. Spitzer and D. F. Klein pp. 178–218. Baltimore: Johns Hopkins University Press.

Luborsky, L., Chandler, M., and Auerbach, A. H. et al. (1971). Factors influencing the outcome of psychotherapy: a review of quantitative research. *Psychological Bulletin* 75:145–185.

Luborsky, L., Singer, B., and Luborsky, L. (1976). Comparative studies of psychotherapies: is it true that "everybody has won and all must have prizes?" In *Evaluation of Psychological Therapies*, ed. R. L. Spitzer and D. F. Klein, pp. 3–22. Baltimore, MD: Johns Hopkins University Press.

Malan, D. (1973). The outcome problem in psychotherapy research. *Archives of General Psychiatry* 29:719–729.

Marholin, II, D., and Phillips, D. (1976). Methodological issues in psychopharmacological research: chlorpromazine—a case in point. *American Journal of Orthopsychiatry* 46:477–495.

May, P. (1968). *Treatment of Schizophrenia: A Comparative Study of Five Treatment Methods.* New York: Science House.

_____ (1976). Rational treatment for an irrational disorder: what does the schizophrenic patient need? *American Journal of Psychiatry* 133:1008–1012.

May, P., and Goldberg, S. (1978). Prediction of schizophrenic patients' response to pharmacotherapy. In *Psychopharmacology: A Generation of Progress*, ed. M. A. Lipton, A. DiMascio, and K. F. Killam, pp. 1139–1153. New York: Raven.

Morris, J. B., and Beck, A. T. (1976). The efficacy of antidepressant drugs. In *Progress in Psychiatric Drug Treatment*, vol. 2, ed. D. F. Klein and R. Gittelman-Klein, pp. 37–54. New York: Brunner/Mazel.

Mosher, L. R., and Keith S. J. (1979). Research on the psychosocial treatment of schizophrenia: a summary report. *American Journal of Psychiatry* 136:623–631.

Ostow, M. (1962). *Drugs in Psychoanalysis and Psychotherapy.* New York: Basic Books.

_____ (1979). *The Psychodynamic Approach to Drug Therapy.* New York: Psychoanalytic Research and Development Fund.

Overall, J. E., and Tupin, J. P. (1969). Investigation of clinical outcome in a doctor's choice treatment setting. *Diseases of the Nervous System* 30:305–313.

Parloff, M. (1975). *Twenty-five Years of Research in Psychotherapy.* New York: Albert Einstein College of Medicine. Department of Psychiatry.

Parloff, M. B., Kelman, H. C., and Frank, J. D. (1954). Comfort, effectiveness, and self-awareness as criteria of improvement in psychotherapy. *American Journal of Psychiatry* 111:343–352.

Paul, G., Tobias, L., and Holly, B. (1972). Maintenance psychotropic drugs in the presence of active treatment programs. *Archives of General Psychiatry* 27:106–115.

Podobnikar, I. (1971). Implementation of psychotherapy by Librium in a pioneering rural industrial psychiatric practice. *Psychosomatics* 12:205–209.

Reich, L. H., and Weiss B. L. (1975). The clinical research ward as a therapeutic community: incompatibilities. *American Journal of Psychiatry* 132:48–51.

Rickels, K., and Catell, R. B. (1969). Drug and placebo response as a function of doctor and patient type. In *Psychotropic Drug Response: Advances in Prediction*, ed. P. R. A. May and J. R. Wittenborn, pp. 126–140. Springfield, IL: Charles C Thomas.

Rifkin, A., Quitkin, F., Kane, J., et al. (1976). Long-term use of antipsychotic drugs. In *Progress in Psychiatric Drug Treatment*, ed. D. Klein and R. Gittelman-Klein, pp. 322–329. New York: Brunner/Mazel.

Rioch, D. M. (1958). Discussion of symposium. In *Research in Psychiatry with Special Reference to Drug Therapy: Psychiatric Research Rep. No. 9*, pp. 68–88. Washington, DC: American Psychiatric Association.

Rush, A. J., Beck, A. T., Kovacs, M., et al. (1977). Comparative efficacy of cognitive therapy and pharmacotherapy in the treatment of depressed outpatients. *Cognitive Therapy and Research* 1:17–37.

Sarwer-Foner, G. J. (1957). Psychoanalytic theories of activity-passivity conflicts and of the continuum of ego defenses. *Archives of Neurology and Psychiatry* 78:413–418.

———— (1960). *The Dynamics of Psychiatric Drug Therapy.* Springfield, IL: Charles C Thomas.

Schoenberg, M., Miller, M. G., and Schoenberg, C. E. (1978). The mind–body dichotomy reified: an illustrative case. *American Journal of Psychiatry* 135:1224–1226.

Schooler, N. (1978). Antipsychotic drugs and psychological treatment in schizophrenia. In *Psychopharmacology: A Generation of Progress,* ed. M. A. Lipton, A. DiMascio, and K. F. Killam, pp. 1155–1168. New York: Raven Press.

Semrad, E., and Klerman, G., (1966). Discussion. In *Psychiatric Drugs,* ed. P. Solomon, pp. 112–120. New York: Grune & Stratton.

Sheehan, D. V., Ballenger, J., and Jacobsen, G. (1980). Treatment of endogenous anxiety with phobic, hysterical, and hypochondriacal symptoms. *Archives of General Psychiatry* 37:51–59.

Strupp, H. (1970). Specific versus nonspecific factors in psychotherapy and the problem of control. *Archives of General Psychiatry* 23:393–401.

———— (1973). Toward a reformulation of the psychotherapeutic influence. *International Journal of Psychiatry* 11:263–327.

———— (1974). On the basic ingredients of psychotherapy. *Psychotherapy and Psychosomatics* 24:249–260.

———— (1975). Psychoanalysis, "focal psychotherapy" and the nature of the therapeutic influence. *Archives of General Psychiatry* 32:127–135.

Tobias, L. L., and MacDonald, M. L. (1974). Withdrawal of maintenance drugs with long-term hospitalized patients: a critical review. *Psychological Bulletin* 81:107–125.

Tseng, W.-S., and McDermott, J. F., Jr. (1975). Psychotherapy: historical roots, universal elements, and cultural variations. *American Journal of Psychiatry* 132:378–384.

Uhlenhuth, E. H., Covi, L., and Lipman, R. S. (1970). Indications for minor tranquilizers in anxious outpatients. In *Drugs and the Brain: Experimental and Clinical Considerations,* ed. P. Black, pp. 203–221. Baltimore, MD: Johns Hopkins University Press.

Uhlenhuth, E. H., Lipmann, R., and Covi, L. (1969). Combined pharmacotherapy and psychotherapy. *Journal of Nervous and Mental Disease* 148:52–64.

Van Praag, H. M. (1972). Biologic psychiatry in perspective: the dangers of sectarianism in psychiatry, 4: some inferred trends. *Comprehensive Psychiatry* 13:401–410.

———— (1979). Tablets and talking: a spurious contrast in psychiatry. *Comprehensive Psychiatry* 20:502–510.

Watt, D. C. (1975). Editorial: time to evaluate long-acting neuroleptics? *Psychological Medicine* 5:222–226.

Weissman, M., Klerman, G., and Paykel, E., et al. (1974). Treatment effects on the social adjustment of depressed patients. *Archives of General Psychiatry* 30:771–778.

Weissman, M., Klerman, G., and Prusoff, B. et al. (1976). The efficacy of psychotherapy in depression: symptom remission and response to treatment. In *Psychological Therapies,* ed. R. L. Spitzer and D. F. Klein, pp. 165–177. Baltimore, MD: Johns Hopkins University Press.

White, R., Davis, H., and Cantrell, W. (1977). Psychodynamics of depression: implications for treatment. In *Depression: Clinical, Biological and Psychological Perspectives,* ed. G. Usdin, pp. 308–338. New York: Brunner/Mazel.

Wolf, S. F. (1965). *The Stomach.* New York: Oxford University Press.

Yager, J. (1977). Psychiatric eclecticism: a cognitive view. *American Journal of Psychiatry* 134:736–741.

Zitrin, C. M., Klein, D. F., Lindemann, C., et al. (1976). Comparison of short-term treatment regimens in phobic patients: a preliminary report. In *Evaluation of Psychological Therapies,* ed. R. L. Spitzer and D. F. Klein, pp. 233–250. Baltimore, MD: Johns Hopkins University Press.

Zitrin, C. M., Klein, D. F., and Woerner, M. G. (1978). Behavior therapy, supportive psychotherapy, imipramine, and phobias. *Archives of General Psychiatry* 35:307–316.

———— (1980). Treatment of agoraphobia with group exposure in vivo and imipramine. *Archives of General Psychiatry* 37:63–72.

3

Will Neurobiology Influence Psychoanalysis?

ARNOLD M. COOPER, M.D.

Neurobiologic research has begun to elucidate brain mechanisms of affective states and behavioral patterns. Discussions of anxiety and sexual identity demonstrate how these researches lead the psychoanalyst to broader views of behaviors that were previously considered entirely psychological in origin. While introspection and extrospection are distinct realms of investigation and conceptualization, they share common boundaries and areas of interpenetration. Psychoanalytic theory is challenged to accord with newer findings in biology and to provide important questions for further research. Neurobiologic advances will continue a centuries-old process of confining the realm of psyche, but there is no danger that mind will disappear.

Psychoanalysis may be characterized as an attempt to decode, that is, interpret, a patient's communications according to a loosely drawn set of transformational rules concerning underlying meanings, motivations, and unities of thought. The analyst does his best to understand the patient's communications as the patient intends them to be, but both patient and analyst are heavily influenced by a theory, or a group of theories, used by both parties. For example, patients have theories about the nature of responsibility and the causal agents of behavior, and these theories may range from extremes of conviction that "everything is my fault" to "nothing is my fault" or from "I intended to do that" to "something made me do that." Patients have theories about the nature of their motivation; some are convinced that all their actions are altruistic, while others believe that their most innocent thoughts are evidence of their murderous intent. Patients have theories about the sources of their behavior; some are firmly convinced that all their actions are explained by the nature of their nurturance, and others are convinced that only a bad fate could explain their lives.

We take for granted that these theories, no matter how firmly held, reflect defensive needs and are to be regarded as an entry to different—we usually imply deeper—aspects of the patient's personality. We also assume that all human beings weave their experience and their capacities into a holistic way of understanding themselves and their world and create a theory that provides some degree of comfort. At high levels, these theories may be philosophies, religions, and life attitudes.

Analysts also have a range of available theories with which we are all familiar. While we share many things in common, it makes a difference whether we see the world through Freud's lens, or Schafer's, Kohut's, Kernberg's, or our own variation of how to view analytic data. The theory will determine how the analyst shapes the patient's material so that he will have the benefit of theory that the patient has; that is, he too will be able to have a holistic, seemingly rational view that will explain the entirety of his patient's behavior and provide the analyst with a bit of needed comfort and confidence in his professional world. Theories also lead us, no matter how we may try to be merely the recipient of the patient's story, to collaborate with the patient in creating a new personal myth, a life narrative more acceptable to analyst and patient. If we believe that the Oedipus complex is central in neurosis, any patient will provide ample opportunity for demonstrating the existence, vitality, and significance of oedipal fantasies. If we believe that preoedipal arrests or fixations are determinants, again it is a rare patient who does not provide adequate opportunity to construct the life story so that preoedipal issues will occupy a central place.

I am not nihilistic about the role of theory. I do not think that theories do not matter; rather I think they matter crucially. But until we have better ways of testing our theories, different theories will coexist, and we will go on, consciously or unconsciously, intentionally or unwittingly, educating our patients to see the world as our theory has already told us the world is. This is inevitable. Because there is a paucity of validating strategies in psychoanalysis, it is important that analytic theories not be out of touch with developing new knowledge in areas adjoining our own area of interest, lest they become idiosyncratic and isolated from the mainstreams of science and humanities. Information from other disciplines may provide a check on our own findings and theories.

The question posed by the title of this paper could be phrased another way: "What does it take to change an analyst's theory?" More precisely, "What are the possibilities that anything found in neurobiology will change the way an analyst hears his patient talking?" It may be instructive to examine the relationship of direct child observation to psychoanalysis, as an example. There has always been and still is a significant group of analysts who have maintained that child research is interesting and even worth knowing for its own sake or for some yet unforeseen purpose but has no relevance to the analytic situation, in which we are interested solely in the psychic reality verbally conveyed by the patient rather than infantile reality observed by the investigator. That is, psychoanalysis in its working mode accepts as data of infancy only the patient's construction of it or our interpretive understanding of the patient's construction of it and not the so-called objective data.

Despite this claim, however, most of us have seen a quiet revolution in analytic theory and practice secondary to the work of investigators as different as Mahler and Bowlby. Whether or not one subscribes to all their views, the data on the central role in development of attachment behaviors and their consequences in separation-individuation have led most analysts to give far more emphasis to these aspects of development in their reconstruction of patient's lives, to give greater weight to the interpersonal and object-relational portions of the developmental narrative, and to look more closely at preoedipal issues than was the case when libidinal and aggressive drives were seen as more simply derived. Furthermore, the recent and ongoing discoveries of the spectacular range of cognitive and affective capacities of the very young infant, with evidence for very early development of capacities for control and for distinguishing self from other, give rise now to new questions concerning the nature of the infant's early tie to the mother. These findings also are leading to suggestions for new theories of the self and different ideas about the so-called symbiotic phase. We do not yet know how these newer findings and formulations will affect the ways in which we listen to our patients' stories, but it is, I think, unlikely that they will leave us unchanged. Similarly, the work of Harry Harlow and the movies of his socially deprived baby monkeys have subtly, but profoundly, altered the way we construct meaningful life narratives when we encounter chronically depressed and anxious and solitary individuals.

Any data, or theories, on development may fade in significance when we encounter seemingly contradictory evidence from the patient, but we know that the evidence from the patient is always the stuff of our interpretation, not the bedrock, and our interpretations will be, and ought to be, in accord with what is objectively known about development. Our confidence in our interpretations will be strengthened by the knowledge that they are in accord with scientific data. Freud, for example, was significantly handicapped in not eventually knowing the data on infant sexual seduction. While his discovery of his error in believing that all neurosis was caused by seduction led to the development of the core of psychoanalysis, the world of psychic reality, it is possible that better information later would have led him to modify the overemphasis he had given to instinct and to alter his theory to find a role for the environment and for the more interpersonal and object-relational modes that were available to him in his practice but were not included in his metapsychology at that time.

Because it is my thesis that neurobiology ought to, probably already does, and surely will influence psychoanalysis, I want first to emphasize the primacy of our effort to listen, as Freud urged, with freely hovering attention, or as Bion said, without memory or desire, or as Kohut said, empathically seeing the world as our patients see it. We should be equally aware, however, of the inherent and inevitable limits to achieving these goals that result from the necessity for an organizing analytic theory. All outside knowledge potentially biases the observer not to hear his patient but to confirm his own a priori knowledge and avoid cognitive dissonance—that great source of anxiety. Knowing that we cannot succeed in achieving "unbiased" listening does not relieve us of the obligation to attempt it.

Many psychoanalysts believe that psychoanalysis can derive useful data only from its own activities, that the scientific development of psychoanalysis depends solely on findings derived from the psychoanalytic situation. It helps if one realizes that what many of us accept as the standard psychoanalytic points of view—whether the stages of libidinal development or the nuclear role of the Oedipus complex or the nature of transference—are not simply derivatives of analytic experience but are amalgams of varieties of analytic experience and other kinds of knowledge. Neurobiologic concepts are built into the core of psychoanalysis. Think for a moment of a few of our core concepts. The pleasure–unpleasure principle is a biologic as well as a psychological concept, whether phrased in Freud's early energic terms—that the individual acts to reduce neural excitation to the lowest level and to maintain homeostasis—or in psychological language—that the individual acts to maximize pleasure and safety and to avoid pain and danger. Those are different ways of phrasing the principle of adaptation, which is at the heart of every consideration of organismic functioning. Much of modern neurobiology can be seen as an effort at the level of the molecule and the cell receptor to understand the ways in which homeostasis, pleasure, and safety are maintained at levels appropriate to the effective functioning of the organism. Even if one chooses to abandon Freud's concept of drive and to accept the psychological concept of wish, as Holt and others have recommended, I think that most of us would agree that we would benefit from a better understanding of the biologic substrate of wishes, their categories, their mixtures, and the regulators that turn them on or off.

Freud did not hesitate to go outside of psychoanalysis for aid in obtaining information useful in forming his concepts. Not only did he model his thinking on the scientific mode of his era, but he looked for specific data. He used the work of the Hungarian pediatrician Lindner to support his libido theory that the sexual drive must be an important part of infantile oral activity even if no overt sexuality, as then conceived, could be demonstrated (Freud 1905). Lindner's description of the infant's evident sensuality while sucking strengthened Freud's conviction about his new theory. He used the data of Sophocles, as described in drama, to support his view that the Oedipus complex was itself a central drama. Freud used his vivid phenomenologic description of the baby's relationship to the mother to support his view of the core constancy of drive aspects of object relations and the nature of transference regression. While Freud gave up his Project, which aimed at making psychoanalysis a branch of, or at least entirely compatible with, neurobiology, he never gave up the desire that psychoanalytic findings should accord with and be affirmed by findings in other sciences and the humanities. In a footnote to his 1912 paper on "The Dynamics of Transference," Freud said,

I take this opportunity of defending myself against the mistaken charge of having denied the importance of innate (constitutional) factors because I have stressed that of infantile impressions. A charge such as this arises from the restricted nature of what men look for in the field of causation: in contrast to what ordinarily holds good in the real world, people prefer to be satisfied with a single causative factor. Psychoanalysis has talked a lot about the accidental factors in aetiology and little about the constitutional ones; but that is only because it was able to contribute something fresh to the former, while, to begin with, it knew no more than was commonly known about the latter. We refuse to posit any contrast in principle between the two sets of aetiological factors; on the contrary, we assume that the two sets regularly act jointly in bringing about the observed result. Endowment and Chance determine a man's fate—rarely or never one of these powers alone. The amount of aetiological effectiveness to be attributed to each of them can only be arrived at in every individual case separately. These cases may be arranged in a series according to the varying proportion in which the two factors are present, and this series will no doubt have its extreme cases. We shall estimate the share taken by constitution or experience differently in individual cases according to the stage reached by our knowledge; and we shall retain the right to modify our judgement along with changes in our understanding. [*Standard Edition* 12:99]

It is in this spirit that we should look at neurobiology today. It may now merit a larger share.

I have suggested a number of ways in which findings of infant observation and ethology already have changed the way we work. Neurobiology, in the broad sense, will almost surely further change some of the ways in which we understand development, affect, learning, sexuality, and the meaning of symptoms. I will mention a few areas of current study in which our growing neurobiologic knowledge may require that we reexamine and perhaps alter aspects of the theories with which we listen to our patients and the ways we teach them.

Research in Anxiety

We know that Freud had an early theory of anxiety that he did not entirely abandon when he developed his later one. According to his original view, anxiety represented psychologically contentless overflow of neuronal excitation, an overflow of blocked and transformed libidinal energy. In this early view, anxiety was not in itself a psychological phenomenon but signaled homeostatic disturbances elsewhere, either in psychological systems or in neuronal function. Freud's second theory of anxiety treated anxiety as part of an evolutionarily evolved biologic warning system, with a signal form of anxiety serving as a mild stimulus for the institution of defense mechanisms in order to ward off more powerful forms of anxiety. Anxiety is part of a biologic fight–flight alerting system, preparing for action to avert dangers either from unconscious impulses or from the environment. It is also assumed that the experience of anxiety is disorganizing and unbearably painful and that it is a major task of the organism to avert that experience.

Psychoanalysis, under the sway of ego psychology and our concern with adaptation, has taken Freud's second theory of anxiety as the basis for our continued thinking on the subject, with various workers constructing lists of the dangers that elicit anxiety. Anxiety in our patients is generally assumed to represent the ego's response to the threatened breakthrough of unacceptable impulses or an anticipated loss of an object necessary for the maintenance of inner stability. In this view, anxiety is always related to psychological content.

Recent neurobiologic findings, however, suggest interesting other possibilities. The discovery of benzodiazepines in 1956 and of benzodiazepine binding sites in the brain in 1977 has led to a series of investigations concerning the biology of anxiety. I will mention only a few of the interesting findings.

One line of research includes the following findings.

1. The locus ceruleus seems to be a regulatory center for neuroexcitatory activity and may serve as a regulatory center for the anxiety level of the organism.

2. Benzodiazepines potentiate the activity of those inhibitory neurons that are responsive to γ-amino-butyric acid (GABA). The inhibitory neurons are specially concentrated in the locus ceruleus, and the activation of these neurons diminishes anxiety.

Another line of research includes the following findings (Crowe et al. 1981).

1. There is increasing evidence that panic attacks differ from generalized anxiety in ways other than simply quantitative. Klein and co-workers have suggested that in certain people panic attacks are a primary event, which secondarily leads to learned anticipatory anxiety and phobic behavior.

2. There is also increasing evidence that panic anxiety is responsive to antidepressant medication.

3. There are not yet confirmed data that many school-phobic children are responsive to antidepressant medication.

On the basis of these kinds of data, one could postulate that there are several different groups of people who are chronically anxious, often phobic, perhaps with intermittent panic attacks, who have developed their anxious personality structure secondary to a largely contentless biologic dysregulation. Whereas psychological triggers for anxiety may still be found, the anxiety threshold is so low in these patients that it is no longer useful to view the psychological event as etiologically significant. One group may have a hyperactive alerting system, related to a failure of GABA activity, resulting in excessive anxiety signaling and breakthrough of anxiety states. These individuals are benzodiazepine responsive. The second group may be understood as suffering a lowered threshold for separation anxiety—the postulated trigger for panic. In effect, this is a return to a version of Freud's early anxiety theory: the trigger for anxiety is a biologic event, as in "actual neurosis," but now the trigger is separation, not dammed up libido. The newer theory postulates that panic is an evolutionarily constructed response to separation, but the mechanism may miscarry and fire independently of appropriate environmental triggers. That neurons mediating separation responses and the creation of panic both seem responsive to tricyclic antidepressants suggests, of course, the psychologically known links of separation and depression. In these two groups of individuals, the presence of anxiety is not an indication of a primary disorder of conflict or self or object relations; these are secondary to the disorganizing effects of anxiety. Furthermore, the biologic dysregulation is not only a developmental event but an ongoing one. These persons are currently physiologically maladapted for maintenance of homeostasis in average expectable environments. Klein claims that individuals with panic disorder who are treated with imipramine cease to have panic attacks but then require psychotherapy to undo the learned antici-patory anxiety and phobic behaviors that were developed as magical efforts to cope with unpredictable panic.

This theory suggests that the psychoanalyst is now confronted with a diagnostic decision in his anxious patient. What portions of the anxiety are, in their origins, relatively nonpsychological, and what portions are the clues to psychic conflicts that are the originators of the anxiety? The neurobiologic theory does not suggest that all anxiety is a nonmental content but rather that a distinction must be made between psychological coping and adaptive efforts to regulate miscarried brain functions that create anxiety with no or little environ-mental input, and psychological coping and adaptive efforts to regulate distur-bances of the intrapsychic world that lead to anxiety and are environment sensitive. Clearly, we have not yet arrived at the point where we can easily make that distinction, but there is good reason to attempt it. In instances in which an underlying biologic malfunction is suspected, there is powerful warrant to attempt a biologic intervention that may then facilitate psychological interven-tions. Let me give an example.

Clinical Vignette

A woman entered treatment describing a history since midadoles-cence of intermittent depression, timidity in relations with men, and very high rejection sensitivity. Any relationship with a man was colored from the start by her expectation that the man would probably leave her. The prospect of desertion would precipitate such anxiety and rage that she was then prone to behave in ways that brought about the rejection she allegedly feared. The patient recalled as a small child always being extremely upset when her parents would go out in the evening, requiring hours before she could calm down. She was mildly school phobic. The patient entered analysis and worked through the consequences of a relationship with a profoundly narcissistic mother who, it became clear, was also chronically depressed. A sister of the mother had been hospitalized with an uncertain diagnosis of schizophrenia. In early latency, the patient had turned from the mother toward the father, whose favorite she was, but the father seemed to go through a profound personality change, presumably a depression, when the patient was about 10 years old. The patient remembers her father becoming extremely withdrawn, going to work, coming home, and watching television by himself. The patient and father began to have tremendous battles when the patient began to date, as the father regularly disapproved of the patient's boyfriends, most of whom were chosen to elicit that disapproval. The father died when the patient was 16 years old, during a period when they were angry at and not speaking to each other, and the patient felt continuing guilt and rage that she had never had the opportunity to make peace with her father.

From the very beginning of the analysis, the transference was characterized by severe anxiety reactions at every disruption of the tie to me. Weekend breaks were extremely difficult, canceled appointments were a crisis, and vacations seemed a major trauma. As the analysis progressed, the patient became generally calmer, was able to pursue her work successfully, began to develop a much higher level of self-esteem, and had somewhat better relationships with men. Despite these improvements, she would episodically revert to the symptoms with which she had entered treatment: a mixed depressive-anxious state with feelings of shame and worthlessness, terrified that she would be rejected by her boyfriend, a female friend, a work supervisor, me, or anyone else. The termination phase of the treatment was difficult but seemed to be successfully negotiated. Two years after termination the patient called me, just before the beginning of my summer vacation. She was already on vacation and was in a state of mixed depression and panic, the kind of feeling with which she had entered analysis. There were no apparent external precipitants other than the preconscious reminder of my vacation time, and she felt extremely discouraged over this uncontrollable state. While her description of her feelings was extremely familiar, this time it occurred to me that she might be describing a recurrent biologic dysregulation and that a search for further psychological content might not be productive. That thought had also occurred to her. Despite much trepidation, she agreed to a trial of imipramine. She responded well to the medication, despite side effects, and stated that she felt relieved and reorganized and had the sense that an outside intrusion into her life, the severe anxiety, had been alleviated. On medication, although she was not free of anxiety, she had a feeling that she was in some way more in control of herself than she had ever been.

The case is suggestive. This woman later decided to return for further analysis to deal with aspects of her conflictual life that had not been successfully analyzed while anxiety and mood dysregulation were, perhaps independently, dominating her ongoing psychological life.

Current research indicates, with varying degrees of certainty, multiple levels—cellular, neural network, and experiential—for the organization and regulation of anxiety and for the development and alteration of pathologic anxiety. The elegant research of Kandel (1979) has elucidated the actual neurochemistry of some forms of learning in the snail, including what may be considered aspects of anticipatory and chronic anxiety. The interaction of the environment and the adaptive responses of the organism can now be partially understood in terms of basic cellular neurobiology. The readiness with which we attempt to affect the patient's self, or his locus ceruleus, through a new relationship or through a new medication has philosophical and ethical connotations, and in the current absence of specific indications for either or both treatments, the treatment choice will reflect individual bias. We are alert to the issue of efficacy. If we can demonstrate that physiologic interventions are more efficient ways to achieve a portion, at least, of the effect we seek—that is, relief of pain and opportunities for new growth—as physicians, we welcome the most effective treatment.

The question may be asked, "Are we as psychoanalysts interested in changing the patient's life or changing the symptom?" Analysts used to find it easy to answer this question. We believed that symptoms were surface manifestations of deep disturbance, as in the rest of medicine, and that the symptom was not the target of our ministrations. In fact, we thought that too easy symptom removal would confront the patient with the task of constructing a new symptom to provide defenses against underlying threatening wishes. This idea of symptom substitution has not been borne out by recent work. Experience with behavior therapy, focal psychotherapies, and pharmacotherapies seems to demonstrate that, contrary to expectation, symptom removal, in many although not all instances, may lead to enhanced self-esteem and possibilities for new experiences and renewed characterologic growth. Most analysts have long realized that excesses of dysphoric affect inhibit the effectiveness of psychoanalysis by fixating the patient on the affective state and limiting the patient's cognitive associational capacity. For the patient whom I have described, I believe, retrospectively, that pharmacologic assistance earlier might have permitted a much clearer focus on her content-related psychodynamic problems and would also have made it more difficult for her to use her symptoms masochistically as proof that she was an innocent victim of endless emotional pain.

I would like to draw another implication from the brief clinical vignette I gave. Most analytic treatment carries with it a strong implication that it is a major analytic task of the patient to accept responsibility for his actions. In the psychoanalytic view, this responsibility is nearly total. We are even responsible for incorrectly or exaggeratedly holding ourselves responsible. It is our job to change our harsh superegos, and it is our job to do battle with unacceptable impulses. However, it now seems likely that there are patients with depressive, anxious, and dysphoric states for whom the usual psychodynamic view of responsibility seems inappropriate and who should not be held accountable for their difficulty in accepting separation from dependency objects, or at least they should not be held fully accountable. There is a group of chronically depressed and anxious patients—perhaps they are part of a depression spectrum disorder, as Akiskal (1983) suggests—whose mood regulation is vastly changed by anti-depressant medication. The entry of these new molecules into their metabolism alters, tending to normalize, the way they see the world, the way they do battle with their superegos, the way they respond to object separation. It may be that we have been co-conspirators with these patients in their need to construct a rational-seeming world in which they hold themselves unconsciously responsible for events. Narcissistic needs may lead these patients to claim control over uncontrollable behaviors rather than to admit to the utter helplessness of being at the mercy of moods that sweep over them without apparent rhyme or reason. An attempt at dynamic understanding in these situations may not only not be genuinely explanatory, it may be a cruel misunderstanding of the patient's effort to rationalize his life experience and may result in strengthening masochistic defenses.

Research in Sexuality

Psychoanalysts have long been torn by arguments over the appropriate attitude toward homosexuality and other gender-deviant behaviors. Neuro-biology will not settle the argument, but advances in neurobiologic under-standing of gender role add intriguing new insights to our outlook on homosex-uality. There is evidence from research with mice that there are two independent brain systems for sexual behavior—one for male behaviors and one for female behaviors, the activity of each depending on genetic, prenatal, environmental, and hormonal influences. It seems that females may be mascu-linized, defeminized, or both, and conversely, males may be demasculinized, feminized, or both. Hofer (1981) reported that

> females whose uterine position was between two males show slight modi-fication of their genitals in the male direction, are more aggressive, do more urinary marking of their cages (a male trait), and are less attractive to males than their litter mates with uterine positions between two females. The implication is that the proximity to males in utero and some sharing of their placental circulation resulted in their being exposed to somewhat more testosterone during the prenatal period. However, it was found that these masculinized females were not defeminized. They were no different in their response to estrogen and they were as capable of all female reproductive functions, including maternal behavior and the raising of young, as their female litter mates who had been together in the uterus. Thus, with

different amounts and timing of exposure to testosterone in male animals, behavior may be feminized without being demasculinized. [p. 273]

Hofer concluded that "a number of sex related behaviors may depend to a certain extent on the presence of testosterone in early development, that both genetic males and genetic females possess the potential for both masculine and feminine behavior traits, and that traits for the opposite sex may be increased or decreased without necessarily impairing the behaviors related to the genetic sex" (p. 273). In other words, depending on the amount of testosterone present in the environment, we can produce effeminate males, fully capable of male sexual function but with female behavioral traits, or we can produce demasculinized males, incapable of male sexual behavior later on even in the presence of testosterone; the converse can be done to females. The fetal mouse brain is exquisitely sensitive to the organizing effect of hormones.

As psychoanalysts, we tend to assume that the presence of effeminate characteristics indicates the presence of a feminine identification and is a result of that identification. The data of neurobiology make us aware that there may be more than one source for effeminate behaviors and that effeminate behaviors may not connect with identifications except in complex secondary ways and may be totally distinct from homosexual tendencies. However, a recent, unconfirmed study by Zuger (1984) suggested that early effeminate behavior in male children is congenital and is the best single indicator of later homosexuality.

Another study was done of a group of genetic males with an enzyme defect that did not permit them to convert available testosterone in utero into an effective genital-masculinizing substance (Imperato-McGinley et al. 1979). Although their brains were exposed to normal intrauterine androgen, they were born with female-appearing genitalia, were given female sex assignment, and were brought up as girls. As these phenotypic females entered puberty, they began to produce their own testosterone and at that time developed normal male genitalia. What makes this group especially interesting is that these individuals seemed to have little difficulty in changing their gender identity and gender role at puberty; of the eighteen studied, fifteen married and showed no evidence of undue stress or distortion of their male role. This result is contrary to the studies of Money and our current wisdom, which conclude that core gender identity is firmly fixed by 18 months and very little affected by later changes of external genitalia. In this group of patients it is as if the fetally hormonally masculinized brain maintained masculine neuronal networks that made later masculine role behavior easily available, overriding the usual psychological influences. Very early, intrauterine patterning of the Central Nervous System seems powerfully determining for later sexual behaviors. In yet another experiment,

> male rats born to mothers stressed during their last trimester of pregnancy by periodic restraint and bright light failed to develop normal male sexual behavior in the presence of receptive females and assumed female sexual

positions when approached by normal experienced males. They were thus demasculinized and feminized as a result of their mother's experience during pregnancy. Treatment of the affected animals with testosterone did not fully correct the deficiencies in male sexual behavior and only served to exaggerate the inappropriate female-type behavior. This means that the alteration was in the *neural systems mediating the behavior,* not in the amount of male sex hormones produced in childhood. Individual animals showed different patterns that were consistent for them. Some were asexual, responding neither to normal females or normal males. Some were bisexual, some only responded with female behavior to males, and some were indistinguishable from normal heterosexual males. [Hofer 1981, p. 180]

These experiments indicate rather conclusively that prenatal experience patterns the brain, at least in mice, and may do so to such a degree that later experience does not significantly alter the early neural patterning. It is a large leap from animal studies to humans, even though there are suggestive data in humans supporting similar conclusions. It seems reasonable, in the light of the studies I have cited combined with earlier psychoanalytic studies, to suggest that there are several pathways to the same end behavior—for example, effeminate behavior in males or perhaps even obligatory homosexuality. The influence either of specific molecules on the brain in utero or of special forms of learning through identification may lead to altered, that is, effeminate, behavior. At this time we have no way of determining the preponderance of biochemical or interactional etiology (both considered biologic) in any individual, nor do we yet know whether it matters in terms of later plasticity. Is the chemically determined effeminate male any more or less likely to give up his effeminacy, if that were desired, than the psychologically determined one? What are the limits of the plasticity of the adult brain? We do not know. Without an answer, it at least behooves the psychoanalyst to be aware that he should proceed with caution. A conviction that all homosexuality is part of a normal range of variability or a conviction that all homosexuality is psychopathologic is unwarranted at this time.

There are now many experiments in human and animal infants that demonstrate the lasting effects of very early life experiences and the powerful shaping of later behaviors by even single early traumas or particular behaviors of the mother. In some instances a fair amount is known about the chemical regulators of these brain changes. At this borderline of neurobiology and psychoanalysis, we are quite in the dark concerning the question of later plasticity of both neural networks and behaviors. Are some of our treatment failures, and endless analyses, a result of the too rigidly prewired brain? It is a potentially convenient excuse, but it is possible that some of these cases represent such neural prepatterning. Again, we need more knowledge before we can usefully address the question; in the meantime, it might be wise to keep the possibility in the back of our minds. One other example illustrates an experience that is becoming increasingly common in the psychoanalytic community.

Clinical Vignette

I recently saw in consultation a 36-year-old male scientist who came to see me for referral to a new analyst because for external reasons he had to interrupt his previous treatment. He gave a classic description of himself as someone with a narcissistic personality disorder: grandiose, self-inflated, full of unfulfilled promise and promises, although innately well endowed and perhaps even potentially brilliant—a brilliance that showed in flashes but never in steady achievement. He was married and had three children; he had married a passive, frightened woman and was himself emotionally detached, remote, and distant. He had entered treatment because he recognized his pattern of making a superb first impression and then disappointing his admirers and himself. He had passed the stage of boy wonder in his early thirties and had begun to worry that he would burn out. He had been in treatment for a few months when he experienced his first clear manic episode, which lasted several months. During the next year he had his first major depression and clearly began a bipolar course. His analyst refused to consider medication, so the patient medicated himself with lithium obtained from a friend, with his analyst's knowledge. His own description of the result was, "The lithium stopped the crazy swings during which I couldn't do any analytic work and was in great danger of either wrecking my life with my financial schemes during my manic periods or killing myself during my depressions. On lithium, I knew I had a severe character problem and needed analysis." The treatment had been enormously helpful, and he was eager to resume.

Possibly, the stress of analysis and the specific address to this patient's characterologic defenses played a role in the appearance of his bipolar disorder. It also seems possible that he would have been untreatable, and would perhaps not have survived, if medication had not been available for the disorder of affect. I cannot think of a significant analytic advantage gained by withholding the medication, and while many transference issues were not resolved at the time he came to me for consultation, there seemed to be no great impediment to his continuing a genuine analysis while taking medication. It was my view that the medication should be properly supervised by a physician, thus probably assuring him better care and interfering with a bit of the narcissistic grandiosity of his conviction that he could do everything himself. This combination of neurobiologic advance and psychoanalytic effort seems at least additive and perhaps even synergistic. Analysts will have to learn how to do this better than we have in the past, developing appropriate criteria for combined treatments.

Discussion

We should not be surprised if advances in neurobiology continue a centuries-old process of confining the realm of mind and psychiatry. It was not very long ago that diseases such as tuberculosis, parkinsonism, tertiary syphilis, and neurodermatitis were considered psychiatric diseases. More recently, syndromes such as Gilles de la Tourette, rheumatoid arthritis, ulcerative colitis, essential hypertension, dysmenorrhea, premenstrual syndrome, and temporal lobe and petit mal epilepsy were considered by some to be psychological in origin and suitable subjects for psychoanalysis, at least in part because the disease course was so obviously event responsive. Current work in personality disorders indicates that some of the behaviors of obsessive-compulsive, explosive, depressive-masochistic, or borderline patients may reflect genetically determined biologic abnormalities that are in part pharmacologically modifiable. As psychoanalysts we should welcome any scientific knowledge that removes from our primary care illnesses that we cannot successfully treat by the methods of our profession because the etiology lies elsewhere or that facilitates our analytic treatment by assisting us with intractable symptoms. We should also not be excessively modest about the contributions we can make to the care of these patients. Psychoanalysis is a powerful instrument for research and treatment, but not if it is applied to the wrong patient population.

It is most unlikely that there will be any direct bridges from neurobiology to the unconscious or to consciousness. Neurobiology explains at a different level than psychology, and knowledge of the brain will not fundamentally alter our mode of inquiry about the mind. What modern neurobiology does is to make it increasingly apparent that knowledge of the brain can help us to refine our knowledge of the mind and, in some instances, by its effects on our theory at its boundaries, it will set different limits to what we consider to be the mind. As Kohut (1978) pointed out, the realms of material observation and experimentation and intrapsychic observation and experimentation are discontinuous. Introspection and extrospection are different processes. Again, what is to be sought is congruence and limit setting on both sides. Psychoanalytic knowledge of unconscious operations poses interesting problems for the biologists and provides important hints for experimental work. The flow goes both ways.

Psychoanalysis requires a theory of development that will help explain the phenomena important to us—the world of internal representations and meanings, the world of attachment and object relations, the world of sexual differentiation, the world of fantasy and wish, the world of intrapsychic conflict, and the modes of learning and the biologic substate that make these worlds possible. We also need far better data, experiments, and theories for understanding the effective agents in the complex undertaking of analysis; neurobiology can help us to understand which of our concepts are unlikely and which are congruent with biologic experimentation. We should be extremely uncomfortable with any theory that is incongruent with neurobiologic discovery. Eric Kandel (1983) recently put the matter very succinctly. He said, "The emergence of an empirical neuropsychology of cognition based on cellular neurobiology can produce a renaissance of scientific psychoanalysis. This form of psychoanalysis may be founded on theoretical hypotheses that are more modest than those applied previously but that are more testable because they will be closer to experimental inquiry" (p. 1282). I think Freud would have been pleased by this prospect.

References

Akiskal, H. S. (1983). Dysthymic disorder: psychopathology of proposed chronic depressive subtypes. *American Journal of Psychiatry* 140:11–20.

Crowe, R., Pauls, D., Kerber, R., and Noyes, Jr. R. (1981). Panic disorder and mitral valve prolapse. In *Anxiety: New Research and Changing Concepts*, ed. D. F. Klein and J. Rabkin, pp. 103–116. New York: Raven.

Freud, S. (1905). Three essays on the theory of sexuality. *Standard Edition* 7:135–243, 1953.

_____ (1912). The dynamics of transference. *Standard Edition* 12:99–108, 1958.

Hofer, M. A. (1981). *The Roots of Human Behavior*. San Francisco: W. H. Freeman.

Imperato-McGinley, J., Peterson, R. E., Gautier, T., et al. (1979). Androgens and the evolution of male gender identity among male pseudohermaphrodites with 5–2-reductose deficiency. *New England Journal of Medicine* 300:1233–1237.

Kandel, E. R. (1979). Psychotherapy and the single synapse: the impact of psychiatric thought on neurobiologic research. *New England Journal of Medicine* 30:1028–1037.

_____ (1983). From metapsychology to molecular biology: explorations into the nature of anxiety. *American Journal of Psychiatry* 140:1277–1293.

Kohut, H. (1978). Introspection, empathy and psychoanalysis: an examination of the relationship between the mode of operation and theory. In *Search for the Self*, vol. 1, ed. P. Ornstein, pp. 205–232. New York: International Universities Press.

Zuger, B. (1984). Early effeminate behavior in boys: outcome and significance for homosexuality. *Journal of Nervous and Mental Disease* 172:90–97.

PART II
Dynamics of Psychopharmacotherapy

4

Adverse Response to Neuroleptics in Schizophrenia

DONALD B. NEVINS, M.D.

Negative therapeutic reactions to neuroleptics in schizophrenic patients are examined from the psychoanalytic perspective through case examples. Intrapsychic changes resulting from this medication, ordinarily considered beneficial, are shown, in some cases, to be disruptive of schizophrenic functioning and organization and potentially to endanger the continuation of medication itself. Changes are described that affect defenses, object relations, psychotic restitution, use of external reality, body image and cognition, and the symbolic significance of medication. Alterations in narcissistic ego states and disruption in preconscious processes, superimposed upon defective ego functioning, are used as explanatory concepts. These interact with transference-based responses; in some cases, important psychodynamic issues emerge amenable to transference interpretations. Further study of intrapsychic changes may be useful in delineating a previously inexplicable response, understanding symptom formation, recognizing shifts in the patient–psychotherapist relationship, and forestalling premature cessation of medication.

Neuroleptic medications are important in the treatment of schizophrenia. These medications reduce psychotic symptoms, the rate of recidivism, and the length of hospitalization (May 1968). Moreover, relapses occur more frequently when these drugs are discontinued (Group for the Advancement of Psychiatry 1975). Some patients complain, nevertheless, of side effects, not attributable to medical factors, but due to disagreeable changes in mental state. They stop medication and become overtly psychotic.

    A review of the literature on adverse psychological effects accompanying neuroleptic administration in schizophrenia is noteworthy in part because of the scarcity of papers despite frequent empirical observations of patients' subjective complaints along these lines. In three recent major reference works on drug treatment (Ban 1969, Kalinowsky and Hippius 1969, Klein and Davis 1969) and in a comprehensive overview of schizophrenia (Bellak and Loeb 1969), there is little mention of negative or undesirable, nontoxic psychological responses. In contrast, there are vast numbers of investigative reports cataloguing physiologic and biochemical variations, social and descriptive alterations, and medical side effects. It seems that the psyche of the schizophrenic, which is after all the target of the psychotropic medications, has been neglected. There is, furthermore, a scarcity of articles bearing directly on the intrapsychic factors leading to discontinuation of these medications, although in clinical medicine such factors are well recognized (Blackwell 1973). Recently, Van Putten (1975) has drawn attention to manic-depressive patients who discontinue lithium during stressful life crises.[1]

According to the available reports, depressive reactions in schizophrenic patients have been noted after long-term neuroleptic medication (Cohen et al. 1964) and in approximately half the schizophrenic patients whose acute psychotic symptoms had been controlled by phenothiazines (Bowers and Astrachan 1967). Sarwer-Foner (1957, 1960, Sarwer-Foner and Ogle 1956) observed adverse "paradoxical" responses to neuroleptics and considered these as based on modifications in defensive activity. Physiologic interference with motor activity, especially when utilized as a major behavioral defense against passive feminine identifications, were psychologically threatening and accompanied by a "paradoxical" increase in anxiety. Also noted were an intensification in depression, changes in body image, and transference reactions, whereby the drug was regarded as an assault or seduction by a powerful doctor. Azima (1957, 1959, Azima and Sarwer-Foner 1960) considered drugs to primarily affect drive systems. As a result, predominantly aggressive impulses emerge: these being facilitated by inadequacies inherent in the schizophrenic's defenses—splitting, withdrawal, and projection. Kline (1956) observed a weakening of "defense mechanisms" that results in the expression and recognition of disturbing underlying emotions.

Clinical Observations

Examining case material obtained in ambulatory treatment from the psychoanalytic perspective shows that intrapsychic changes, even those that reflect apparent improvements, can in themselves be disruptive and give rise to regressive alterations in schizophrenic personality organization and func-

---

[1]Since this article was written, Van Putten, Crumpton, and Yale (1976) have described a group of chronic schizophrenics who habitually refused medication. There was a significant association of drug refusal with grandiosity. The findings were interpreted by these authors to mean that some schizophrenics may "prefer" an ego-syntonic grandiose psychosis to a relative drug-induced normality.

tioning—alterations potentially endangering the continuation of medication itself. An appreciation of these intrapsychic changes may be useful in forestalling premature cessation of medication, as well as in understanding the more general issues of noncompliance in the patient–psychotherapist relationship. The latter is especially important in view of the increasing use of depot medication (Groves and Mandel 1975).

Changes in Defenses

Changes in defensive activities occur as an accompaniment or result of neuroleptics. This may be particularly true with such primitive defenses as denial.

C., a 26-year-old schizophrenic man, denied that he did not have a job or vocational skill and that his father, a former art teacher, was now dead. His father was replaced by his "father who art in heaven," and through a psychotic identification, the patient believed himself to be Jesus Christ. Indeed, he did then have a job and a skill, if not a mission. With medication, the sudden distressing awareness developed that he was not the Savior. He was now unlike his dead father and developed a poorly tolerated grief reaction. He felt guilty in that by not possessing a job or skill he would be a failure to his father. The subjective experience and complaint, however, were focused on the medication: it made him feel tired and depressed and caused him to become withdrawn.

As I inquired further into his objection to the medication, C. expressed a desire to know me better. He wished I was his friend and thought I was unhappy and alone. Why, he asked in a sad and plaintive manner, was I "saturating [him] with Prolixin?" This, he felt, only necessitated his drinking excessive amounts of coffee to "counteract" the medication (otherwise he would "disappear") and led to memories of his father's alcoholism and to beatings he had suffered at his father's hands. During those beatings, he had longed for his father to leave, or to sober up with coffee so the alcoholic state would go away.

He began to blame me for causing him to feel fatigued, "slowed down," and withdrawn. How could I "predict" his response to medication? I was cruel for causing him to suffer. The psychotic belief emerged that the medication was an "input from the spiritual," "someone pressing on . . . squashing my skull." "Heavenly powers" were using the therapist . . . to reach him. The medication "slowed" him down and made him feel "tired and depressed," which was particularly frightening because he then became the "center of the universe: If I'm the slowest moving object . . . things circle around me." This state enabled his father to locate and make contact with him. He recalled having once "predicted" his father's death and felt that he was now being punished: "Things I've done are coming back to haunt me." He believed he was being punished for killing insects (animals) as a child and decided to become a vegetarian. With trepidation he asked whether I ate meat. If so, he was nervous about animals that I had killed. I was murderous and my own body, containing dead animals (bodies) might kill me or, in fact, I might be dead.

I interpreted his fear of being harmed and punished by the medication, his concern for my safety, and his guilt in relationship to his father's death. C. became a vegetarian and initiated vocational-rehabilitation training in food preparation—rather than "waiting for another lifetime." He continued to take medication and his complaints about the medication, while they persisted, were expressed in a less punishing manner. There was improvement in his feelings of depression, lassitude, and in his fears of being slowed down.

Another schizophrenic patient, M., denied he was ill despite multiple hospitalizations. Instead, he maintained the delusional belief that he was in charge of weather control for an entire metropolitan area. Abruptly, feeling unprepared, panicky, and overwhelmed, he complained bitterly that "Thorazine makes me aware I am ill." In a similar manner, changes occur in repressive defenses, bringing about awareness of previously unconscious thoughts and fantasies. In another schizophrenic patient, R., the neuroleptics were accompanied by memories of adolescent pedophilic activities whenever he would now be in the company of younger men; medications "caused perverted thoughts," he said.

A response to medication, by virtue of reduction in motor outlet or activity, can bring about a heightening of passivity, feelings of helplessness, and an increase in feminine homosexual ideas (Sarwer-Foner 1960). This is especially a problem when motor activity has been utilized as a major behavioral defense or when passivity has been a major characterologic feature. In addition, when the drug is regarded as a magical substance, a further increase in passivity is fostered.

A., a 21-year-old schizophrenic man, had been unemployed and dependent upon his parents for support. Unable to engage in social relationships without disorganizing panic, he maintained a withdrawn, autistic existence, one in which he would "carry on my own thoughts . . . that's my life." A major portion of his day was spent actively and compulsively participating in sports and maintaining the grandiose belief he was a nightclub entertainer who awaited discovery. Toward his father, he held the paranoid psychotic identification: "He's like me, I'm like him: He's nervous around people. He can read people too much. I can feel his feelings, but don't know why he can't handle it. Dad doesn't want me to work. Dad likes to have me by him, for his security so he can have something to do. I humble myself."

Administration of Stelazine was followed by feelings of laziness, bodily fatigue, and fears of physical immobility. His body felt heavy ("can't shake it"); he shaved his moustache and stopped playing sports. He was a "lazy person anyway; this makes it worse." The medications were "killing some-thing in my body." Furthermore, medications were a magical "crutch [to] rely on ... not you." His thoughts felt slowed down: The medications "control me. Make me dwell—not get off [unpleasant] thoughts. All of a sudden they hit me. Don't know where from. Off the wall. Things I'm thinking aren't me." He began awakening in the morning feeling "pinned down—with nothing to do other than fight for my life. Toward evening he feared for his safety and before falling asleep he would compulsively check his windows and closets for the presence of robbers. He believed he would be mugged because he was the smartest person in the world and because he intimidated others by "seeing things in them that they could not see in themselves. I stare at people and make them look at themselves." (This belief has interesting transference implications.) He had fantasies of either being pushed out a window or being commanded to jump or be shot: "Take your pick; I'd get shot." He also feared that he would be required to submit to being stabbed, tortured, crucified, and forced sexually to perform fellatio by a gang of Hell's Angels while they shit on him. He began to feel like a woman and prayed, "If you're going to take me, take me in my sleep."

Therapeutic sessions were punctuated by A.'s impressions of singers and movie stars. At times, he would assume their affectations and postures, or even stand up and enact a brief dance or choreography routine. His father admired show business and took him on trips to Las Vegas and Broadway and introduced him to famous people. His attempts to entertain me were a form of acting out within the transference. In response to my interpretation of his behavior, he voiced complaints that I, and the medica-tion, forced him to "jump hoops." In association to this, he had the image of having to passively submit to being pinned up against a wall and having a man shoot arrows at him.

Following a series of clarifications of his sense of reality in relationship to me and my continued presence, and following interpretations directed at his passivity, fears of being harmed by the drugs, and having to submit to my demands, A. resumed athletics and moved out of his parents' home. Both his delusional fears of personal harm and complaints directly referable to the medication subsided.

It should be emphasized that these changes in defensive structures are experienced by the schizophrenic as sudden, and as an interference with automatic modes of functioning. There are accompanying feelings of powerless-ness, helplessness, and loss. In these patients, and in those described below, there are also complaints of sudden unfamiliar feelings of self and changes in the self.

Changes in Object Relations

Use of medication may lead to symptomatic improvement in the sense of reality and reality testing (Bellak and Loeb 1969). It may also lead to decreases in hostility, belligerence, uncooperativeness, social isolation, and withdrawal; along with these changes, the use of medication may bring about a lessening of autistic behavior (Klein and Davis 1969) and of narcissistic preoccupations. Such changes may result, however, in secondary, or subsequent, interference with areas of functioning previously nonconflictual, or not recognized.

C.'s characteristic style of relating to women was to be superficially involved in a number of sexual affairs at any given time. With Prolixin he would complain of a change in and loss of "sexual drive." Further examination revealed that as he developed more sustained relationships with women he began to recognize them as separate from himself. He would now, however, experience fears of merger during sexual intercourse and the subjective experience of not being involved in, or a part of, the sexual act. In addition, instinctual regression and conflict emerged, as did a more direct expression of aggressive drives. He would: "Try to get my mind in a romantic frame of mind. [Begin] stroking a girl. What comes out [is] now it's time to feel her butt up. Wasn't thinking of dirt—or of eating my dandruff, but that's what it comes down to." He feared he "might become violent— like choking [or] cremating mother" and become a woman himself: "Feel I am a witch. I'm not the only one. I'm running into other girls too." The result was an inability to have an erection, and counteravoidance of the sexual act. This same individual was no longer able to pick up male hitchhikers. Formerly, once he had picked up a hitchhiker he would be unaware of that person's physical presence and would proceed without concern or distraction. Now he became apprehensive of the desire to place his hand upon the hitchhiker's leg, stimulating the emergence of partially repressed and frightening homosexual thoughts and feelings. I interpreted his conflict over sustaining close relationships, including one with me, and his fears of submitting and being harmed by me. He developed more prolonged, passive relationships with women, who now functioned as maternal figures, and he regained his sexual potency.

In another schizophrenic male, H., the institution of Trilafon was associated with cessation of the need for compulsive autoerotic masturbation. At the same time, however, masturbatory activity was regarded as "freaky" and his penis as without feeling and not a part of himself. Because heterosexual activities had always been frightening, he now felt "sexless" and depressed.

Thus, with partial reintegration of personality organization and abandonment of a more regressive narcissistic position, previously repressed impulses, as well as the invocation of defensive depersonalization, can emerge. This produces anxiety, instinctual regression and conflict, deneutralization of aggressive drives, and interference in previously unaffected drive discharge or secondarily autonomous functions.

Interference with Psychotic Restitution

Neuroleptics may interfere with psychotic restitutive symptoms.

A schizophrenic man, T., attributed to medication his lack of energy and alertness, diminished awareness, and inability to relate to others. Further exploration revealed the lack of a former sense of omniscience in controlling traffic lights, clouds, and the sun. T. now believed that when he approached another automobile's rear bumper or when he shifted his clutch he could no longer trigger the traffic light green. Clinically, the psychiatrist would judge this as a decrease in ideas of influence, that is, a positive therapeutic response. This was experienced by the patient, however, as a debilitating loss of energy and as an inability to influence or reestablish relationships with other persons. Similarly, being unable to bring out the sun or move the clouds meant that he was no longer the "center of the universe" nor the main authority on anything or anyone, including himself. Consequently, he felt incompetent, retarded, and depressed: "Prolixin rips off my power to open up the sky. I need to have more influence over it than it has over me."

Bodily Harm

To the patient, the use of medication may represent bodily harm with an accompanying loss of powers.

J., a 27-year-old paranoid schizophrenic man and a former construction worker, had a history of publicly disruptive behavior, jailings, physical abuse of girlfriends, repetitive hospitalizations following discontinuation of medication, exhibitionism, and recurrent psychotic episodes involving great feats or bursts of physical activity. On one such occasion he was apprehended by the Coast Guard after swimming out 2 miles into the Pacific Ocean on his way to Asia in order to locate his girlfriend. Injectable Prolixin Enanthate was experienced as producing a weakened condition with subsequent diminished energy and inability to "boast" or have an erection. He was no longer able to "walk through anyone," became increasingly dependent upon his girlfriend, who opposed the medication, and had recurrent dreams in which the medication would incarcerate and kill him. He abruptly terminated treatment and eloped with his girlfriend.

K., a 24-year-old schizophrenic male, through his facility with and access to primary-process material, gained local notoriety as a palm reader. In a clandestine manner he taught palmistry and developed a following; at the same time he worked as a junior executive in his father's business. He sought psychiatric treatment following the birth of a son, and the development of insomnia and overt psychotic thoughts. The administration of Stelazine was followed by an inability to perform previously practiced (even in the overtly psychotic state) palm reading. This was experienced as being "absent minded," "dissipated," "forgetful," and "not having the powers I once thought I had." He became depressed.

Approximately one month later K. noted that Stelazine was a pill like his wife's oral contraceptive. He believed, as a consequence, that he could no longer father a child. He feared becoming "dependent" on an "artificial" pill. He began to vomit in attempts to reduce the impact of the pills. This behavior, he remarked, was like that of his mother who suffered from chronic stomach ailments. He feared adult responsibilities and became panicky when, alone in the presence of his infant son, he felt like a child himself. At this point, he dreaded both working at his father's office and continuing his psychotherapy appointments. When his father was away, K. would secretly sit at his father's desk and have a "power trip." At other times he had fantasies of blowing up corporate buildings. He feared that his thoughts and behavior would now be revealed. Similar competitive feelings emerged toward me. He recalled that when he practiced palmistry, he "would not have to draw attention" to himself directly. He possessed a "gift" that would make people come to him. Everyone, including doctors, were "awed" by his powers. "People told me you tell me more than my psychiatrist." He feared I would now condemn him for being a "witch doctor," and, as a consequence, he would be punished: "Fear whatever I do to others. [Will] have it done to me. When I open up others I'm opening up myself." He would now suffer bodily mutilation ("get blown apart into twenty pieces"). Stelazine dosage at the time was 20 milligrams. His brain would be "opened up [for a] blood letting."

My interpretation of his punitive castration fears, his psychotic elaboration fantasies of body damage, and his conflicts over competitive strivings in relationship to me were followed by a reduction in his fears about medication, psychotherapy, work, and fatherhood. He did not resume palm reading but became more involved with his job and family.

Interference in the Use of External Reality

Neuroleptics may interfere with the schizophrenic's attempt to use external reality, especially interpersonal relationships, to ward off psychotic conflicts and further psychotic disintegration. An example is patient C., whose numerous sexual encounters permitted a warding off of disorganizing underlying homosexual conflicts. K., the palmist and local guru, who experienced a decreased facility in retrieval of primary-process material, could no longer turn to his following and "make them come to me," and was less able to resolve conflicts in this manner. Similarly, a male schizophrenic patient, W., used absurd humor (including condensation, displacements, and fragmentation of thought) to permit relationships with women. Neuroleptics interfered with access to primary-process thinking and, as a consequence, his appeal diminished. He could no longer turn to women and utilize them to prevent further psychotic disorganization.

Symbolic Significance

The medications may have major symbolic significance.

S., 22-year-old college coed, whose father was a chemist, had an initial response to Stelazine characterized by a clinical improvement of both schizoid withdrawal and difficulty in concentration, as well as abatement of hallucinations and delusional thoughts. Medication came to represent, however, submission to her father's influence, and her own personal failure and loss of self. She viewed herself as evil, unlovable, a peasant, and a "basket case." Soon she began to arise late in the morning and developed accusatory auditory hallucinations. That she was taking a chemical and that her father was a chemist symbolically brought her in closer contact with him, the individual against whom she measured herself. This served to increase her feelings of guilt, worthlessness, and self-punishment—feelings elaborated in a psychotic manner. She believed the medication was intended to "disrupt" and control her thinking. Cognition, an area of major importance to S.'s sense of self, was now threatened. She could no longer think for herself ("I don't think, therefore I'm not"), and she began having feelings of dissolution. There was difficulty in both separating herself from her father and in distinguishing between father's will and her response. I became an agent of her father, and the medication was seen as intended to "kill" her. Furthermore, medication became equated with her mother's alcoholism. S. believed that by taking medication she would become a prostitute and defended against this concern with the paranoid belief that the medication I gave her would result in her being "crippled," like her brother's wife who was paralyzed (without feeling) from the waist down.

Interpretations were directed at reality testing, ego boundaries, and autonomous functioning. Although there was subsidence of overt paranoid thoughts and hallucinations, she complained the medication made her feel "empty," without feelings, and less capable in handling her studies. She terminated therapy when she left home to resume college study.

Alterations in Body Image

Neuroleptics, by virtue of their direct pharmacologic effects on peripheral tissues and their functioning, may cause changes in body image and distortions in the sense of reality, thus imposing added reality tasks on the schizophrenic's already defective or weakened ego. Frequently these changes are elaborated in a psychotic manner. For example, O., a schizophrenic man, complained that the medication caused him to become withdrawn. Further examination revealed this sequence: neck muscle stiffness, weightiness to the neck, God coming down on me, the fear of God, withdrawal. Blurred vision in another schizophrenic, L., was magnified into a more global problem with perception: "Something is always wrong with how I see things." Ego boundaries then became less distinct and his tears became the result of another's sadness. At the same time, his powers increased to the point of "penetrating" vision and "extrasensory perception." Muscle stiffness in another schizophrenic was felt as a being encased inside the body; it led to social isolation. To yet another, sedativeness was "brain damage."

Incorporation into Schizophrenic Cognition

Furthermore, when bodily changes are combined with idiosyncratic schizophrenic cognition, utilizing primary-process thinking and predicate logic (Arieti 1955), they assume an even greater psychological meaning. A 26-year-old schizophrenic man, E., while on low doses of injectable depot Prolixin Decanoate (25 mg 1M every 2 weeks) would complain of fatigue and incessantly requested a prescription for Ritalin to give him more energy. He believed the injectable Prolixin *Deca*noate would result in infiltration of a chemical substance into the body causing it to *decay* and age. He also feared, through a psychotic identification with his deceased alcoholic father, who had been further wasted by cancer, that he himself would, like his father, decay. He had observed that Ritalin was given to hyperactive schoolchildren who themselves were young. Through the identity of predicates, the identity of subjects emerged: receiving Ritalin became identical to the attribute of being young. To him, this youthfulness would counter the psychotic body image distortion and decay brought upon him by the Prolixin Decanoate.

Discussion

Sudden intrapsychic changes brought about by chemical alterations in schizophrenic personality organization, though facilitative, can also be disruptive. Neuroleptics have characteristics that 1) pharmacologically alter peripheral somatic processes (for example, in their effects on the autonomic nervous system) and 2) psychotropically affect the functions of the central nervous system—the ongoing central program is altered. This paper is primarily concerned with this disruption of the ongoing central program. These medications alter both physiologic and psychologic frames of reference. This alteration interacts with both preexisting defective (Beres 1956) and weakened (Hartmann 1953) ego functioning; a sudden rate of change from a formerly stable, though pathologic, personality organization occurs. As a result, a disorganizing unfamiliarity is produced.

   This report is not intended to describe the positive therapeutic changes in psychotic symptoms or social functioning attendant on neuroleptic usage, nor their psychophysiologic effects. Nor does it refer primarily to the medical side effects of neuroleptics, such as those affecting extrapyramidally mediated motor functioning or autonomically mediated cholinergic or adrenergic changes, although any of these changes can be stressful and may be psychotically elaborated. In my opinion, however, dosages can be adjusted to deal with these problems, and most patients do not stop medication because of medical side effects alone. Finally, I am not describing those complaints that are incorporated into a preexisting delusional system and become attributed to medication—paranoid delusions, for example, that the medication is poison. Also not included in this study are complaints which serve to externalize and provide a focus for regressive behavior and schizophrenic disorganization: complaints of the medication's causing, for example, oversedativeness or difficulty in arising in the morning, which may reflect instead, a progressive state of withdrawal or the stressful ego-fragmenting transition from sleep to wakefulness. In either instance, discontinuation of medication or lowering of dosage would neither alter psychopathologic changes nor decrease complaints.

   These medications have been hypothesized as helpful agents in diminishing levels of disproportionate perceptual input and central nervous system arousal or activation (Lehman 1974). Furthermore, they may exert beneficial effects by reducing cognitive distortions brought about by inclusion of irrelevant stimuli, overinclusive thinking (Cameron 1946), or by the inability to maintain a major set (Shakow 1962). Adverse responses may, however, be produced, because of an interference in the adaptive value (though limited) of the organism's ongoing stabilized (though pathologic) state.

   If schizophrenic interference is likened to the interruption of an ongoing computer set, with both persistence and diversion from the program (Callaway 1970), then certain parameters of functioning are aided by a medication which would reduce this interference (such as by alteration in stimulus barrier), while other parameters may be differentially and variably affected. Neuroleptics have been postulated to increase (perceptual) sensory filtering by delaying EXIT from a program. That is, a reduction of the ongoing program's vulnerability to environmental interference by delaying premature EXIT may allow an increased time for perceptual sensory filtering. However, as Callaway (1970) points out, the operation of one program may inhibit the running of other programs.

   I propose that the major adverse effects of these drugs are that other personality functions, other programs, are differentially affected. What is suggested by the negative response to medication is that alterations are produced in narcissistic ego states and disruptions occur in preconscious processes, including access to primary-process content. These interact with transference-based responses to receiving the medication. Furthermore, in some cases, as economic and adaptive shifts occur, conflictual reactions become displaced onto the therapist and psychodynamically central issues emerge that are amenable to transference interpretations.

Affects not only signal danger but give an appraisal, of adaptive value, of the state of the organism (Pribram 1967, Rapaport 1953)—a how-am-I-doing? Medicated schizophrenics frequently complain of "feeling not myself," "zombie feeling," "I can't feel," "strange," "changed," "altered," and so on. The medicated schizophrenic feels himself to be unreal; a state of depersonalization is produced.

The concept of ego feeling is relevant here. According to Federn (1950), ego feeling is the feeling of uninterrupted bodily and mental relation. This includes motor and sensory memories concerning one's own person and the somatic organization or unity of ordered perceptions of one's body, with respect to both time and content. These medications appear to produce a discontinuity of preexisting ego feeling. The ego unit or self is changed. According to Schilder (1950), the body ego is the continuing awareness of one's body. The neuroleptics produce discontinuities here as well. These discontinuities can occur independently or may precede a psychotic elaboration of body image distortion. The unique paradox of the ego is, according to Federn, that it is subject and object in one, "The ego knows itself, feels and encounters itself. . . . The ego is the feeling of it*self*" (1950, pp. 8–9, my italics). It is not surprising that when we engraft this unfamiliar feeling onto the schizophrenic's weakened ego (for example, defective synthetic functioning, Nunberg 1931)—which already has a tendency to disorganize—both the unity of the organism is stressed and other significant disturbances in functioning occur.

Neuroleptics produce narcissistic changes which are defensive in nature and result in depersonalization. As Jacobson (1971) points out, these states of depersonalization "represent attempts at solution of narcissistic conflict. . . . The conflict develops within the ego and has its origin in struggles between conflicting identifications and self images" (p. 160). Furthermore, the state of depersonalization in schizophrenics is "a defense of the ego which tries to recover and to maintain its intactness by opposing, detaching, and disowning the regressed, diseased part" (p. 164). This can occur in reaction to a bodily part or be displaced onto the neuroleptic medication. The feeling of estrangement or depersonalization can then represent a rejection by the patient of the medication. It is defensive and hypochondriacal in nature and directed against further narcissistic regression.[2]

To the extent that there are two elements—medication-induced perceptual change in the feeling of unreality and psychotic defensive depersonalization—it

---

[2]Tausk (1919) has described a related phenomena in the sequential development of the *influencing machine*, though here the emphasis is on the patient's body. Hypochondriacal internal alteration is followed by rejection, experienced as estrangement, and leads to construction of the influencing machine, which is a summation of these alterations projected outward as a hostile power.

may be an important task of psychotherapy to differentiate one from the other. When the two become confused and further psychotically elaborated (as for example in a grandiose, hypochondriacal, or punitive manner), a stressful state is produced which may culminate in discontinuation of medication. Moreover, neuroleptics appear to produce abrupt, massive interruption of grandiose pre-occupations and of the associated pleasurable omnipotent feelings—especially when considered in relation to the nature reconstitutive process. Concurrent psychotherapy having to do with narcissistic changes and the sense of loss may be particularly important in this phase.

Furthermore, if we examine ego functions (in contrast to feelings of self, body image, ego feeling, sense of reality, etc., Spiegel 1959), a major problem of the schizophrenic's weakened ego is the regressive alteration of ego functions, including extreme forms of defensive activities (Arlow and Brenner 1969). A medication which produces sudden substantial changes in perception, body image, and grandiosity would affect not only feelings of self, but also such other ego functions as object relations, regulation of drives, synthetic-integrative functioning, and defenses. The latter by their very nature in psychoses are primitive and "unreliable" (Arlow and Brenner 1969, p. 11). The disruption in K.'s relationship with his father—and following the panic occasioned by the emergence of his poorly tolerated aggressive feelings, and the interference in his ability to continue working—is a good example.

Jacobson (1967) has drawn attention to the use of objects and reality for defensive purposes to control psychotic conflict. As a result of weaknesses in boundaries between psychic representation of objects and the self, a regressive narcissistic relationship to objects can permit an externalization of conflicts. In some of my patients this appeared to have been interrupted by medication. As an illustration, K., the palm reader, could neither control his hostile impulses when he felt displaced by his newborn son, nor, owing to changes in precon-scious ego state, externalize conflicts toward his following by projective identi-fication. He lost his powers, could no longer control himself, and became both agitated and depressed.

Federn (1950) described *preconscious falsification* as the process whereby preconscious ego states lose the cathexis of their boundaries and fail to function automatically; on the other hand, ideas seem imposed upon, or taken away from, the schizophrenic. Medications in some patients appear to enhance preconscious falsification. The occurrence of perverted thoughts in patient R. is an example, as is the change in preconscious states occasioned in the palm reader, K.

In this paper I have sought to describe a number of intrapsychic changes that occur during the administration of neuroleptic drugs. Unless these are recognized (and within the context of the therapeutic relationship), the schizo-phrenic patient experiences these changes as *due* to the medication, and *on this basis* may discontinue the medication or undergo considerable confusion and morbidity.

References

Arieti, S. (1955). *Interpretation of Schizophrenia.* New York: Brunner/Mazel.

Arlow, J. A., and Brenner, C. (1969). The psychopathology of the psychoses: a proposed revision. *International Journal of Psycho-Analysis* 50:5–14.

Azima, H. (1957). Psychoanalytic action of rauwolfia derivations. In *Psychopharmacology Frontiers* (International Congress of Psychiatry, Proceedings of the Psychopharmacology Symposium, Zurich, 1957), ed. N. S. Kline, pp. 281–284. Boston: Little, Brown.

_____ (1959). Effects of rauwolfia derivatives on psychodynamic structures. *Psychiatric Quarterly* 33:623–635.

Azima, H., and Sarwer-Foner, G. J. (1960). Psychoanalytic formulations on the effect of drugs in pharmacotherapy. In *International Symposium on the Extrapyramidal Reactions and Neuroleptics, Montreal, 1960,* ed. J. M. Bordeleau, pp. 507–518. Montreal: Editions Psychiatrique, 1961.

Ban, T. (1969). *Psychopharmacology.* Baltimore: Williams & Wilkins.

Bellak, L., and Loeb, L. (1969). *The Schizophrenic Syndrome.* New York: Grune & Stratton.

Beres, D. (1956). Ego deviation and the concept of schizophrenia. *Psychoanalytic Study of the Child* 11:164–235. New York: International Universities Press.

Blackwell, B. (1973). Drug therapy: patient compliance. *New England Journal of Medicine* 289:249–252.

Bowers, M. B., Jr., and Astrachan, B. M. (1967). Depression in acute schizophrenic psychosis. *American Journal of Psychiatry* 123:976–979.

Callaway, E. (1970). Schizophrenia and interference: an analogy with a malfunctioning computer. *Archives of General Psychiatry* 22:193–708.

Cameron, N. (1946). Experimental analysis of schizophrenic thinking. In *Language and Thought in Schizophrenia,* ed. J. S. Kasanin. Berkeley: University of California Press.

Cohen, S., Leonard, C. V., Farberow, N. L., and Shneidman, E. S. (1964). Tranquilizers and suicide in the schizophrenic patient. *Archives of General Psychiatry* 11:312–321.

Federn, P. (1950). *Ego Psychology and the Psychoses.* New York: Basic Books.

Group for the Advancement of Psychiatry (1975). *Pharmacotherapy and Psychotherapy: Paradoxes, Problems and Progress.* Vol. 9, Rep. No. 93. New York: Group for the Advancement of Psychiatry.

Groves, J. E., and Mandel, M. R. (1975). The long acting phenothiazines. *Archives of General Psychiatry* 32:893–900.

Hartmann, H. (1953). Contributions to the metapsychology of schizophrenia. *Psychoanalytic Study of the Child* 8:177–198. New York: International Universities Press.

Jacobson, E. (1967). *Psychotic Conflict and Reality.* New York: International Universities Press.

_____ (1971). *Depression.* New York: International Universities Press.

Kalinowsky, L. B., and Hippius, H. (1969). *Pharmacological, Convulsive and Other Somatic Treatments in Psychiatry.* New York: Grune & Stratton.

Klein, D. F., and Davis, J. M. (1969). *Diagnosis and Drug Treatment of Psychiatric Disorders.* Baltimore: Williams & Wilkins.

Kline, N. S. (1956). Pharmacology. Publication No. 42 of the American Association for the Advancement of Science, Washington, DC, p. 87.

Lehmann, H. E. (1974). Physical therapies of schizophrenia. In *American Handbook of Psychiatry,* vol. 3, ed. S. Arieti, 2nd ed., pp. 652–675. New York: Basic Books.

May, P. R. A. (1968). *Treatment of Schizophrenia.* New York: Science House.

Nunberg, H. (1931). The synthetic function of the ego. In *Practice and Theory of Psychoanalysis,* vol. I, pp. 120–136. New York: International Universities Press, 1948.

Pribram, K. H. (1967). Emotion: steps toward a neuropsychological theory. In *Neurophysiology and Emotion,* ed. D. C. Glass, pp. 3–40. New York: Rockefeller University Press.

Rapaport, D. (1953). On the psychoanalytic theory of affects. *International Journal of Psycho-Analysis* 34:177–198.

Sarwer-Foner, G. J. (1957). Psychoanalytic theories of activity-passivity conflicts and of the continuum of ego defenses. *Archives of Neurology and Psychiatry* 78:413–418.

———— (1960). Recognition and management of drug-induced extrapyramidal reactions and "paradoxical" behavioral reactions in psychiatry. *Canadian Medical Association Journal* 83:312–318.

Sarwer-Foner, G. J., and Ogle, W. (1956). Psychosis and enhanced anxiety produced by reserpine and chlorpromazine. *Canadian Medical Association Journal* 74:526–532.

Schilder, P. (1950). *The Image and Appearance of the Human Body.* New York: International Universities Press.

Shakow, D. (1962). Segmental set. *Archives of General Psychiatry* 6:17–33.

Spiegel, L. A. (1959). The self, sense of self, and perception. *Psychoanalytic Study of the Child* 14:81–109. New York: New York Universities Press.

Tausk, V. (1919). On the origin of the "influencing machine" in schizophrenia. In *The Psychoanalytic Reader,* ed. R. Fliess, pp. 31–64. New York: International Universities Press, 1948.

Van Putten, T. (1975). Why do patients with manic-depressive illness stop their lithium? *Comprehensive Psychiatry* 16:179–183.

Van Putten, T., Crumpton, E., and Yale, C. (1976). Drug refusal in schizophrenia and the wish to be crazy. *Archives of General Psychiatry* 33:1443–1446.

5

The Effect of Lithium on Manic Attacks

FELIX F. LOEB, JR., M.D.
LORETTA R. LOEB, M.D.

This paper describes a predictable relation between our manic-depressive patients' blood lithium levels and particular changes in their conscious and unconscious mental processes (i.e., their thoughts, wishes, fantasies, inclinations, and feelings). These changes were, in turn, predictively related to specific changes in these patients' overt manic symptomatology.

Because each of our patients' manic episodes was *heralded* by a marked increase in unconscious or conscious phallic sexual thoughts, feelings, and behaviors, and because this increase *preceded* any observed deterioration in ego or superego functioning, we hypothesize that a *primary* increase in our patients' phallic instinctual drives *secondarily* overwhelmed the capacity of their egos to defend against these drives, and that this, in turn, resulted in the development of our patients' overt manic symptoms.

Psychoanalysis (or psychoanalytically oriented psychotherapy) made our patients consciously aware both of their previously unconscious phallic sexual thoughts and impulses, and of their defenses against them. This new awareness enabled our patients to recognize when their, now conscious, phallic sexual impulses and thoughts became inappropriately intensified; and this, in turn, permitted them to avoid overt manic episodes by counteracting these inappropriate inclinations with increased doses of lithium.

Psychopharmacologic treatment with lithium dramatically alleviates the psychopathologic symptoms in patients suffering from manic-depressive psychosis without producing significant adverse *psychological* changes. This makes one wonder if the blood lithium levels in manic-depressive patients receiving lithium might correlate predictively with specific changes in their conscious and/or unconscious mental processes, and if these changes in mental processes might, in turn, lead to the changes seen in their overt clinical symptomatology. In this chapter, we try to shed light on this question by reporting on the relations between our manic-depressive patients' blood lithium levels, their conscious and unconscious mental processes (i.e., their thoughts, wishes, fantasies, inclinations, and feelings), and their manic symptoms. We observed these relations in the psychoanalysis (or psychoanalytic psychotherapy) of seven manic patients who were taking lithium. We shall describe three of these patients.

Review of the Literature

Kraepelin (1896) proposed the name *manic-depressive insanity*. He discounted the importance of psychic causality because usually there were no precipitating events. Krafft-Ebing (1906) documented that a general excitation, including sexual excitation, existed in mania. He felt the sexual instinct was not simply recklessly manifested, but was present in "actual abnormal intensity"; this was the basis of the sexual delusions in mania. Sexual affects completely swayed the imagination and behavior of these patients: In men, at the height of mania, he observed obscenity, exhibitionism, open onanism with pelvic movements of coitus, great excitation at the sight of women, and demands for coitus which could lead to sexual attacks on women. In severe cases, he noted ethics and willpower lost their controlling influence entirely, whereas in milder cases restraint was still possible.

Abraham's (1911) manic patient's sexual instinct began with "great violence" in his sixth year when he was caught and punished for masturbating (p. 139). During adolescence, he continued to masturbate, but showed little interest in girls. During his first manic attack, at age 28, his sexual interest turned to women, and, "Nearly every night a sexual excitement used to overtake him with sudden violence" (p. 142).

Freud (1921) said that a mania may emerge from a melancholia because the patients' "ego ideal might be temporarily resolved into their ego after having previously [in the instance of melancholia] ruled it with special strictness" (p. 132). Later, Fenichel (1945) said that in mania the ego has freed itself from the superego's pressure, resulting in release of an abundance of mostly oral impulses. He recognized, however, that the ". . . hypergenitality of the typical manic" (p. 408) did not readily fit into this oral model. He also observed, ". . . a manic behavior may be rationalized or idealized" (p. 410). Fenichel felt that, because the periodicity of mania seemed at times unrelated to external precipitants, purely biological determinants were involved.

In discussing elations, including mania, Lewin (1950) stated that in all his cases except for one, the oral triad was used to defend against external stimuli pertaining to the oedipal situation. Lewin cites a case in which a hypomanic patient has a blank dream with orgasm that was equivalent to the avoidance of sexual ideas.

According to Ostow (1962), the libido in mania is turned away from the love object and redirected narcissistically, toward either the self or objects representing the self, and there is an intensification of sublimation activities. In 1971, Freeman found that patients who otherwise had little genital drive became very sexually active during acute manic episodes. When they were unable to immediately satisfy their needs, they became aggressive. Van Putten (1975) studied six manic-depressive patients who developed acute manic attacks after they stopped taking lithium. Each, respectively, felt marvelous, participated in wild sexual parties, danced a great deal (some in the nude), and kissed people at random. Some of the women became illegitimately pregnant. Shopsin's (1979) manic patients also had an insatiable sexual appetite which led to abounding energy, sexual preoccupations, and indiscriminate sexual acts.

A dampening of sexual fantasies and activities in three prisoners who were given lithium was noted by Sheard and colleagues (1975). Sheard and colleagues (1977) showed that lithium reduced assaultive behavior in young male aggressive offenders. This was accompanied by a significant increase in their serum luteinizing hormone without any significant change in serum testosterone. They felt that because their results showed that lithium had an effect on the system that regulates gonadal hormones, there was a possibility of lithium effects at other sites sensitive to androgens or luteinizing hormones, possibly in the central nervous system.

There is agreement in the literature that MHPG (3-methoxy-4-hydroxy-phenyl-ethylene glycol), a breakdown product of norepinephrine that is excreted in the urine, is a biochemical marker for state changes in subjects with affective disorders (Pickar et al. 1978). The precursors of MHPG are considered to be responsible, in part, for the excessive behavioral activation in mania. Deleon-Jones and colleagues (1982) reported a case of a 43-year-old woman whose father was a presumed manic-depressive. She belonged to a subgroup of subjects who suffer from a subsyndromal affective disorder during their premenstruum. During her premenstrual phase her MHPG levels were considerably higher than they were during her follicular and luteal phases, and these elevations coincided with the severest manifestations of her symptoms. These elevations did not occur during cycles when she was receiving lithium.

Clinical Material

Patient R.

R., a 32-year-old male biochemist, sought help with his manic-depressive illness and his poor marital relationship. In the fall of his 29th, 30th, and 32nd years, he had had to be hospitalized for uncontrollable attacks of anxiety, anger, insomnia, flight of ideas, clang associations, and grandiose ideas. His third hospitalization lasted only a week because, for the first time, he was diagnosed as manic-depressive and placed on 2,100 mg of lithium per day. R. had never had delusions or hallucinations, and related warmly. After discharge, R. began twice-a-week psychotherapy; 6 months later, he began four-times-a-week psychoanalysis, which lasted almost 1,000 hours. During the analysis, except for the time of his single manic attack, he was maintained first on 1,200 mg and then 1,800 mg of lithium per day; the therapeutic level of his blood lithium varied between 0.6 and 1.2 mEq/L.

Initial History. R.'s attractive mother was volatile, but "lax and inconsistent." When the patient was 5 years of age, after his father's infidelity led to a divorce, R.'s mother, who was dressed in a sheer nightgown, said R. was now the "man of the house." Then for years R. obsessed whether or not he caused the divorce. At age 8, he discussed his "elated and depressed" feelings about the divorce with a girlfriend. R. said his sexual explorations with this girl were less important to him than her emotional support.

Repressed History Recalled During the Analysis. R. recalled inspecting his stepmother's genitals through her negligé when he was aged 8. At age 12, he undressed his sleeping stepmother, kissed her breasts, and felt he could have won her away from his father. During adolescence, R. avoided sexual feelings by dating only "unattractive women." When aged 22, R. became jealous of his best friend's affair with his stepmother, and precipitously married a 28-year-old woman. Six months later, R. had an affair, "because he was lonely"; paradoxically, his sexual activity with his wife increased. This was R.'s first, though unrecognized, manic attack. During each of his three subsequent attacks, R. made inappropriate sexual advances to women and wrote to his mother about his intimate sexual life.

Psychoanalysis of R.'s Manic Breakdown while on Lithium. The analytic process and technique (including parameters) are mentioned only when pertinent to the purpose of this paper.

Retrospectively, the first indication of R.'s impending manic attack occurred in the forty-sixth hour: R. said a secretary, M., told him she was lonely, and he was tempted to share his own "loneliness" by having an affair with her. The patient learned later that this early symptom, "loneliness," represented a defensive euphemistic rationalization of his then pathologically increasing, unconscious sexual inclinations. For the next few weeks R. felt what he called "pressured," "laughed too often and too loud," had difficulty sleeping, and abstained from sexual intercourse with his wife. He later learned that by abstaining he was trying to keep unconscious his then increasing sexual desires. Although R. was taking his usual 1,200 mg of lithium daily, his blood lithium level fell below its therapeutic range to 0.54 mEq/L. R. increased his lithium dose to 1,500 mg per day, but over the next 2 weeks, he became "pressured" by obsessive romantic fantasies about M. and began masturbating several times a day.

Soon R. told M. of his "romantic" thoughts about her, but he was unaware of any *sexual* thoughts or feelings for her. R. was being threatened by increasing sexual impulses, but his ego was still able to defend against these impulses with isolation, rationalization, and idealization.

In spite of his taking 1,500 mg of lithium daily, over the next 5 days R.'s blood lithium level fell below 0.40 mEq/L. He then began making love several times a day instead of his usual three times a week. Over the course of the next several days he developed all of his other manic symptoms and was hospitalized. In the hospital R. repeatedly phoned M. to ask her to have intercourse. R. was no longer able to idealize M., and he was no longer able to isolate and rationalize his sexual desires for her. He was now acting out these impulses. After 4 days on 2,700 mg of lithium, R.'s blood lithium level rose to 1.2 mEq/L, his manic symptoms subsided, and he was discharged.

The next day R. resumed analysis and said, "I am pleased; the hospitalization prevented me from having a sexual affair with M. My usual sexual reticence is a protection against my sexual urges, which become intense and out of control when I become manic. Now that my lithium is almost doubled, I am able to handle these feelings." R. remained energetic and jocular, but behaved appropriately. His thoughts slowed down, and he began sleeping all night. Then he stopped masturbating, and began making love only once a day. Within a few days, R.'s desire for intercourse with M. was forgotten, and he visited her "to communicate," "for approval," or because he was "lonely" and "in love." R. was again isolating and rationalizing his sexual urge, and idealizing M.

A month later, R.'s blood lithium level rose to 1.8 mEq/L; his lithium dose was lowered from 2,700 to 1,800 mg/day. He was maintained on this dose during the rest of his analysis.

Four months later, R. began having intercourse regularly with M. Then, when M. went away for a week, R. became "pressured"; he stopped having intercourse with his wife. He said he could not have sex with his wife because she did everything else for him, such as housekeeping and cooking. He now realized he had been isolating the affectionate feelings he had for his wife from the erotic feelings he had for M. In M.'s absence, both sets of feelings became directed toward his wife, and he became anxious and sexually inhibited. R. next remembered that at the time of his parents' divorce, after his mother, dressed in a sheer nightgown, told him he would now have to be the man of the house, he had "panicked while swimming," fearing that "a fish might nibble his feet." After this, he had felt "pressured," became restless, had trouble sleeping, and began obsessing whether or not he was responsible for the divorce.

Over the course of the analysis, R. had the following dreams, associations, and recollections, which led him to understand his unreasonable childhood fear that a fish might bite him. R. dreamed: "I am resting in the woods near a sexy girl who is another man's wife. I can't eat with, or have sex with her, or I will get my brains beat out." He had the following associations: (1) When little, he had seen his grandfather, who had always been nice and kind, beat the brains out of a cat for chasing a squirrel. (2) He had been unable to express anger at his best friend for having an affair with his stepmother. (3) R. recalled that, after his stepfather caught him masturbating and criticized him for it, he had feared his sexual feelings for his mother and sister and had kept them at a distance. Subsequently, R. got angry at his analyst for having interrupted therapy for a few days. R. then dreamed, "Someone who resembled both you [his analyst] and my father caught me in bed with my mother and chased me away." After working on this dream, R. realized he was angry at his analyst, not because his analyst missed sessions, but because R. felt that his analyst, like his father and stepfather, was critical of him for having sexual feelings for his mother, sister, and daughter. In a later hour, R. had the following fantasy: "I have a general feeling of arousal that is spreading from my penis, and I am/was worried that it will reach my head. Then it does, and I leap about the room. Finally, I am back on the couch with a flower in my hand, like a corpse." He said the fantasy meant he was afraid that his analyst would kill him if he became aroused. Later R. had another dream: "I went to M.'s house where there were some men who took my wallet, car keys, and pants. I fought to get them back." He associated that he feared being emasculated for his affair with M. and for his sexual feelings for his stepmother and his daughter. After making the preceding connections, R. understood that his childhood fear of being bitten on the foot by a fish had concealed his fear that his "father might cut off his penis for having sexual desires for his mother and for causing the divorce." R. now understood that his early fear of castration had prevented him from becoming aware of his sexual feelings and had kept him from acknowledging his intensified sexual impulses during his manic attacks.

R. had always felt that he had had affairs to obtain "love" and "approval," so that he could dissipate his "pressured, lonely feelings" and raise his low self-esteem. But, after R. understood his fish phobia, he began to notice that M.'s *love and praise* did not relieve his "pressured, lonely feelings" or raise his self-esteem; whereas *sexual intercourse* with her did. He was now able to remember that during his manic attack he had consciously wanted sexual intercourse with M., and he realized that before and after his attack he had concealed this sexual wish from himself behind ideas of love, affection, approval, and loneliness. Now R. understood that in the past he had defended against recognizing his "pressured" sexual urges by rationalizing them and calling them "loneliness," or "a need for love and approval." He had disguised his desire for intercourse by euphemistically calling it "loneliness" or "love," in the same way he had, as a child, disguised his masturbation by calling it "climbing a pipe."

R. could now see that he was provoking his daughter to anger—just as he had his mother, his sister, his wife, and M.—to push them away so he would not have to acknowledge his sexual feelings for them. R. then had a nightmare: "I'm in a damaged ship's hold. Water rushes in, and I try to keep it sealed up." He associated that he ". . . feared being swamped by sexual desires." He then had a dream of a wall—a blank dream (Lewin, 1950). In addition to the oral meanings Lewin described, the dream represented a defensive barrier against his phallic inclinations.

During termination, R. stated he had feared and overcontrolled his sexual impulses, not only because they were incestuous but because he feared they might make him give up all productive work to engage in constant sexual activity. Five years after the analysis, R. was doing well at work, and was having no marital problems. He jokingly said that he was still on lithium and was living an ordinary, dull life—with no affairs and no manic attacks.

Patient V.

In his first visit, V., a 25-year-old single male, complained of difficulty controlling his sexual desires around women and of a need to masturbate five times a day. He was anxious, laughed incessantly, had a flight of ideas, and used denial. He alternately behaved seductively or frighteningly toward his (female) therapist. No hallucinations, delusions, or ideas of reference were present, nor were deficits found in his proverb interpretations or judgment. He had experienced undiagnosed manic episodes and periods of depression frequently since age fifteen.

In early childhood, V. had been easily excited sexually when given a bath; and in the second grade, he had to hide his erections when talking to an attractive teacher. After age 12, women dominated his thoughts, and he masturbated incessantly. V. felt that his mental problem began at age 4 when his fingertip was bitten off by a dog after he thought he had won his Nanny away from her husband. Shortly thereafter, he was dressed in girls' underwear because his clothes got wet. At 14, V. began running away and using street drugs. Although he had given his mother a hard time, his father never disciplined him.

V.'s aggressive sexual behavior necessitated a 2-year hospitalization at age 16. At 20, V. again became confused, sexually threatening toward females, and grandiose. He was again hospitalized. His Rorschach responses were to female anatomy, primal scene material, and rape. After discharge, V. got a job in a factory. At 24, he began demanding "instant" sexual gratification from his girlfriend. Soon his impulsiveness and grandiosity returned, and he was again hospitalized. In the hospital, he frequently entered the women's unit and, when he could not obtain sexual gratification, he complained and became unruly.

At age 25, V. began four-times-a-week, analytically oriented psychotherapy. After a month, the diagnosis of manic-depression was made, and V. was started on lithium. Three days after his blood lithium level rose above 1.5 mEq/L, his onanistic frequency decreased, he inhibited his sexual feelings toward his female therapist, his wild gaze and inappropriate laughter subsided, he could sit still and talk without a flight of ideas, and his "enjoyment of food," which was always absent during his manic attacks, returned. During V.'s next 25 days on lithium, he shaved off his beard, took off his earring, improved his hygiene, and organized his clothing.

To control V.'s manic symptoms, his blood lithium had to be maintained between 1.5 and 1.8 mEq/L and monitored two to four times a week. The intensity of V.'s hypersexuality was inversely related to his blood lithium level. When he forgot to take his lithium, his blood lithium level would fall, and his erotic feelings and fantasies toward his therapist would increase. He would euphorically describe feeling "handsome and masculine" and having sexual feelings "running down his legs," which he wanted to satisfy immediately. When V.'s blood lithium level was in the therapeutic range, he had an empty, "no more energy" feeling, felt "ugly and unattractive," and was pleased to have affectionate instead of erotic feelings toward his therapist, whom he then saw as a mother figure. V.'s therapist learned that when his thoughts turned to sex, his blood lithium level had fallen.

The relation between V.'s blood lithium level, his unconscious psychodynamics, and his manifest symptoms can be illustrated by two typical episodes in which his blood lithium level fell. In the first episode, V. developed lithium toxicity, and his lithium had to be discontinued. His blood lithium level fell to 0.82 mEq/L, and he developed manic symptoms. He began masturbating five or more times a day, became sexually demanding and impulsive, could not keep his thoughts on a single subject, and then stopped sleeping. In therapy, V. talked incessantly and crudely of his wish to have intercourse with his therapist. Lithium therapy was resumed. When, after 3 days, V.'s blood lithium level returned to its therapeutic level, his thoughts slowed down and he was again able to sleep. After a few more days, V.'s wild sexual fantasies became confined to his dreams, and he began to express guilt for the erotic fantasies he had experienced and acted on during his attack. He again idealized his therapist and felt her to be "like a mother." Although it "embarrassed" him, V. could now discuss his sexual feelings with his therapist without feeling he must immediately act on them.

In the second episode, V.'s blood lithium level fell in spite of the fact that he was taking his regular dose of 2,700 mg of lithium each day. He began masturbating incessantly and feared he would lose control of his unrelenting sexual attraction for his therapist. Next he became agitated, spoke rapidly of an impulse to put out his eyes, and readily agreed to be hospitalized. Over the course of the next 2 weeks, V.'s lithium dose was slowly increased; as his blood lithium level gradually came back up to its therapeutic level, his manic symptoms subsided. Following discharge, V. spoke of having become "oversexed," and that this had made him feel "guilty" and had "driven him crazy."

In this manic attack, like in others, V. had the impulse to put out his eyes *only* when he was going into, or coming out of, the attack. Going into a manic attack, when V.'s blood lithium level dropped to between 0.82 and 1.5 mEq/L, his formerly unconscious, unacceptable phallic sexual impulses became conscious as fantasies, and he wanted to punish himself for them by putting out his eyes. Once V.'s blood lithium level dropped below 0.82 mEq/L, he began acting out his sexual fantasies without experiencing guilt, and he no longer expressed the wish to put out his eyes.

When threatened by his sexual feelings for his therapist, V. would try to push her away by provoking her to anger, or he would "turn himself off" by thinking she was "full of shit" or "smelled like a fish." He then remembered that, when he was 14, he had vomited when he observed his sister's menstrual flow. He realized that since that time he had, from time to time, stopped himself from becoming sexually aroused by thinking of menstruation or defecation.

Patient X.

Before beginning lithium therapy, X., a 39-year-old, married, manic-depressive woman, had had seven severe manic breakdowns. Once on lithium, her manic attacks had been much fewer, shorter, and milder. She began weekly psychoanalytic psychotherapy to improve her poor marital relationship. She was plainly dressed, shy, and prudishly refused to discuss her sexual history. She had no memories of her thoughts or actions during her manic attacks. By refusing to use the couch, X. controlled herself and her therapist as she had controlled her family.

After a year of therapy, after X. became aware of her unconscious, transferential distrust of her therapist, she spontaneously lay down on the couch and, unaware that her fly zipper was open, she recounted with pleasure the many times during her manic attacks when she had enticingly, "wantonly and indiscriminately" seduced men. Following her manic attacks, X. had become guilty and had repressed these hypersexual episodes.

Subsequently, X. acknowledged she had been unconsciously using erotic transference feelings toward her therapist to resist remembering the unacceptable sexual thoughts, feelings, and actions she had experienced during her manic attacks. She had originally forgotten these sexual experiences because they reminded her of frightening sexual fantasies she had had as a child toward her dominating and impetuous father.

One year after psychotherapy ended, X.'s husband reported that his wife had become calmer, more sexually open with him, and less shy with friends.

Discussion

Our seven patients had manic attacks while both in analysis (or psychoanalytically oriented psychotherapy) and on lithium. This permitted us to observe and analyze the development and resolution of their manic episodes in detail. We made the following relevant observations:

1. At the onset of each manic attack, *prior to* developing manifest manic symptoms, our patients' blood lithium levels fell, and there was a marked increase in the overt manifestations of their usually unconscious, phallic[1] sexual fantasies and impulses. *After a time,* our patients' increasing unconscious sexual urges and phallic-type fantasies seemed to overpower their ego defense mechanisms and to produce the symptom of hypersexuality, which was manifested by increased unconscious sexual thoughts and feelings followed by inappropriate, sexually motivated behavior and the other symptoms of mania. It should be stressed that prior to undergoing psychoanalysis or psychoanalytic psychotherapy, our patients were not *consciously* aware that their phallic sexual fantasies and inclinations were increasing prior to their developing hypersexual behavior.

2. During their manic attacks, when we brought our patients' blood lithium levels back within their therapeutic ranges, *initially,* the overt manifestations of their unconscious phallic sexual fantasies and inclinations diminished; *then,* their premanic ego defense mechanisms came back into operation; *finally,* their manic symptoms ceased.

3. During the development of our patients' overt manic attacks they used increasingly regressive defense mechanisms to try to keep their increasing phallic sexual inclinations and fantasies out of consciousness.

4. Psychoanalysis (or psychoanalytically oriented psychotherapy) made our patients consciously aware both of their previously unconscious phallic sexual inclinations and thoughts, and of their defenses against them. This new awareness enabled them to recognize when their, now conscious, phallic sexual impulses and thoughts became inappropriately intensified; and this, in turn, permitted them to avoid overt manic episodes by counteracting these incongruent inclinations with increased doses of lithium.

Because each of our patients' manic episodes was *heralded* by a marked intensification of their unconscious or conscious phallic inclinations, and because this intensification *preceded* any deterioration in their ego or superego functioning (such as their using more primitive defense mechanisms), we hypothesize that a *primary* increase in our patients' phallic inclinations and wishes *secondarily* overwhelmed the capacity of their egos to defend against these tendencies; this, in turn, resulted in the development of our patients' overt manic symptoms. *We thus hypothesize that the primary and underlying, though most often kept unconscious, psychological disturbance in manic-depressive illness is a biologically determined increase in phallic sexual instinctual drive* (Moore and Fine 1968) *and not a primary weakening of ego or superego functioning. This biologic determinant is counteracted by lithium therapy.* We do not mean to

---

[1]By "phallic" or "phallic phase" we refer to the developmental phase in which other urges *begin* to be subordinated to the primacy of the genitals (Freud 1938, pp. 154–155). This process is not completed until the subsequent genital phase. We do not mean to imply by the term any of the other meanings Freud had given it.

imply by this hypothesis that we feel there is a one-to-one, direct causal relation between manic patients' increased phallic sexual instinctual drives and their manic symptoms. Rather, we feel that this relationship must be the consequence of a sequence of as yet unknown, complex interactions among multiple neurophysiological, biochemical and psychological variables.

In addition to the preceding hypothesis, the following alternative hypotheses could also explain our observations: (1) Certain types of ego weakness result in the emergence or intensification of otherwise well-defended or well-sublimated phallic sexual inclinations. (2) Some unknown factor or factors result in both the intensification of phallic sexual inclinations and the subsequent ego weakness. Although we cannot rule out the possibility that further observations may prove one of the two latter hypotheses to be more correct, at present we find the first hypothesis to be the most useful clinically. It best corresponds to our clinical observations that as manics go into manic attacks, they regularly manifest an intensification of their phallic sexual thoughts, feelings, and behaviors long before they show any signs of ego weakness. In a direct and relatively uncomplicated way, the intensity of our patients' unconscious or conscious phallic interests and inclinations could successfully be used clinically to predict how their egos would function subsequently. For example, when the level of their phallic sexual inclinations and wishes increased, one could predict that soon their level of ego functioning would diminish. One could successfully predict that they would soon begin to use more and more primitive defenses in an effort to sustain their faltering integration and control and that eventually their relation with reality would be compromised.

Abraham (1911), Fenichel (1945), Freeman (1971), Krafft-Ebing (1906), Lewin (1950), Shopsin (1979), and Wolpert (1981) all found heightened phallic sexual activity in patients suffering from mania. We are in agreement with Fenichel (1945) and Jacobson (1971), who felt that biologic factors were causative in mania. Jacobson's (1971) patients were able to observe, with intact egos and insight, the onset of manic attacks, which they felt to be somatic in origin (pp. 104, 173). Other authors, Deleon-Jones (1982), Sheard and colleagues (1975, 1977), and Van Putten (1975), each observed that lithium reduced patients' sexual thoughts and activities and/or that lithium was related to, or had an effect on, the systems that regulate gonadal hormones. Because each of our patients' manic episodes was heralded by an increase in sexual thoughts, feelings, and behaviors, *we feel that in manic patients, causative biological factors result in their having periodically intensified unconscious phallic sexual wishes and inclinations, which can somehow be counteracted by lithium.*

During their acute manic episodes, our patients' phallic sexual needs were markedly increased, whereas their oral requirements and anal demands were significantly diminished. When acutely manic, they showed little or no interest in food, and they neither displayed nor sought admiration and affection. They ceased to express oral-dependent longings for their love objects, and they demanded "instant" sexual gratification.

Abraham (1911) clearly documented his manic patients' hypersexuality, but he did not feel that this hypersexuality was a cause of the illness. Abraham could only have conducted analysis on his patients during their remissions. At other times, without the use of lithium, his manic patients could not have lain still on his couch. During such relative remissions, manic-depressives display those oral and anal symptoms that led Abraham to believe that these patients must have had causative, traumatic experiences—fixations—at the late oral and early anal stages of development. Our observations of manic patients on lithium suggest, instead, that the oral-anal characteristics Abraham observed are the result of a defensive regression away from the overwhelmingly traumatic, phallic impulses our patients began to experience intermittently in their phallic-oedipal phase of development. During remissions, the manic unconsciously remembers, and overdefends against, his previously intensified conscious or unconscious phallic sexual wishes and inclinations. He characteristically uses regressive anal or oral defenses to channel his unacceptable instinctual drives into obsessive-compulsive symptoms and character traits. Our patients' oral-anal symptoms were clearly a consequence of their using regression as a defense against their periodically overwhelming and frightening phallic impulses. For example, before and after R.'s psychotic episode, his elaborate ego defense mechanisms, through a defensive regression, concealed his phallic sexual impulses behind oral-anal, obsessive-compulsive symptoms and character traits. Wolpert's (1981) observation that some manic-depressive patients display other than oral-anal symptoms also contradicts Abraham's conclusion.

Like our manic patients, Lewin's (1950) elated patients defended against a genital-oedipal conflict by regressing to a pregenital, oral level. Lewin, however, saw elation as a defense—denial, whereas we see mania as the manifestation of an instinctual drive that is defended against. The dynamics of elation in people who are not manic-depressive might, therefore, be different from the dynamics of elation in patients who are manic-depressive.

Rangell (1968), Glenn (1974), and others state that the concept of an actual neurosis contains a "kernel of truth" (Glenn, p. 183). Although Freud (1925) did not deny the existence of mental conflicts in patients with actual neuroses, he felt "that the symptoms of these patients are not mentally determined or removable by analysis, but they must be regarded as direct toxic consequences of disturbed sexual chemical processes" (p. 26). Our observations support Wolpert's (1977) contention that manic-depressive psychoses are genetically determined, actual neuroses (p. 584). We suspect that lithium treatment combats this actual neurotic process, not by increasing the manic's ability to use ego defense mechanisms, but by counteracting certain unknown, "disturbed sexual chemical processes" that increase his phallic instinctual drive. Once the strength of the sexual instinctual drive is reduced to manageable proportions, either by lithium or by a naturally occurring remission, the manic is again able to use his prepsychotic, neurotic defense mechanisms to realistically and appropriately channel his libidinal strivings.

According to Wolpert (1981), some manic-depressive psychoses are purely psychologically determined, some are purely physiologically determined, and some are determined by both psychological and physiologic factors. Yet, according to Pollock (1977), manic-depressive patients suffer from two diseases. One is the manic-depressive illness, which can be treated with lithium; the other is the obsessive-compulsive personality, which can be treated by analysis. We agree with Pollock, but also feel that the manic-depressive's personality is itself significantly determined by his having had abnormally intense, conscious or unconscious phallic wishes and inclinations, which clashed with his environment during his phallic phase of development and later came into conflict with his superego.

Although the adult syndrome of manic-depressive illness is not seen before puberty (Anthony and Scott 1960, Thompson and Schindler 1976), we agree with Anthony and Scott and Feinstein and Wolpert (1973) that the disease can exist as a psychodynamic entity in childhood. Our manic-depressive patients did not display unusually intense oral or anal inclinations or behaviors before their phallic phase, but during that phase they did exhibit unusually intense phallic sexual desires and preoccupations. These intense sexual wishes and preoccupations exaggerated our patients' oedipal conflicts and led them to regress, defensively, to their earlier oral and anal inclinations and defenses. Their oral and anal preoccupations and behaviors then persisted throughout the latency phase.

Neither R. nor V. displayed exceptionally intense oral or anal inclinations before the age of 5, but both exhibited intense sexual strivings as children. Beginning at age 4, R. "climbed the plumbing" to masturbate. When R. was 5 years of age, his mother, dressed in a sheer nightgown, told him he was the man of the house. Following this, R. became "pressured" and restless, had difficulty sleeping, started to obsess whether or not he was responsible for his parents' separation, and became afraid to go swimming lest a fish bite his feet. At age 8, R. told a girlfriend of this continuing obsession and tried to look at his stepmother's genitals. V. said his childhood had been filled with sexual stimulation and that he had been easily aroused. At age 4, V. was bitten by a dog and fantasied that this was a punishment for his sexual desires. In the second grade, V. had had to hide his frequent erections.

To defend against these intense phallic wishes and inclinations, both patients regressed to their oral and anal levels. During latency, R. used the anal defense mechanism of isolation to separate his erotic feelings for his stepmother from his affectionate feelings for his mother. To avoid seeing his mother as sexually attractive, R. repressed that his mother was affectionate, caring, giving, and accommodating, and imagined her instead to be (orally) distant and rejecting, and (anally) overcontrolling. "Every day" during latency, R. did something (anally) "sadistic" to anger his mother so that she would "keep her distance." During the analysis, he dreamed he was picking his nose and eating what he got out, to disgust his mother and push her away. R. felt semen, like feces, was dirty; and he compulsively washed his penis after intercourse. V. would deliberately "turn himself off" by thinking that a girl "smelled like a fish" or that she was "full of shit." Only when on lithium was V. able to interrupt his phallic pursuits and show any interest or enjoyment in eating.

Our patients staunchly defended against remembering the lustful sexual activities, thoughts, and feelings they experienced during manic attacks. Before his manic attack, R. had neurotically inhibited his phallic sexual wishes and inclinations and idealized (Glover 1938) the objects of his instinctual drive. He had rationalized euphemistically that his attachment, both to his wife and M., was based on "loneliness," "love," and "a wish for approval." During his manic attack there was no such rationalization or idealization; he wanted only to attain the pleasure and release of orgasm with women. As R.'s defense of idealization was analyzed, he gradually became conscious of his primitive phallic needs, which he had hidden from himself behind his so-called "need for love and approval." As Freud (1921) said, ". . . wherever we come across an affectionate feeling it is successor to a completely 'sensual' object-tie . . ." (p. 138).

Our data corroborate Jacobson's (1971) observation that manic-depressive patients suffer from an instability of self-esteem, which is readily damaged by frustrations of their overdependent attachments to overvalued love objects (p. 231). Our data, however, do not support her conclusion that this instability of self-esteem is the result of a primary ego weakness. Instead, our patients' self-esteem was readily damaged by frustrations of their dependent attachments to defensively idealized love objects, because our patients were made overly dependent on their love objects by their intense, unconscious phallic wishes and inclinations.

Unlike their increased phallic behavior, the increased aggressive behavior our patients displayed during their manic attacks did not appear to be *primarily* biologically determined. Instead, aggressive behavior occurred when phallic sexual impulses were not immediately gratified (Freeman 1971, McDevitt 1983). R. became inappropriately aggressive during his acute manic attack, not simply because he lost or was slighted by an object, but because when he lost an object, his intense sexual desires could not be immediately gratified by that object. Between their acute manic episodes our patients sought to contain their unconscious phallic wishes and inclinations by aggressively provoking loved objects to anger.

Following their manic attacks, our manic patients often considered the excessive sexual feelings, thoughts, and behaviors they had experienced during their manic attacks to be improper or indecent, and they became guilty. This guilt led them to punish themselves with self-deprecatory thoughts and self-destructive behaviors, and to complain of feelings of depression. For example, when coming out of a manic attack, V. often had the impulse to put out his eyes. Object losses rarely preceded our manic-depressive patients' depressions. Their depressions appeared to be endogenous. When our patients did suffer actual losses, they usually went into mourning, but did not become depressed. Thus, manic-depressive depressions are different psychodynamically from the melancholiac depressions described by Freud (1915b). When depressed, like in melancholia, our manic-depressive patients' anger was turned inward upon themselves, but, unlike in melancholia, their anger was not directed toward an introjected object that had been ambivalently loved and then lost. For example, when the mother of one of our manic patients died, the patient went through a normal mourning process without developing any manic or depressive symptoms.

Freud (1924b) differentiated neurotics from psychotics, showing that their respective egos relate differently to reality. He pointed out that the neurotic's ego attempts to resolve a conflict between his id and reality by first suppressing a piece of the id, and by then ignoring, without disavowing, a piece of reality; the psychotic's ego attempts to resolve this same conflict by first disavowing a piece of reality that does not correspond to his id wishes and by then actively remodeling or replacing this piece of reality with a wished-for fantasy—a hallucination. This model applies to schizophrenic psychoses, but cannot, without modification, be applied to all psychotic conditions. Unlike the schizophrenic, who has a primary disturbance of ego functioning with a resultant defect in thinking and reality testing (Arlow and Brenner 1973, p. 156), the manic's ego does not initially disavow and detach from a piece of reality (Freud 1924a). It first goes through a characteristic phase of hypercathecting the external world—of displaying extravagant object love.

We shall elaborate this model, which Freud used to differentiate neurotics from (schizophrenic) psychotics, to explain the progressive development of a manic attack. Between manic attacks, the manic's ego seems to function like a neurotic's, and he uses neurotic defense mechanisms to resolve conflicts between his id and reality. He first defends against his instinctual impulses and then ignores an aspect of his outer reality while maintaining a realistic view of, and adaptation to, his outer world (Freud 1924b). We hypothesize that a manic attack is precipitated when this relatively good, neurotic adaptation is disrupted by certain, as yet unknown, biologic determinants that cause the manic's phallic libido to pathologically intensify. We assume that this increasing id instinctual drive then pressures the manic's ego for release and thereby throws the psychological equilibrium of his ego—the balance between the forces of his id, his superego, and the outer world—out of balance. This disequilibrium is then experienced by the manic as anxiety, which acts as a signal to his ego and motivates him to intensify his neurotic defense mechanisms against the increasing "pressure" of his id (A. Freud 1936). For a time, this increase in ego defensiveness may reestablish the manic's intrapsychic equilibrium and reduce his anxiety.

If, however, we assume that the manic's phallic libido continues to increase until it becomes so intense that his *neurotic* defense mechanisms can no longer keep his heightened libido in psychological equilibrium with his superego and with reality, the manic state worsens. The disequilibrium is experienced by the manic as anxiety, which motivates his ego to try to reestablish intrapsychic equilibrium by resolving the conflict between his id and his superego and reality. The manic's ego tries to do this, first, by discharging his excessive phallic libido in verbal symptoms. If these symptoms do not relieve the anxiety, the manic's ego goes on to try to discharge the remaining phallic libido in nonverbal symptoms. These two successive, but overlapping, forms of motor behavior are seen clinically. They aim both to gratify the manic's phallic needs in the outer world and to adapt the outer world to the manic's phallic needs. The manic's typical primary-process play with (on) words begins with his making sexual and aggressive puns and jokes, and progresses to his having pressure of speech, flight of ideas, neologisms, and finally word salad. For a time this play with words may relieve the manic's anxiety. However, if the manic's phallic impulses are too intense, this verbal form of discharge proves inadequate. The manic must also act out (A. Freud 1968) his phallic sexual wishes and fantasies nonverbally. He may become so hyperactive with his real objects that he cannot sleep or sit still to eat. Verbal and nonverbal behavior during this phase of his manic attack exceeds the usual limits set by his superego (Freud 1927), but remains within the boundaries of reality set by his ego.

This defensive acting out may permit the manic to maintain his intrapsychic equilibrium. However, if, as we hypothesize, the manic's phallic libido continues to increase, his acting-out behavior may become so intolerable to people around him that they will no longer accommodate to his needs. Then the manic's phallic needs will become frustrated, and his ego will again fall into disequilibrium. Since now neither the manic's neurotic defenses nor his verbal and nonverbal acting-out behaviors are adequate to relieve his anxiety, the manic adds to his repertoire of defense mechanisms some of the psychotic defensive measures. The first is to deflect his phallic libido away from his internal representation of the now unyielding external world and to redirect it narcissistically—toward his self-representation. This process is manifested clinically in the pathognomonic symptom of mania—exaggerated self-esteem to the point of delusional grandiosity, accompanied by an exuberance of pleasurable affect to the point of euphoria. If the strength of the manic's phallic instinctual drive overcomes this first extreme defensive measure and prevents it from alleviating his anxiety, the manic turns to his most radical defense mechanism. He disavows that portion of his intrapsychic representation of the outer world that does not yield to his wishes, and replaces it with a fantasy that corresponds to his wishes. Only now, at the peak of mania, after the manic's attempt at discharging his excessive phallic libido on his own self-representation has failed, does the manic patient experience hallucinations.

In summary, as our patients' manic attacks developed, the ego defense mechanisms they used against their increasing phallic wishes and inclinations became more and more regressive (Freud 1900, p. 548). First they used their usual *neurotic defense mechanisms* to modify their *thought processes*. Then they employed *verbal and nonverbal motor actions* in an effort to gratify their increasing phallic needs in reality (Freud 1924b). Finally, they attempted to gratify their phallic needs in fantasy by *distorting their psychic representations—their thing representations—of reality* (Freud 1915a). Not all manic patients regress to the same extent, and a given manic patient will regress to different levels in different manic episodes.

After the peak of a manic attack has passed, whether spontaneously or due to lithium therapy, the manic's regressive defensive operations and overt symptoms begin to disappear. The symptoms that were the last to appear are the first to go; those that appeared first are the last to go.

Thus, within the context of Freud's structural model, the development of symptoms in a typical manic attack corresponds to what one would expect if one were to assume that the *underlying cause of these symptoms is an increasing phallic sexual instinctual drive within the id.*

Freud (1921) assumed that mania is the consequence of the overcoming of a formerly too-strict superego against which the ego rebels, but our findings suggest that a too-intense phallic libido underlies mania, and that the need to control this too-intense libido impels the manic-depressive to develop a too-strict superego. A depression ensues when the force of this superego exceeds what is required. A manic attack results when this too-strict superego is overwhelmed by phallic desire.

Psychoanalysis (or psychoanalytically oriented psychotherapy) did not reduce the frequency or intensity of our manic-depressive patients' periodic episodes of intensified phallic sexual desires, but such therapy did make them consciously aware both of these previously unconscious impulses and of their defenses against them. This new awareness enabled our patients to prevent overtly psychotic manic episodes by increasing their lithium dosage whenever they noticed an inappropriate intensification of their phallic sexual desires.

References

Abraham, K. (1911). Manic-depressive insanity. In *Selected Papers of Karl Abraham*, pp. 137–157. New York: Basic Books, 1953.

Anthony, J., and Scott, P. (1960). Manic-depressive psychoses in childhood. *Child Psychology and Psychiatry* 1:53–72.

Arlow, J., and Brenner, C. (1973). *Psychoanalytic Concepts and the Structural Theory.* New York: International Universities Press.

Deleon-Jones, F., Val, E., and Herts, C. (1982). MHPG excretion and lithium treatment during premenstrual tension syndrome. *American Journal of Psychiatry.* 139:950–952.

Feinstein, S., and Wolpert, E. (1973). Juvenile manic-depressive illness. *Journal of the American Academy of Child Psychiatry* 12:123–136.

Fenichel, O. (1945). *The Psychoanalytic Theory of Neurosis.* New York: W. W. Norton.

Freeman, T. (1971). Observations on mania. *International Journal of Psycho-Analysis* 52:479–486.

Freud, A. (1936). The ego and the mechanisms of defense. In *Writings*, vol. 2, pp. 1–200. New York: International Universities Press, 1966.

———— (1968). Acting out. In *Writings*, vol. 7. pp. 94–109. New York: International Universities Press.

Freud, S. (1900). The interpretation of dreams. *Standard Edition* 4 & 5.

———— (1915a). The unconscious. *Standard Edition* 14:159–215.

_____ (1915b). Mourning and melancholia. *Standard Edition* 14:237–258.

_____ (1921). Group psychology and the analysis of the ego. *Standard Edition* 18:132–138.

_____ (1924a). Neurosis and psychosis. *Standard Edition* 19:148–153.

_____ (1924b). The loss of reality in neurosis and psychosis. *Standard Edition* 19:183–187.

_____ (1925). An autobiographical study. *Standard Edition* 20:584.

_____ (1927). Humour. *Standard Edition* 21:159–166.

Glenn, J. (1974). The analysis of masturbatory conflicts of an adolescent boy, with a note on actual neurosis. In *The Analyst and the Adolescent at Work,* ed. M. Harlev, pp. 164–189. New York: Quadrangle.

Glover, E. (1938). A note on idealisation. *International Journal of Psycho-Analysis* 19:91–96.

Jacobson, E. (1971). *Depression.* New York: International Universities Press.

Kraepelin, E. (1896). *Psychiatrie.* 7th ed. Leipzig: Barth.

Krafft-Ebing, R. (1906). *Psychopathia Sexualis.* Chicago: Login Bros., 1929.

Lewin, B. D. (1950). *The Psychoanalysis of Elation.* New York: *Psychoanalytic Quarterly, Inc.* 1961.

McDevitt, J. (1983). The emergence of hostile aggression and its defensive and adaptive modifications during the separation-individuation process. *Journal of the American Psychoanalytic Association* 31:273–300.

Moore, B., and Fine, B. (1968). *A Glossary of Psychoanalytic Terms and Concepts.* New York: American Psychoanalytic Association.

Ostow, M. (1962). *Drugs in Psychoanalysis and Psychotherapy.* New York: Basic Books.

Pickar, D., Sweeney, D., Maas, J., and Heninger, G. (1978). Primary affective disorder, clinical state change, and MHPG excretions. *Archives of General Psychiatry* 35:1378–1382.

Pollock, G. (1977). Foreword. In *Manic-Depressive Illness,* ed. E. Wolpert, pp. 1–2. New York: International Universities Press.

Rangell, L. (1968). A further attempt to resolve the problem of anxiety. *Journal of the American Psychoanalytic Association* 16:371–404.

Sheard, M., Marini, J., and Giddings, S. (1975). Lithium in the treatment of aggression. *Journal of Nervous and Mental Disease* 60:108–118.

_____ (1977). The effect of lithium on luteinizing hormone and testosterone in man. *Diseases of the Nervous System* 38:765–769.

Shopsin, B. (1979). *Manic Illness.* New York: Raven.

Thompson, R., Jr., and Schindler, F. (1976). Embryonic mania. *Child Psychiatry and Human Development* 6:149–154.

Van Putten, T. (1975). Why do patients with manic-depressive illness stop their lithium? *Comprehensive Psychiatry* 16:179–183.

Wolpert, E., ed. (1977). *Manic-Depressive Illness.* New York: International Universities Press.

_____ (1981). On the nature of manic-depressive illness. In *The Course of Life,* vol. 3, ed. S. I. Greenspan and G. H. Pollock, pp. 443–452. Madison, CT: International Universities Press.

Zilboorg, G. (1941). *A History of Medical Psychology.* New York: W. W. Norton.

6

Medication and Transitional Phenomena

ROBERT HAUSNER, M.D.

Winnicott's concept of transitional phenomena is employed as a means of further understanding the effect of medicine and the medication-giving process itself. Particular facets examined include the "soothing" function of medication, the placebo effect, and medication compliance, as well as countertransference difficulties encountered in administering the medicine. Medication as a transitional object is viewed largely as a creation along the self-object interface, with the "potential space" between patient and therapist recapitulating aspects of the original dyad. This usage of medicine as a transitional object, or its ultimate abandonment as such, is presented in terms of the vicissitudes of internal object relations, with clinical case examples to clarify particular issues.

The usage of medication is predicated on its pharmacologic effect, and an alteration in mental status following the administration of a psychoactive drug is thus generally considered to be pharmacologically induced. It is well recognized, however, that other factors may be involved in both the prescribing and taking of a drug. For example, placebo effects may appear that are unrelated to the intrinsic properties of the medication, or so-called noncompliance may develop because of meanings that may be attached to the drug, the therapist, and/or the process of medicine giving itself. The prescription of medication therefore should prompt an ongoing examination of meanings surrounding the process, and such an examination obviously is essential to a psychoanalytic psychotherapy or an analysis proper (Ostow 1979).

What follows is an exposition of a particular set of meanings involved in medicine giving, meanings that hark back to an earlier stage of development and are reexperienced in the therapeutic setting. The concept of a transitional object (Winnicott 1951) provides the basis, I feel, for understanding many of the phenomena associated with the administration of medicine, including aspects of the placebo effect and noncompliance already mentioned. Winnicott's particular genius led him to consider the intrapsychic processes involved in the universal experience of self-object differentiation and the phenomena that may be observed as part of this. The process of separating self and object is necessarily a complex and extended one, such that a transitional (or intermediate) state is encountered in which the boundaries between the two are not only indistinct but also moot and unchallenged. In accordance with this, certain inanimate objects during this period may be imbued pari passu with properties reflecting the transitional state. Winnicott thus referred to the substance of *illusion* and the natural distortions that occur in the initial experiencing of "not-me" objects. As he emphasized, such an experience is universal, not necessarily pathologic, and may persist into adult life, for example, in artistic or religious choice and creation.

Recognition of transitional phenomena, when they extend into the treatment situation, may help provide a focus for understanding and managing aspects of the therapeutic process itself (Horton 1974, Volkan 1973). It is noteworthy that despite broadening the concept of a transitional object to include various facets of the treatment milieu, little consideration seems to have been given to medication—or to the medication-giving process—in regard to transitional relatedness and associated phenomena. This is understandable to some extent insofar as psychoanalysis proper is concerned, in that medications are seldom administered as part of the treatment. It is less understandable with regard to psychoanalytic psychotherapy, in which pharmacologic intervention is much more common.[1] The prescription of medication in itself may evoke significant countertransference (Levy 1977) or, at the least, some unease over indications, timing, general appropriateness, and interference regarding the therapeutic process. The sense that medications represent a nonhuman intrusion into the psychotherapeutic relationship (Searles 1976)—that they may vitiate or denigrate the process—may be partly responsible for the lack of exploration in this area. Nonetheless, the not-infrequent use of psychoactive medication in such a treatment setting necessitates its being examined as yet another feature of the therapy. When the concept of transitional phenomena is then introduced, not only may medication effect be understood better but so may the therapeutic interaction.

In regard to overt interaction, medication giving comprises one of the few phenomena in which a concrete object related to the therapist is possessed by the patient; it is the only one in which the object is actually ingested by the patient. This situation may immediately be recognized as an implicit repetition of the early maternal dyad: something is received from the mother and becomes part of the infant, thus satisfying an inchoate need. The orality of this process,

---

[1] An extended case report (Schlierf 1983), highlighting some aspects of medication's usage as a transitional object, provides a notable exception to the paucity of material on the subject.

though, is enriched by an additional perspective. Unlike milk, medication passes through an intermediary stage in which it is possessed; this possession is derived from the therapist but is nonetheless the patient's. As such, it occupies the transitional region (me/not-me; external/internal) that Winnicott began to explore. Although he stressed the creative act of the infant itself in the formation of a transitional object—to the detriment, perhaps, of environmental influence, as Brody (1980) mentioned—Winnicott certainly recognized that transitional objects are "created by the infant and at the same time provided from the environment" (1951, p. 241). In this respect, medication is a possession uniquely situated so as to be endowed with qualities emanating from the patient himself or herself, qualities involving both internalized self- and internalized object representations. There are several clinical manifestations of this, and an attempt will be made next to delineate and expand upon some of them.

Soothing Function

In his original description of the transitional object, Winnicott emphasized its being a defense against anxiety, a "resting place" in the continuous task of keeping inner and outer realities separate yet related. This function is fundamental and has been used as an important criterion for evaluating transitional object usage (e.g., Horton et al. 1974). There are various ways in which this may be encountered clinically, one of the more obvious being a patient's wanting medication "just in case. . . ." The medication may rarely, if ever, be taken but offers the illusion of security in the face of anticipated anxiety. As a 30-year-old female stated, several months after beginning psychoanalytic psychotherapy, "I just need to have it on the shelf. I can look at it and know that I can have it if I need it." The unconscious illusion of the maternal breast is obvious (terms that Winnicott used to describe the original transitional object); yet the employment of medicine in this manner may also be construed as a symptom: it represents an unconscious wish for the breast as well as the need to defend against it, to keep it "at arm's length." When anxiety (particularly of the depressive type) becomes overwhelming, then the medication is more powerfully cathected with qualities of the part object/breast and is taken in. One patient, who twice had asked for tranquilizing medication minutes before the end of sessions that marked my taking temporary leave, reflected 2 years later on this behavior and observed, "It's a way of having you when you're not here." Kahne (1967) stressed the revival of transitional phenomena when the ego is threatened by separation from a significant contemporary object; the separation may be fantasized or literal. An example of the latter may also be seen in the following case, the general circumstances of which are probably quite commonplace:

A 28-year-old woman (Mrs. S.), hospitalized 4 years previously and diagnosed as paranoid schizophrenic, entered twice-weekly psychoanalytic psychotherapy with her previous regimen of both an antidepressant and an antipsychotic. During the therapy, she was rediagnosed as having a narcissistic personality disorder with paranoid features, largely due to an idealizing transference pattern with the concomitant presence of an unconscious archaic "grandiose self." The antidepressant was slowly tapered off owing to questionable indication for usage, and the antipsychotic (perphenazine) was reduced over 1½ years from six to three tablets per day. Following a brief leave-taking, the therapist was confronted in the return session with a broadly smiling and ostensibly pleased patient, who indicated that she had had a "swell time" during the hiatus. Several minutes later, Mrs. S. casually mentioned that she was taking six tablets of perphenazine a day. A number of factors soon became apparent with regard to her self-adjusted dosage, including the wish to return to a less troubled time in the therapy (when she was on six tablets per day) and the need to combat lack of control by turning passive into active and identifying with the aggressor-therapist. Of more immediate pertinence, however, were her numerous allusions to the feeling of "safety" attained with the extra medication, coupled with her practice during the therapist's absence of always keeping the medication on her person. Both of these phenomena ceased with the therapist's return.

As with the child's transitional object, the medication is kept near the patient so as to provide a sense of safety in the therapist's absence; in Brody's terms, the patient is "receiving from its nearness a reassurance of some kind . . . [and] having it at hand seems to help him feel intact" (1980, p. 592). The medication has acquired magical and illusory properties, assuming the omnipotence that the therapist had previously been invested with unconsciously as part of an idealizing transference (Kohut 1968). Some of the renewed importance of the medication may also be understood in terms of the separation's being experienced by the patient as a precursor to loss. In such instances, "we can sometimes see the exaggeration of the use of a transitional object as part of *denial* that there is a threat of its becoming meaningless" (Winnicott 1971, p. 15). Technically, interpretations in this case were made over time and pertained to the medicine's fantasized soothing power and its ability then to reduce the patient's anxiety. This led to exploration of the equivalence of therapist and medication and eventually to assimilable direct transference interpretations without the need for an intermediary object. Recognizing the medicine as a transitional object and its intrapsychic vitality for the patient may thus enable the therapist not only to "reach the patient" (Searles 1976) but also to advance the analytic work itself.

The above case example touches upon another aspect of the original transitional object as defined by Winnicott: "It must never change, unless changed by the infant" (1951, p. 233). The wish-fulfilling nature of this quality of the object, as well as its defensive function, is apparent. In some instances, both the dosage of medication and the specific type (including the trade name) must continue to be the same. This is undoubtedly a familiar phenomenon to most clinicians who occasionally utilize medication. On a fundamental level, it appears to represent a facet of the infantile narcissistic perfection that Freud alluded to in stating that "man has . . . shown himself incapable of giving up a satisfaction he had once enjoyed" (1914, p. 94). The transitional object, so profoundly a self-object, must remain unaltered: Its concrete constancy may serve as an anchor in a sea of seemingly changing objects, while providing a vehicle for the continuation of archaic omnipotent and self-soothing fantasies. As Winnicott noted, transitional object usage implies "some abrogation of omnipotence . . . from the start" (1951, p. 233) by the user, with the transitional object itself carrying the omnipotence; the user unconsciously partakes of this and in the process wards off annihilative or depressive anxiety.

The immutability of the transitional object may be seen most prominently in certain patients treated in institutional settings, in which they may have several different therapists, each of whom remains for a year or so. In such cases, the transitional object may degenerate into a fetish object (Greenacre 1969) whose only function is to defend against castration fear or its equivalents (fragmentation, annihilation, and the like).

A 50-year-old female, treated in a psychiatric outpatient clinic by six succeeding therapists over the span of 12 years, was exceedingly resistant to any attempts to change either the dose, type, or number of her medications. She was initially on three different drugs whose pharmacologic effectiveness and indication for usage were questionable. Although one of her medications, the anticholinergic, was able to be discontinued, she has been on the same two medications (thioridazine and diazepam) for 4 years. An earlier attempt to substitute thioridazine was met with greatly increased anxiety, leading a medication consultant to reassure her that "we would continue them [her medicines], if necessary, for the rest of her life." Several of the therapists remarked upon her resistance to medication change in the following terms: "One of her greatest fears [is to] change her medications without which she knows she will be hospitalized"; "She feared *loss* [italics mine] of her medicines"; "She felt she could not do without her medications." In the final session before her transfer to her current psychiatrist, it was noted that the patient "made sure several times that the new therapist will not take away her medicines." Nearly all the therapists have recognized that there exists a need for the medication apart from its pharmacologic value, and changes in the regimen (as prompted by concerns over unnecessary polypharmacy) have been attempted with caution and a sense of process.

In such instances, what probably serves initially the partial function of a transitional object (possibly even for the therapist, as elaborated below) ultimately deteriorates into a fetish object, losing the vitality and depth of the intermediate zone upon repeated permanent leave-takings of the mother/therapist. To avoid this, the therapist must return in a "good-enough" time, "before longing turns into trauma" (Deri 1978). Within institutions, the therapist may not only leave but also be supplanted by another and yet another, and so the repetition of separation inherent in the object relationship itself is defended against by means of the degenerated transitional object qua fetish object. As expected, the tenor of the object relationship within the therapeutic hours is often rigid and seemingly one-dimensional, reflecting the patient's internal object world. Accordingly, countertransference commonly leads to frustration, disappointment, and a sense of "settling" for treatment with a fixed medication. The therapist sometimes may be able to use such experiences, particularly in light of projective identificatory mechanisms and techniques designed to bring them into therapeutic focus (Langs 1976, Ogden 1982).

Placebo Effect

Closely related to the soothing function of the transitional object is the placebo response. In strictly medical situations, it is well recognized that the physician's positive attitude toward and reassuring tone regarding medication may produce a beneficial response. In these circumstances, the doctor seems to become the conveyor of omnipotent and omniscient wishes arising from the patient's need to be healed: The disruption in the continuity and integrity of the body ego may be thought of as recreating needs appropriate to the original "holding environment" (Winnicott 1960b). This primitive idealization entails the establishment, however transitory, of an archaic self-object in the form of the doctor. The original state of fusion with the mother is now reintroduced in the form of an unconscious wish for merger, which itself is promoted by such conventions of the doctor–patient relationship as the pact of confidentiality (unity of the dyad), the injunction that "doctor knows best," and ultimately the laying on of hands (concretely breaching body boundaries and, in doing so, reinstating the careful holding and touching of infancy). Separation from the doctor would then create significant trauma while this unconscious infantile transference is in full sway, and transitional object usage becomes more likely to occur. Medication thus develops into the vehicle for omnipotent healing attributed unconsciously to the doctor. The patient *believes* in the medicine, creates a vitality for it that derives both from within the patient and from socioculturally derived attributes of the doctor and the doctor's medical appurtenances.

Similar principles apply to the therapist–patient relationship, perhaps to an even greater degree: the mind itself may be construed unconsciously as a symbol of the individual self, such that a disturbance within the mind ipso facto necessitates repair. The therapist is, of course, enlisted in the repair process, becoming the bearer of the patient's wishes for omnipotent healing. Indeed, Greenson (1965) considered object hunger an important factor in the development of transference reactions in general and cited the mobilization of "early longings for an omnipotent parent" as a central feature of the working alliance.

Medication as a transitional object preserves this omnipotence even in the absence of the therapist-parent, as in the following case example:

Ms. L., a 37-year-old female, was referred for medication consultation because of intractable depression that had recurred frequently over the past 5 years. She was engaged actively in twice-weekly insight-oriented psychotherapy (of 4 years' duration) but had recently found herself reluctant to attend sessions when most depressed. This coincided with a somewhat critical transference perception by the therapist. It was decided that a trial of antidepressant medication might be useful, mostly because of the presence of depressive vegetative signs. The consultant described the nature of the medicine in detail, including the expected 10- to 14-day delay of onset. Nonetheless, within 2 or 3 days, the patient reported feeling better, which she initially attributed to the medication. On associating to the alteration in feeling-state, the patient recalled that she had also been depressed when she first saw her therapist but had experienced a "lifting" of the despondency shortly after the initial visit. The patient then referred to the "hopes" that she held for the medicine and observed that she had had similar hopes for the therapist following the first visit. Further associations led to her uncovering a fantasy that the consultant would be capable of "getting rid of" her depression and that the medication he prescribed would be the means of accomplishing this. The despondency returned shortly thereafter, eventuating in an unsuccessful medication trial.

In this case, there seems to have been a degree of splitting between the therapist and the consultant. The therapist received transference projections of the bad internal object, and the consultant was initially the recipient of projected idealized internal object representations (as was the therapist 4 years earlier). The wish for an omnipotent and omniscient healer, which could be readily elicited, had provided the basis for transitional object usage in the form of medicine. The transitional object in this sense may also be understood as a means of defending against individuation, with a simultaneously greater capacity in unconscious fantasy to manage the "healer" as the patient "assumes rights over the object" (Winnicott 1951). As the constellation of fantasies surrounding the wish became increasingly conscious, these primary-process modes of operation became progressively more subject to secondary-process mechanisms and eventually resulted in aborting the placebo effect. This is in keeping with Winnicott's understanding that transitional phenomena antedate reality testing and are not challenged, so that secondary process scrutiny may negate their very existence. Such a process, I feel, is not necessarily restricted to those with an abnormal development or an arrest in development but may appear under a variety of conditions in which the need for a transitional object is re-evoked. The mere presence of primary process mechanisms need not indicate severe psychopathology, as can be attested to by dreams, art, and elements of free association itself.

Certain variations of the placebo response may be seen more frequently than others are. It is well recognized, for instance, that a change in medication regimen may lead to transference and/or countertransference issues. In cases in which medication is restarted or increased after a period of constant dosage, further questions arise regarding the need for a transitional object by the patient, the therapist, or both. Such a situation may occur when the patient seems to become "sicker" during a phase of the therapy, that is, when regression occurs. Whatever the overt form of regression may be—deepening depression, loosening of associations, increased paranoia—reversion to a transitional object will be more likely if there is a separation, so to speak, between the patient and the therapist. Although actual separation from the object-therapist is the most easily identifiable stimulus (as with Mrs. S., cited previously), more subtle "separations" may, I feel, be even more significant. These separations may be considered in metaphoric terms, as is the case during the establishment of the first "not-me possession," so as to include processes such as disillusionment, frustration, empathic disruption, and lack of continuity within the therapeutic milieu. Whether within the patient or the therapist, these conditions may lead to a search for an "object equivalent" (Stevenson 1954), in which object hunger is transformed into transitional object hunger with the concomitant risk of ultimate transformation into a fetish object. Medication thus may be prescribed or increased (or requests for medication accepted) in an unconscious attempt to reduce the intrapsychic discord resulting from the greater cathexis of bad internal object representations. Again, an area of illusion develops within which a transitional object is created, providing a buffer against the threatening bad internal part object. In this case, the principal characteristic of the transitional object is not play or exploration of the transitional zone so much as denial of separation from or loss of the (self) object. Under these circumstances, the medicine may at times be seen to "work," that is, to alleviate anxiety. What may be less clear is the extent to which the effect is pharmacologic, as opposed to intrapsychic.

Another common presentation of the placebo effect and transitional object usage is encountered when the patient has been on medication for some time and the therapist then attempts to decrease or discontinue it. Although the patient might be judged to be ready "pharmacologically" for this, he or she may manifest a good deal of reluctance and renewed anxiety, and the process is often an extended one. Some patients may consciously recognize the value of the medication apart from its pharmacologic action. One patient with anxiety attacks, Ms. D., spoke of her medication in the following manner:

> I know there must be something psychological about it. I can take it and . . . almost immediately feel calmer. Maybe it's knowing that I've taken something that will work. I know it takes time—an hour—before it's digested! This doesn't happen all the time, though. Sometimes it doesn't really help at all.

Another patient had been on the antidepressant desipramine with questionable benefit and had actually told the prescribing psychiatrist about its dubious effect. Despite this, she was extremely hesitant to discontinue the medicine and noted, "I think I need it as some security." This theme was repeated a number of times with the relatively new therapist, the patient seeming to cling to the drug even after her internist informed her that it might be responsible for her rapid heart rate. Such a phenomenon may in fact be expected in those who need a transitional object. Like the original transitional object, it cannot be relinquished by fiat and is a process that takes time, one in which there develops concomitantly a greater or lesser degree of object constancy associated with "a sense of trust or of confidence in the environmental factor" (Winnicott 1967, p. 371). Barkin (1978) pointed out that when maternal representations are unstable or when soothing functions are not adequately internalized, transitional object usage may persist. On experiencing the persistence of medication taking in certain patients, one is again impressed by the deeply unconscious transference perception of the therapist as a mother and by the therapeutic process as recapitulating aspects of the early self-object interface.

Of course, these problems of continuing medication often have little relevance to transitional phenomena. A change in medication regimen may be resisted, for example, secondary to castration anxiety attendant on the fantasied usage of a more "potent" agent. A decrease in dosage may unconsciously be construed by the patient as a loss of interest by the therapist, as an indication of withdrawal in general, or even as a demand by the therapist that the patient "improve" (with a host of associated fantasies leading to their own resistances). In some situations, the patient may use medication as a means of protecting the therapist and the therapeutic relationship, particularly as a defense against overwhelming anger. One patient, a 59-year-old woman with a schizoaffective disorder, would become increasingly enraged at her therapist for extended periods and sometimes became nearly uncontrollable. During these periods, she would angrily talk about leaving for another country and would refer to the therapist as a torturer. This might persist for a number of sessions and would be marked by repeated statements such as "If it weren't for the medicine, I wouldn't even be here!" The fantasies surrounding medication in this case may be regarded as a vehicle for splitting good and bad aspects of the therapist as experienced by the patient, with defensive displacement and rationalization most prominent. It also contributed, however, to her continuing in therapy, while at the same time proving to be a powerful resistance against considering more positive aspects of the therapist that could not be readily integrated with negative perceptions. In any case, transitional object usage did not appear to play a significant role intrapsychically for this patient, although the medication itself had major defensive and resistive functions.

In a sense, the discontinuation of medication (for those who utilize it largely as a transitional object) may contain precursor elements of termination itself as well as characteristics of the termination phase in general, attesting further to the medicine's objectlike qualities. Conflicts leading to anxiety and secondary defenses may be re-evoked, particularly in regard to dependence, separation, mourning, and disappointment. When medication is no longer available, the patient must somehow deal with the loss of illusion involving an externalized, idealized maternal imago. The patient is now confronted, so to speak, with the therapist as a whole object, which naturally entails major developmental tasks. Many of these tasks, as Bergman (1978) emphasized, revolve around separation and symbiosis, issues integral to both the rapprochement subphase and transitional phenomena. Of course, this does not exclude oedipal factors from being transferred onto the medication taking, particularly if an actual triangular element is present (for example, a prescribing doctor separate from the therapist). The ramifications of this, however, are beyond the scope of this chapter.

I feel it should be stressed that the placebo phenomenon does not exclusively or even predominantly require transitional object usage. There is evidence that placebo reactors may be a distinct group with particular character pathology (e.g., Lasagna et al. 1954, Linton and Langs 1962), and features of those who respond to placebo may indeed include traits such as a tendency toward somatization with somatic preoccupations and greater dependency longings. Such traits, though, have not been found consistently in the literature, and so the placebo response may be seen to transcend diagnostic lines, much as conversion reactions have been noted to do (Rangell 1959). With this in mind, Wolf's classic study of the placebo reactor (1959) concluded:

> Placebo reactions depend upon the particular circumstances prevailing at each administration. Relevant among these would be the nature of the symptom being treated, the motivation of patient and physician, the nature of the test agent, its mode of administration and the life situation of the subject at the time he is tested. [p. 700]

One medical researcher thus suggested that "given the appropriate circumstances each one of us has the makings of a placebo reactor" (Parkhouse 1963, p. 308). Within this context, these "appropriate circumstances" may at times, I believe, involve an unconscious reconstruction by the patient of the "omnipotent healing matrix," an aspect of the holding environment, in which medication maintains the illusion of the matrix, an illusion that harks back to the universal transitional phase and of which we all may partake under "the strain of relating inner and outer reality" (Winnicott 1951, p. 240). In fact, it is quite understandable that the placebo response is so varied and widespread: culturally sanctioned facets of the doctor–patient relationship not only provide but also reinforce the unchallenged intermediate area of transitional object usage.

Medication Compliance

In using the term *compliance,* the physician is referring to the degree of the patient's cooperation regarding a medication regimen. It is now well recognized that such cooperation may be more than merely a function of what the patient understands about the medicine and that unconscious factors may also be important. Nevins (1977) approached this issue in terms of a patient's defensive structure, and I wish to extend the discussion to include aspects of transitional object usage.

It is interesting that the medical term for adhering to a drug regimen implicitly refers to the doctor as an omnipotent rule giver. As just emphasized, this may contribute significantly to the development of a positive placebo effect, but it should also be evident that conflicts and structural distortions related to an omnipotent object would naturally be activated as well. The very concept of compliance includes the process of "fitting in," of acting according to the wishes or commands of another. Indeed, Winnicott used the term in discussing the False Self system (Winnicott 1960a). This "system" may be viewed as the conceptual precursor to the spectrum of narcissistic personality disturbances, in that issues of omnipotence, self-esteem, and an inner sense of emptiness are so prominent in both.

Reference to Winnicott's schema of compliance within the False Self system may at first seem only peripherally related to the subject at hand, but I feel that the allusion is apt. Although difficulties with medication compliance are certainly not restricted to those with narcissistic personality structure, the metaphoric use of True and False Selves implicitly entails related themes of "inner" and "outer," "internal" and "external" (Winnicott describes the False Self as hiding the True Self). Under certain conditions, particularly when a therapeutic alliance has not been established, medication may be accepted, but as a form of compliance akin to the Winnicott usage. Instead of a unity within the dyad, a partaking of the "healing matrix," there remains a division that is difficult to bridge and in which the proffering of medicine is construed as an environmental demand. In such instances, the medication appears to be experienced as a foreign object and not a transitional object; it is felt to intrude into the intermediate zone between the patient and the therapist and is not imbued with the vitality of a transitional object precisely because the actual object (the therapist) is not sufficiently cathected. Medication giving thus becomes more the province of the external than the self-object interface, with also a greater possibility of the patient's investing it with intrusive qualities. This is reminiscent of Winnicott's description of the mother who is not good enough and gives rise to False Self anlage, insofar as "she substitutes her own gesture which is to be given sense by the compliance of the infant" (Winnicott 1960a, p. 145).

If these conditions prevail and are not recognized by the therapist, the therapeutic milieu itself will be endangered. The administration of medicine is then analogous to maternal impingement (Winnicott 1956), the delicate potential space between patient and therapist suddenly being filled with material from without, as opposed to arising from the unconscious merger–separation process of the two. In a separate paper on the origin and nature of cultural experience, Winnicott (1967) alluded to a particular danger "that this potential space may become filled with what is injected into it from someone other than the baby. It seems that whatever is in this space from someone else is persecutory material, and the baby has no means of rejecting it" (p. 371). Indeed, persecutory fantasies—of being poisoned, controlled, deadened, and the like—commonly emerge when medicine is given early in the course of the treatment. One patient, who in her second session readily spoke of a "need for support" by the therapist while recognizing conflicts over the need itself, seemed quite relieved when told that neither lithium carbonate nor any other psychotropic drug seemed indicated (a trial of lithium or an antidepressant had been suggested by a relative). The patient's apparent relief was commented upon, and after a period of silence, she observed: "There is a very fine line between being cared for and being controlled." The potentially intrusive persecutory therapist and "his" (or her) medicine (containing aspects of the bad internal object) produce fantasies of being controlled. Because the transitional zone between the patient and the therapist is most fragile at the beginning of a therapy, it may be seriously disrupted if the administration of medicine becomes a "substituted gesture" that intrudes upon this potential space. Similar mechanisms may underlie Freud's suggestion, in "On Beginning The Treatment" (1913), that interpretations not be made until "an effective transference . . . a proper rapport" is established (p. 139); that is, the therapist may introduce material into the potential space with which the patient may create only when it is judged that the patient will not experience it as an intrusion. One is led to wonder whether the rule of relative abstinence by the therapist toward the beginning of treatment (in psychoanalytic psychotherapy or psychoanalysis per se) is a general expression of this and is determined not only by a need to collect information and a desire to promote the transference neurosis but also by the therapist's sense of when it is "safe" to make a gesture of his or her own that the patient will not feel as an impingement (and thereby produce premature transference expectations involving projected aspects of the internalized bad object).

If these projective mechanisms are used to an extreme during treatment, the external object-therapist may be experienced as overwhelmingly bad. This is frequently encountered as a profound transference distortion among those with preoedipal disorders, so that the therapist becomes the superego-aggressor in projected form (Rosenfeld 1978). In these instances, a patient on medication may cease to take it or may consider it to have lost its effectiveness. This might be understood as an example of defensive displacement but should in no way negate the medication's use as a transitional object whose existence depends on the projection of the internal object's aspects. In a sense, this change in medication taking can be viewed as a repetition of earlier infantile trauma, for as Winnicott (1951) noted, "After a persistence of failure of the external object the internal object fails to have meaning to the infant, and then, and then only, does the transitional object become meaningless too" (p. 237). The original failure is, of course, reexperienced as part of the patient's transference expectations. However, rather than the internal object's becoming meaningless, it seems more accurate to describe the process as a potential overwhelming of the object's more positive valences by negative ones. The transitional object then becomes overwhelmed secondarily, resulting in its devaluation or outright abandonment. The more medication functions as a transitional object, the greater will be the correlation between the patient's perception of it and his or her perception (conscious or unconscious) of the therapist. Within the broad range of the narcissistically derived disorders (encompassing narcissistic personality proper, borderline states, psychosis, certain affective conditions, and the like), experiencing the illusion–disillusionment process in therapy is repeatedly traumatic. If the trauma is not catastrophic, more medicine may be requested as part of the transitional object's soothing function or as a defensive maneuver (and not necessarily or primarily because of any specific pharmacologic effect expected by the patient). Only when such trauma in the therapeutic setting becomes unmanageable does medication seem to be devalued or discarded, and then usually in the context of severe regression in ego function.

A 22-year-old male, Mr. G., was engaged in weekly and then twice-weekly psychoanalytic psychotherapy within a long-term inpatient setting. Beginning at the age of 16, he had experienced intermittent severe depression associated with auditory hallucinations (generally of a persecutory nature). Between these overt depressions were periods of low-grade despondency without hallucinations but with a sense of inner "emptiness" and meaninglessness. He had been repeatedly hospitalized and variably diagnosed as paranoid schizophrenic, schizoaffective, atypical bipolar (manic-depressive), and borderline personality, but had been treated only with neuroleptics. There apparently had been no previous attempts at involving the patient in a transference-based/insight-oriented therapy. Mr. G. himself was adamant about not wanting to be placed on a neuroleptic, indicating that the side effects were always distressing (and portraying the psychiatrists who gave him the medicine as being sadistic). The therapist agreed not to use a neuroleptic but, in view of the patient's marked depression with profound vegetative signs, suggested antidepressant medication, which the patient immediately accepted (the therapist noted that the patient "avidly" took him up on the suggestion). Mr. G. also spoke of wishing that something could relieve him of his depression and at one point referred to the therapist's "understanding" of what he was experiencing.

Within 2 days of starting the antidepressant, the patient expressed to the staff his feeling of not being depressed any longer, and at the next session 2 days later, he spoke of feeling "more normal." He attributed his altered mood to the medication, and the therapist did not challenge this assessment, despite recognizing that the change in mood could not have been pharmacologically induced because of the rapidity of its onset. No antidepressant blood level had been drawn so soon after starting the medication, when the initial dosage was 100 mg of amitriptyline per day.

Shortly thereafter, however, at a dosage of 150 mg per day, antidepressant levels were at the lowest end of the therapeutic range (that is, amitriptyline 0.09 mcg/ml and its breakdown product, nortriptyline, 0.05 μg/ml, with the therapeutic range being 0.05–0.20 μg/ml and 0.02–0.24 μg/ml, respectively). Elements of idealization and wish-fulfillment regarding the therapist also emerged during that session (for example, the patient remarked, "I think you know how I'm feeling" and, later, "You really know your medicine.") This overt idealization of the therapist continued through several sessions, during which time the medication was ostensibly effective. Over the succeeding weeks, however, repeated references were made to his "uncaring" parents, and homicidal anger began to emerge directed toward them. This coincided with the erratic reappearance of depressive features, and the patient would occasionally wonder aloud whether more medicine was needed. At this time, amitriptyline dosage was 250 mg per day, with antidepressant blood levels well within therapeutic range (amitriptyline 0.14 μg/ml and nortriptyline 0.13). Despite the therapeutic rise in antidepressant levels, depressive complaints and symptomatology increased. Eventually, interpretations were made concerning the patient's anger toward the therapist, related to feelings that the patient "needed more" from him. Disappointment, frustration, and at times rage reactions emerged during these sessions, punctuated intermittently by urgent requests for more medication "to make me feel better!" Finally, within a 1-week period, the therapist gave notice of brief leave-taking and then the patient's father unexpectedly died. Mr. G. shortly thereafter refused any medication and left the facility.

Both the placebo effect and transitional object (medication) hunger in the face of perceived deprivation by the actual object are illustrated here. In accordance with the principle of multiple function (Waelder 1936), the transitional object serves in a soothing capacity while also defending against a relationship with the object per se (now threatening as part of the transference distortion). The transitional object may then be rejected only when aspects of the good internal object projected into the transitional object are overwhelmed by projected aspects of the bad internal object (a process intensified by the transference and, in this case, overdetermined). Descriptively, the potential space may be conceived as contracting during this process, with an ultimate collapse of the space coincident with the abandonment of the transitional object. Although other facets of the case are worthy of scrutiny, such as the nature and function of the initial overt idealization, they would entail too great a digression from our discussion of transitional phenomena.

Countertransference

Certain countertransference difficulties regarding medication have previously been mentioned in passing, and I now wish to expand on this. Just as medication may serve a soothing function for the patient, so may it for the therapist, particularly when the patient is severely disturbed or regressed. In such cases, a degree of disequilibrium may develop within the therapist and is even to be expected. Ogden emphasized that a part of the therapist's response to the patient's transference is an induced identification with an unconscious aspect of the patient and that

> this identification on the part of the therapist represents a form of understanding of the patient that can be acquired in no other way ... it is not possible to analyse the transference without making oneself available to participate to some degree in this form of identification. [Ogden 1983, p. 236]

At times the induced identification may be with the self component of the patient's internal relations and at other times with the object component. In any event, the therapist's own self-representation (conscious and unconscious) becomes subject to distortion secondary to the projective identificatory process. Searles described aspects of this as "symbiotic relatedness" (1961), referring to the self-object dedifferentiation that must be reinstated as part of the therapeutic process per se.

This blurring of the self-representation and of the self-object interface itself may cause a basic anxiety on the part of the therapist. Under these circumstances, medication may be prescribed or increased as an unconscious means of soothing the *therapist's* anxiety. Multiple determinants of this might indeed be involved, for example, the need to delimit more clearly self-object boundaries and an inability to utilize projective-incorporative processes therapeutically (Levy 1977), but I wish to emphasize that the therapist's resorting to medication may represent his or her own usage of it as a transitional object. As with the child's (and the patient's) use of the transitional object, it is closely related to anxiety arising out of self-object differentiation, particularly the loss of the illusion of control over one's own self. Although the child may turn to a transitional object in response to the "loss" of the mother (as a narcissistically invested part of the self) and the therapist may turn to one in response to projections onto the self, both entail a disturbance of self homeostasis as well as efforts to restore the previous equilibrium. Medicine may then be used as a means of alleviating anxiety, presumably the patient's.

A 27-year-old single female was referred to a crisis center by her therapist because of her mounting anxiety prior to the therapist's vacation. She initially was pacing and chain-smoking but spoke slowly and deliberately: "There's a bomb. I know there's going to be a nuclear attack. . . . Something terrible is going to happen." She went on to speak of her anger at her boyfriend and doctor, of being told that it was time to begin planning for discharge from her halfway house, and of wishing that she had the courage to commit suicide by taking "a bunch of pills." In conjunction with the recommendation of a supervisor who was immediately available, the crisis center therapist interpreted the "bomb" as being inside her, in that she felt she might do something terrible or that something terrible might happen to her. During the first meeting, the therapist reported feeling "somewhat anxious" but nonetheless believed that the patient would be able to benefit from specific interventions. The patient was also asked at this time whether she wished to have medication, but she refused it because "the relief is only temporary."

Because of a miscommunication between the crisis center staff and the patient's ongoing therapist, she mistakenly was informed that the therapist would see her later in the evening. When the patient was then told that this understanding was an error, she immediately became more angry and agitated, throwing an ashtray against the wall while reiterating suicidal wishes and fears of being left alone. She spoke of wanting to leave the clinic and was again asked whether she wished to have medication (again refused). By this time the crisis therapist had spent nearly 3 hours with the patient and in reviewing the case was struck by her own feelings of helplessness and fear. She repeatedly experienced feelings of wanting to go home but was afraid to leave the patient alone or have the patient go home, "afraid something terrible would happen." Fantasies of forcing medicine on the patient, of "pouring it down her throat," were entertained and then consciously worked over, with the therapist eventually recognizing that the wish to medicate was based not necessarily on the patient's need for medication but on the therapist's need to feel less helpless and anxiety-ridden.

The crisis therapist's experiencing of the patient's own feeling-state of helplessness and fear, including the fantasy that "something terrible might happen" with which the patient initially presented, is a testament to the power of the projective identificatory process. The therapist's anxiety as a result of the patient's projection, as well as the content of the projections involving helplessness and the loss of the "illusion" of control, may lower the threshold at which transitional objects are used for defensive purposes. It is of more than incidental interest that when medication is given under conditions such as this, the therapist not infrequently feels "calmer" almost immediately (similar to the feeling described by Ms. D., the patient with anxiety attacks cited earlier). The therapist's newly found calm underscores the identification with the patient and the engagement in a transitional form of relatedness via medication.

In the context of a longer term therapy, an unconscious need by the therapist to maintain a union with the patient may also catalyze the transitional function of medication prescribing. Like the patient's reaction to disruption within the therapeutic field, a therapist might likewise react to subtle or not-so-subtle signals that are felt to comprise or presage a disturbance of the wished-for union. In certain instances, as Searles (1959) and Levy (1977) emphasized, a therapist's unconscious conflicts over regressive yearning for symbiotic relatedness may prompt him or her to introduce medications, which precludes or forestalls a patient's departure from this mode of relatedness. In other cases, the reemergence of primary-process material may be construed as evidence of a patient's "worsening." Aside from the function or content of the primary process, its very presence may be felt by the therapist as undesirable or even distressing. This appears to be a fairly common phenomenon, and certainly understandable in view of our expectation and commitment to convert primary into secondary process. If the primary process and its associated meanings are sufficiently disturbing to the therapist, then the need to separate out and "distance" oneself from the patient will become that much greater. Rather than desiring a continued union, the therapist may experience a spectrum of feelings from vague discomfort to conscious repulsion during the hours, frequently preceded by a sense of anticipatory dread. Under these circumstances, medication may be considered in an unconscious effort to isolate and concretize the source of disturbance. In this respect, the usage of medicine seems to entail fantasies of separation and demarcation in which highly defensive functions predominate over those involving transitional relatedness.

A crucial element in whether the therapist will use medication as a transitional object or a defensive tool, therefore, is the extent to which he or she can tolerate and use the primary process rather than experience it as a disruption of the therapist–patient unit. This unit is an implicit condition of any meaningful therapeutic relationship. The therapist's ability and willingness to engage in the union while concomitantly "suspending" himself or herself to observe and comprehend the process provides an essential fulcrum for therapeutic movement. As Loewald (1970) noted in regard to the analytic process, "Our object, being what it is, is the other in ourselves and ourself in the other. To discover truth about the patient is always discovering it with him and for him as well as for ourselves and about ourselves" (p. 65). This expected state of therapist–patient unity will naturally be disrupted repeatedly, with the patient and/or therapist (depending on the need of each) possibly turning to medication as a transitional means of retaining that unity. As noted above, the therapist may additionally use medicine as a defensive means of emotionally disengaging from the patient, and so in some instances, medication prescribing becomes a symptom that embodies compromise-formation (representing a wish for continued union with the patient as well as a defense against it). In either case, medicine may ostensibly be employed to avoid "unnecessary or undue regression" or to enable the patient to continue to be "workable," with the result that the therapeutic work itself may be aborted (Langs 1973). In fact, medication sometimes is necessary; the principal purpose of the foregoing is merely to emphasize the multiply determined nature of medication prescribing and its therapeutic ramifications for both patient and therapist.

Finally, in this regard, questions arise about the therapist's use of medicine to, in essence, mollify the patient so as to avoid some of the labor of the therapeutic task. This may be done quite consciously and certainly has its precedent in the mother's offering of the blanket when her child is distraught. As Tolpin observed in regard to the transitional object, "since it 'bolsters' the functions that are so wearing for the mother to perform it is not surprising that she too accepts the restorative powers of the blanket with relief and cooperates with her child's need for it" (1971, p. 328). The difficulties and dangers of this with respect to medication are perhaps too obvious: aside from pharmacologic side effects (some, such as tardive dyskinesia, being quite treatment resistant), the very aims and focus of therapy are distorted. The patient's need is not necessarily for the transitional object but for aspects of the object (therapist) itself, with the analysis of this need prematurely truncated. Certain fundamental needs to restore feelings of well-being and safety, for example, may evoke wishes that the object provide this (Sandler and Sandler 1978). Transference manifestations involving repetition and defenses against the repetition of these wishes then constitute a crucial element of the treatment. When the therapist, for whatever reason, substitutes a potential transitional object (medication) for the object itself (himself or herself), the source of well-being and security may become invested in the medication, with attendant displacement, distortion, and potential undermining of the therapeutic process itself. Brody (1980) alluded to the frequent "collusion" of the mother in sustaining a child's attachment to the transitional object, and it seems that the therapist needs to guard against such collusions lest they produce pathologic and unanalyzable attachments to the transitional object/medication. This activity by the therapist constitutes a form of seduction, leading in turn to a greater likelihood that the therapeutic potential space will secondarily be constricted and the transitional object be transformed into a fetish object. This is in line with Dickes's (1978) observation that the parents of children with fetish objects may encourage the cathexis of inanimate objects rather than themselves and in so doing decrease their own anxiety. According to Dickes, this anxiety is closely related to the mother's conflicts over the child's needs, and so inanimate object usage is encouraged to avoid direct interaction in which needs are more specifically addressed (such "emotional disengagement" was referred to earlier as a potential defensive stimulus for a therapist's using medication). There appear to be sufficient therapeutic difficulties related to medicine's transitional objectlike qualities without having the additional complexity of the medicine's being administered *because* of the putative advantages of these qualities.

Conclusion

It is hoped that the foregoing has provided a framework, however preliminary, for the examination of medication taking and prescribing in light of transitional phenomena. It may be necessary to emphasize that this perspective is not necessarily applicable to all situations in which medicine is involved and, conversely, that it is not solely a certain type of pathology that is under discussion. Rather, I consider it to be a commonly encountered clinical entity, with poorly delineated distinctions (at this point in our knowledge) between who may use medication more as a transitional object and who may not. Indeed, there are valid questions whether medication's usage as a transitional object need be pathologic in itself. This would seem a logical outgrowth of Winnicott's original depiction of transitional phenomena as universal. Nonetheless, in an addendum to his original thesis (1971), Winnicott acknowledged in greater depth the possible psychopathology manifested in the area of transitional phenomena. Instead of cleanly dichotomizing, it seems wisest to consider the processes surrounding medicine giving as potentially involving transitional phenomena and to be attuned to their causes and ramifications within the analytic process.

There is one final, intriguing question with regard to psychoactive medicine and the benefits it may effect or promote. There seems little doubt that psychotropic drugs may be of significant value, if carefully evaluated, in ameliorating the intensity of psychic distress in a given individual. What has always been less clear is the drugs' long-term pharmacological benefit and whether the pharmacologic activity itself is primarily responsible for desired change over time. This is an exceedingly complex topic, with particular arguments and approaches beyond the scope of this discussion. But what must be added to it are the heuristic elements related to medication in its role as potential transitional object. Those therapists who have occasion to use medications are well aware of how important it may be to the patient as perceived by the patient. When this importance stems from its use as a transitional object, it is then invested with a vitality that in itself, over time, may promote psychic structuring. Because the medicine is both an external entity and the recipient of profound internal fantasies/representations and instinctual drives, it may serve as a buffer when one or the other (external or internal) becomes overly threatening to the ego. If instinctual demands become overwhelming, then a greater cathexis may develop to that part of the medicine representing external reality, and vice versa. In this fashion, as Copolillo (1967) observed, "The transitional object insures continuing optimal autonomy to the ego and allows impulses to emerge only to the degree that they will participate in structuralization and serve adaptation" (p. 243). The promotion of psychic structure by a transitional object was also emphasized earlier by Kris (1955), who spoke of the illusion inherent in a transitional object as constituting one of the earliest stages in neutralization and thus preparing the way for identification. Tolpin (1971) expanded on this aspect of the transitional object and used Kohut's concept (1971) of transmuting internalization to postulate that "the transitional object is thus normally neither missed, mourned, nor repressed because it is not really lost. Its functions have been internalized" (p. 330). Is this what occurs as well when medication, in the form of a transitional object, is taken in the course of a psychotherapy? May its ultimate discontinuation, and a portion of the benefit that was felt to accrue, be secondary to internalization of the transitional object's tension-regulating properties? It seems worthy of further examination, for medication at times may have a therapeutic action over and above its pharmacologic effect, one that supplements and is contingent upon the continued relation with the object-therapist. In this sense, medication assumes an intrapsychic function parallel to its pharmacologic one, and "medication effect" must then be conceived in terms of unconscious mental mechanisms as well as designated biochemical processes.

References

Barkin, L. (1978). The concept of the transitional object. In *Between Reality and Fantasy: Transitional Objects and Phenomena*, ed. S. A. Grolnick, L. Barkin, and W. Muensterberger, pp. 513–536. New York: Jason Aronson.

Bergman, A. (1978). From mother to the world outside: the use of space during the separation-individuation phase. In *Between Reality and Fantasy: Transitional Objects and Phenomena*, ed. S. A. Grolnick, A. Barkin, and W. Muensterberger, pp. 147–165. New York: Jason Aronson.

Brody, S. (1980). Transitional objects: idealization of a phenomenon. *Psychoanalytic Quarterly* 49:561–605.

Coppolillo, H. P. (1967). Maturational aspects of the transitional phenomenon. *International Journal of Psycho-Analysis* 48:237–246.

Deri, S. (1978). Transitional phenomena: vicissitudes of symbolization and creativity. In *Between Reality and Fantasy: Transitional Objects and Phenomena*, ed. S. A. Grolnick, L. Barkin, and W. Muensterberger, pp. 45–60. New York: Jason Aronson.

Dickes, R. (1978). Parents, transitional objects, and childhood fetishes. In *Between Reality and Fantasy: Transitional Objects and Phenomena*, ed. S. A. Grolnick, L. Barkin, and W. Muensterberger, pp. 307–319. New York: Jason Aronson.

Freud, S. (1913). On beginning the treatment. *Standard Edition* 12:121–144.

_____ (1914). On narcissism: an introduction. *Standard Edition* 14:67–102.

Greenacre, P. (1969). The fetish and the transitional object. *Psychoanalytic Study of the Child* 24:144–164. New York: International Universities Press.

Greenson, R. (1965). The working alliance and the transference neurosis. *Psychoanalytic Quarterly* 34:155–181.

Horton, P. C. (1974). The mystical experience: substance of an illusion. *Journal of the American Psychoanalytic Association* 22:346–380.

Horton, P. C., Louy, W. J., and Coppolillo, H. P. (1974). Personality disorder and transitional relatedness. *Archives of General Psychiatry* 30:618–622.

Kahne, M. J. (1967). On the persistence of transitional phenomena into adult life. *International Journal of Psycho-Analysis* 48:247–258.

Kohut, H. (1968). The psychoanalytic treatment of narcissistic personality disorders. *Psychoanalytic Study of the Child* 23:86–113. New York: International Universities Press.

_____ (1971). *The Analysis of the Self: A Systematic Approach to the Psychoanalytic Treatment of Narcissistic Personality Disorders*. New York: International Universities Press.

Kris, E. (1955). Neutralization and sublimation: observations on young children. *Psychoanalytic Study of the Child* 10:30–46. New York: International Universities Press.

Langs, R. (1973). *The Technique of Psychoanalytic Psychotherapy*. Vol. 1. New York: Jason Aronson.

_____ (1976). *The Bipersonal Field*. New York: Jason Aronson.

Lasagna, L., Mosteller, F., von Felsinger, J. M., and Beecher, H. K. (1954). A study of the placebo response. *American Journal of Medicine* 16:770–779.

Levy, S. T. (1977). Countertransference aspects of pharmacotherapy in the treatment of schizophrenia. *International Journal of Psychoanalytic Psychotherapy* 6:15–30.

Linton, H. B., and Langs, R. J. (1962). Placebo reactions in a study of lysergic acid diethylamide (LSD-25). *Archives of General Psychiatry* 6:53–67.

Loewald, H. W. (1970). Psychoanalytic theory and the psychoanalytic process. *Psychoanalytic Study of the Child* 25:45–68. New York: International Universities Press.

Nevins, D. B. (1977). Adverse response to neuroleptics in schizophrenia. *International Journal of Psychoanalytic Psychotherapy* 6:227–241.

Ogden, T. H. (1982). *Projective Identification and Psychotherapeutic Technique.* New York: Jason Aronson.

_____ (1983). The concept of internal object relations. *International Journal of Psycho-Analysis* 64:227–241.

Ostow, M., ed. (1979). *The Psychodynamic Approach to Drug Therapy.* New York: Psychoanalytic Research and Development Fund.

Parkhouse, J. (1963). Placebo reactor. *Nature* 199:308.

Rangell, L. (1959). The nature of conversion. *Journal of the American Psychoanalytic Association* 7:632–662.

Rosenfeld, H. (1978). Notes on the psychopathology and psychoanalytic treatment of some borderline patients. *International Journal of Psycho-Analysis* 59:215–221.

Sandler, J., and Sandler, A. M. (1978). On the development of object relationships and affects. *International Journal of Psycho-Analysis* 59:285–296.

Schlierf, C. (1983). Transitional objects and object relationship in a case of anxiety neurosis. *International Review of Psycho-Analysis* 10:319–332.

Searles, H. F. (1959). Integration and differentiation in schizophrenia: an over-all view. In *Collected Papers on Schizophrenia and Related Subjects,* pp. 317–348. New York: International Universities Press, 1965.

_____ (1961). Phases of patient-therapist interaction in the psychotherapy of chronic schizophrenia. In *Collected Papers on Schizophrenia and Related Subjects,* pp. 192–215. New York: International Universities Press, 1965.

_____ (1976). Transitional phenomena and therapeutic symbiosis. *International Journal of Psychoanalytic Psychotherapy* 5:145–203.

Stevenson, O. (1954). The first treasured possession. *Psychoanalytic Study of the Child* 9:199–217. New York: International Universities Press.

Tolpin, M. (1971). On the beginnings of a cohesive self. *Psychoanalytic Study of the Child* 26:316–352. New Haven, CT: Yale University Press.

Volkan, V. (1973). Transitional fantasies in the analysis of a narcissistic personality. *Journal of the American Psychoanalytic Association* 21:351–376.

Waelder, R. (1936). The principle of multiple function. *Psychoanalytic Quarterly* 5:45–62.

Winnicott, D. W. (1951). Transitional objects and transitional phenomena. In *Through Paediatrics to Psycho-Analysis,* pp. 229–242. New York: Basic Books, 1975.

_____ (1956). Primary maternal preoccupation. In *Through Paediatrics to Psycho-Analysis,* pp. 300–305. New York: Basic Books, 1975.

_____ (1960a). Ego distortion in terms of true and false self. In *The Maturational Processes and the Facilitating Environment,* pp. 140–152. New York: International Universities Press, 1965.

_____ (1960b). The theory of the parent–infant relationship. *International Journal of Psycho-Analysis* 41:585–595.

_____ (1967). The location of cultural experience. *International Journal of Psycho-Analysis* 48:368–372.

_____ (1971). *Playing and Reality.* New York: Basic Books.

Wolf, S. (1959). The pharmacology of placebos. *Pharmacology Reviews* 11:689–704.

7

Pills as Transitional Objects

STEVEN A. ADELMAN, M.D.

Combining psychotherapy with psychopharmacology is a clinically challenging endeavor. In the psychopharmacology of the borderline patient, pills may function as transitional objects. This point is derived from a review of the literature, and illustrated by clinical material from three case studies. Recognition of the transitional properties of pills may aid therapists in making sense of many clinical phenomena and in developing effective treatment strategies. Other psychodynamic concepts may be useful in understanding the complex integration of psychotherapy and psychopharmacology.

Psychiatric syndromes and therapies are frequently classified as being either biological or psychological. This dichotomy does not do justice to the multidimensional nature of most mental disorders. Van Praag (1965), Schoenberg, Miller, and Schoenberg (1978) and Docherty and colleagues (1977) have suggested that the mind–body dichotomy is a spurious one. Studies by Karasu (1982), Klerman (1975), and Rothschild (1981) indicate that psychotherapy and psychotropic medication may be additive, and possibly synergistic, in their combined effects. Nonetheless, the Group for the Advancement of Psychiatry Report 93 (1975) suggests that in clinical practice many psychiatrists limit themselves to a single, predominant therapeutic modality based on either a psychological or a somatic orientation. In an effort to promote a more holistic and clinically comprehensive approach to mental illness, Karasu has called for an "integrative model of psychopharmacology for the 1980s."

The multi-axial diagnostic scheme of *DSM-III* has heightened clinical awareness that disorders of state or "clinical syndromes," found on Axis I in *DSM-III*, frequently coexist with disorders of trait, the Axis II personality disorders. Many patients' disorders represent an amalgam of state (Axis I) and trait (Axis II) features. This point was elegantly demonstrated by Pope and colleagues (1983), who found that of thirty-three patients who met *DSM-III* criteria for borderline personality disorder, seventeen (51 percent) had a possible or probable concomitant diagnosis of major affective disorder.

Treating such complex patients is a challenge even to the most experienced clinicians. The literature offers little that is germane in formulating a clinically useful rationale for integrating psychotherapy and pharmacotherapy in the treatment of patients with personality disorders who have concomitant Axis I diagnoses. The studies of combining psychotherapy and pharmacotherapy in the treatment of depression by Klerman (1975) and Luborsky, Singer, and Luborsky (1976) frequently ignore the dynamics of using medication and do not specify the characterologic traits of the patients studied. The psychoanalytic literature is nearly devoid of references to the use of medication in the course of psychoanalysis or psychoanalytic psychotherapy. Pharmacologic studies by Cole (Cole and Sunderland 1982) and Soloff (1981) on drug treatment of the character disorders ignore psychodynamic factors. Van Praag (1965) and Linn (1964), who do address dynamic aspects of using medication in psychotherapy, deal in generalities and do not address specific diagnostic groups or invoke particular dynamic concepts.

In order to understand the nature of the complex transaction that occurs when a psychotherapist uses medication, one must apply psychodynamic principles to the clinical situation. I hope to demonstrate the usefulness of this notion by limiting the discussion to a narrow group of patients, those with borderline personality disorders, and to a specific psychodynamic concept. The psychodynamic concept I have found most applicable is Winnicott's conceptualization of the transitional object and transitional phenomena. After a review of the literature, I present case reports to illustrate the existence of transitional phenomena in the psychopharmacotherapy of the borderline patient.

Review of the Literature

Tablets and Talking

The first papers that address the use of medication in psychotherapy appeared in the psychiatric literature in the early '60s. Sarwer-Foner (1960), Ostow (1962), and Bellak (1966) attempted to explain the medications' modes of action in terms of primary effects on theoretical psychological mechanisms. Winkelman (1960) and Savage (1960) worried that the use of medication adversely affected the transference by stirring up patients' concerns over issues of castration, homosexuality, and oral gratification. Regarding countertransference, therapists employing medication were alleged to fear their patients (Sarwer-Foner), to be managing their own anxiety (Savage), or to be giving up on therapy by turning to medication (Levy 1977). Ostow (1962), however, claimed that medications were indispensable for helping difficult patients make use of psychotherapy. The 1975 GAP *Report on Pharmacotherapy and Psychotherapy* maintains in its literature that there is no systematic evidence that medication interferes with psychotherapy.

Van Praag and Schoenberg and associates have confidently announced that psychotherapy and psychotropic medication should be used together. Extein and Bowers (1979) recommend that state and trait disorders be treated sequentially in patients who manifest symptoms of both types of disorder. Docherty and colleagues invoke the useful concept of "biomodal relatedness" to explain why there has been such difficulty in integrating psychotherapy and psychopharmacology. Psychotherapists and psychopharmacologists employ vastly different concepts in understanding the patient and his problem. The former view the patient as a "disturbed person" ("subject-subject mode"), the latter view him as a "diseased organ" ("subject-object mode"). These authors suggest that integrating these different modes of relatedness is stressful to psychiatrists, but argue that optimal care is achieved when the patient and his problem are regarded holistically and not reduced to either mode.

Most authors who advocate the integration of psychological and biological treatment modalities advocate the development of a collaborative doctor–patient relationship in which decisions regarding medication are made conjointly (see Havens 1968; Irwin 1974). Gutheil (1982) has most clearly articulated the need for "participant prescribing" and has coined the useful term "pharmacotherapeutic alliance." Ostow (1962) suggests that when the idea of medication is introduced into a psychotherapeutic treatment, it should be presented as something for patient and therapist to explore and understand together. Rothschild advocates eliciting patients' fantasies concerning the meaning of initiating drug treatment, increasing dosage, and the implications of improvement. Gutheil finds that the introduction of medication into a psychotherapy in this way becomes a rich source of therapeutic material, a focus around which issues of transference, control, and helplessness are played out and addressed.

Transitional Phenomena

Winnicott (1953) recognized that infants and young children develop intense attachments to inanimate objects. He considered this a healthy, universal phenomenon. Stevenson (1954) and Greenacre (1977) have expanded Winnicott's original observations, and subsequently the concepts "transitional object" and "transitional phenomena" have been used to understand adult psychology by Grolnick, Barkin, and Muensterberger (1978), Johansen (1983), Kafka (1969), Kahne (1967), and Modell (1963, 1968).

Winnicott labeled the transitional object (TO) the first "not-me possession," which emerges in the context of a "good enough mother," who cares for the child and is comfortable with the child's moves toward autonomy. The TO, usually a blanket or piece of cloth, is typically selected by the infant but may be provided by the parents at an opportune moment. The mother accepts the child's use of the TO. It may be viewed as a breast substitute, and frequently the child fondles and smells the TO while sucking his or her thumb. The TO is often indispensable at bedtime. Only the infant may change the TO, refusing imposed substitutes. A child sometimes abuses or neglects a TO; however, he virtually never destroys it. Stevenson (1954) noted that others learn not to insist that the child give up the TO. Frequently it is given up when, diminished in size, it is gradually replaced by toys. Brody (1980) points out that decreased use of and need for the TO is a consequence of healthy development.

The TO serves as a bridge between inner experience and external reality; although it is objectively separate from the infant, it is imbued with tremendous individual significance. As the child's purview of the external world increases, he clings to the TO to temper frustration and gain mastery over new and frightening situations. The TO, with its "reassuring illusions" (Greenacre 1977), promotes separation at a critical time in development.

Winnicott (1953) and Greenacre point out the soporific qualities of the TO. Greenacre, who has described the relationship between TOs in children and fetishes in adults, has described adult patients who manifest a "pill fetish." These are persons whose daily ritualistic use of bedtime medication is parallel to the child's use of the TO. Greenacre labels this psychological need for a reassuring pill "pseudoaddiction." Both Winnicott and Stevenson have commented that the true addictions in adulthood may originate in childhood transitional phenomena.

Sheard (1963) and Gutheil described positive transference to the actual medications with which their patients were treated. For these patients, medications take on the attributes of a person. Gutheil found this phenomenon to be most striking on inpatient units when there was turnover of psychiatric residents. The new residents' attempts to alter their patients' medication regimens typically met with an intense and almost incomprehensible resistance from the patients. Gutheil posits that to these patients medications represented their recently departed physicians, whose loss they were actively mourning. Although he does not label it as such, Gutheil is clearly describing the way in which medications can function as TOs. Schlierf (1983) describes the psychotherapy of a patient with anxiety neurosis for whom pills played the role of a transitional object that promoted the formation of mature object relationships. In fact, transitional phenomena appear to be most prominent in the therapy of patients with primitive character structures.

Transitional Phenomena and the Borderline Patient

Modell (1963, 1968) finds similarities between the borderline's relationship with other people and the child's relationship with transitional objects. In psychotherapy the therapist is imbued with qualities that emanate from the patient, thus functioning as a TO. The borderline patient fails to appreciate the therapist for what he is; instead, the patient defines the therapist according to his own needs. Modell views this transitional state of relations as a way-station between primitive narcissism and mature object relations. Therapy with the borderline patient, therefore, consists of the therapist's tolerating, and some-times interpreting, the patient's use of him as a TO. This fosters the patient's growing autonomy, promoting ultimate recognition of the therapist as a sepa-rate person.

Arkema (1981) reports that borderline patients frequently have a history of prolonged attachment to TOs. Fintzy (1971) hypothesizes that the borderline patient is able to maintain a normal facade because of the existence of secret TOs. In psychotherapy with a borderline child of latency age, Fintzy shows how therapeutic work with the child and his TO promoted more adaptive relation-ships. Fintzy raises the interesting possibility of the therapist purposefully introducing a TO into therapy in order to foster psychological growth.

Clinical Correlation

It appears that the borderline patient's relationship to the world is "transi-tional" in nature; that is, external reality is clouded and colored by the patient's internal state. This transitional state of relations is seen quite clearly in the intense, highly ambivalent transferences that characterize psychotherapy with borderline patients. Just as the borderline may use his therapist as a TO, I believe that such a patient will also relate to inanimate objects, particularly pills, provided by the therapist as TOs. This concept of "pills as TOs" may help therapists to effectively integrate medication with psychotherapy. The applica-tion of this concept to actual clinical situations sheds light on much clinical material. The following case reports illustrate these points.

Case 1

Ms. A., a 28-year-old woman with a long history of depression, alcohol abuse, and self-mutilation, was admitted to the hospital for long-term treatment following a serious suicide attempt. She was treated with both antidepressants and psychotherapy. Her psychiatrist deemed the antide-pressant to be ineffective and discontinued it. Ms. A. became enraged at her doctor, complaining that he had no right to deprive her of something that she found important. She was subsequently transferred to a different ward, where her new psychiatrist permitted her to take the lead in determining which drugs were of use to her. Before long, she was on a cumbersome regimen that included three different p.r.n. medications. Ms. A. made use of her different medications at times of stress. Although the medications had similar pharmacologic properties, Ms. A. imparted to each of them a unique identity and discriminated between the different medications according to her own idiosyncratic notions. As Ms. A. began to change, her treatment team identified and addressed her "transitional" pattern of medication usage by repeatedly pointing out to her that her requests for medication were actually statements expressing her desire to be nurtured at times of stress. Slowly she outgrew her reliance on the pharmacologic supports which she could call upon around the clock. By the time of discharge, her medication regimen was simplified and met objective needs.

The case of Ms. A. illustrates that the treatment team's tolerance of her intense "transitional" attachment to medications facilitated her ability to utilize the psychotherapeutic milieu. Ms. A.'s use of medication became a focus of treatment only when she was able to examine herself and her actions with more objectivity than she possessed at the start of her hospitalization. In this case, the patient's growth toward mature object relations paralleled her ability to give up her p.r.n. medications, which had become cherished transitional objects.

Case 2

Ms. B. is a 20-year-old college student, who has been in outpatient psychotherapy for 5 years. Because of her affective lability, stormy inter- personal relations, and tendency to resort to magical thinking, she has been diagnosed as a mixed personality disorder with borderline and schizotypal features. When Ms. B. first presented at age 15, she was in the throes of an acute psychotic episode. Her therapist treated her with chlorpromazine and saw her weekly in psychotherapy. Some time after her therapist's first vacation, she admitted to ongoing hallucinations of flashing orange lights. She associated these lights with a friend who had recently moved away. Several months later, when the hallucinations had stopped, she told her therapist that she had begun to see the lights during his vacation. This led the patient and therapist to address separation issues. Eventually, they recognized that the flashing orange lights represented the orange chlorpro- mazine pills, which, both in reality and in their hallucinatory equivalent, served as transitional objects during the therapist's absence.

This patient's psychotic symptom symbolizes the "transitional" significance of her medication. The pills and her hallucination helped her recall both her friend and therapist. This case suggests that some patients are highly aware of the physical attributes of the pills they ingest. Similarly, young children are typically cognizant of subtle physical properties of their TOs. In order to facilitate understanding of therapeutic material, psychopharmacotherapists might find it useful to acquaint themselves with the physical properties of the actual pills they prescribe.

Case 3

Ms. C. is a 30-year-old woman with a severe borderline personality disorder and recurrent episodes of major depression. She has been treated with psychotherapy and antidepressants for three years. One and a half years ago, she began treatment with her current therapist. He became aware of her propensity for transitional relatedness when, prior to terminating with her previous therapist, she sought to meet with her new therapist in order to "ease the transition" and to foster the illusion that her previous therapy was not really ending. Her current therapist was unable to meet with her until termination had taken place. In the first few sessions she insisted on quitting therapy with her new therapist and simultaneously demanded that he renew her previous therapist's prescription for antidepressants. The therapist pointed out her contradictory stance and addressed her need for medication which appeared to be both physiological and psychological. The beginnings of a tenuous working alliance emerged from these initial negotiations, which focused on medication.

After 2 months of therapy the patient appeared increasingly depressed. She was switched to a different medication, and the following week she missed an appointment and began cutting her wrists. She was admitted to the hospital, where she disclosed that for a week prior to her hospitalization she had walked around with a bottle of sleeping pills in her purse, intending to overdose. The pills had been prescribed by her family doctor. Her psychotherapy and pharmacologic regimen were stabilized in the hospital, and breaking with standard hospital practice, her inpatient administrative psychiatrist saw to it that her discharge prescriptions were filled out by her therapist. By using the therapist in this way, the inpatient psychiatrist reinforced the idea that the patient's medications embodied special properties that had to do with the therapist.

Shortly after discharge, Ms. C. overdosed on a small quantity of pills prescribed by her family doctor. This occurred 2 days following her therapist's vacation. At this junction, the therapist noted the patient's predilection to overdose on medications prescribed by physicians other than himself, and he suggested that all future requests for sedatives be raised with him. The patient and her family doctor complied. The therapist was becoming aware that he and his pills served as transitional objects. Even when Ms. C. devalued her therapist, she appeared to remain intensely loyal to his medications. Even when the therapist was viewed as "all bad," the pills he prescribed retained some of his previous goodness. Thus, the patient repeatedly made use of another doctor's medications for her suicide attempts.

Later the patient revealed to her therapist that she possessed stockpiles of medication which she kept available in order to overdose at times of great distress. The therapist requested that she flush these pills down the toilet. In the next session, the patient sadly admitted that she had taken his advice and stated, "I feel scared—I lost my security blanket."

As is the case with many borderline patients, Ms. C. thought about her stockpiles of pills and occasionally resorted to using them at times of tremendous stress and frustration. Her cache of pills provided Ms. C. with the "reassuring illusion" (see Greenacre 1977) that she had something she could always turn to in order to soothe herself in a crisis. Her reference to her stockpiles as a "security blanket" confirms that they functioned as TOs. As Ms. C. learned to use her therapist and his medications as TOs, she was able to give up the maladaptive use of her suicide stockpiles. Consequently, her propensity to overdose and to act out self-destructively diminished.

Two months later, as Ms. C. was becoming increasingly self-destructive, she requested that her therapist give her a prescription for a medication with which she had overdosed several months earlier. The therapist pointed out that her request may have represented an attempt to enlist his assistance in her self-destructive behavior. The patient persisted in cutting herself, did not overdose, and was rehospitalized for 7 weeks. Shortly after discharge, the patient took a serious overdose in the context of expressing anger at the therapist's setting limits around telephone calls between sessions. Ms. C. was briefly rehospitalized, and the focus of the hospitalization was to point out her use of suicide as an instrument of anger and manipulation.

Since that hospitalization, the patient has done well for 2 years in ongoing outpatient psychotherapy. The therapist decided to set aside the first few minutes of one of their weekly sessions as a time to talk about medications and to write prescriptions. When the patient brings up medication-related issues outside the standard time, this has generally indicated that medication was being used as a way to talk about other therapeutic issues. On one occasion the therapist questioned the patient about her requesting prescriptions for a sedative two weeks in a row. The patient, who had lost her prescription, became enraged at the therapist for questioning her integrity and intimating that she might be abusing the medicine he prescribed. Ms. C. emphatically stated that she would never think of abusing her therapist's medications and she expressed anger and disappointment that he seemed unaware of this. Ms. C.'s psychopharmacotherapy is currently ongoing.

Transitional phenomena pervade the psychopharmacotherapy of Ms. C. For her, pills have multiple significance: They function as TOs; they become concrete entities with which the transference is played out; and, by virtue of their pharmacologic properties, they address the patient's constitutional deficits.

Discussion

In the context of psychotherapy with the borderline patient, the use of pills parallels the child's use of TOs in the following ways:

1. Reasonable medication trials may take place only when the patient and therapist have at least a rudimentary sense of a therapeutic alliance (i.e., the therapist is viewed by the patient as "good enough").

2. The decision to take medication or to use a particular form of medication needs to come primarily from the patient, encouragement from the therapist notwithstanding.

3. The medication may soothe the patient during times of stress and at bedtime. This may derive from the medication's representation of the therapist as well as from its primary pharmacologic properties.

4. The therapist, at times, may need to tolerate the patient's idiosyncratic and unconventional use of medications.

5. As therapy progresses and the patient's object relations mature, concomitant changes may take place in the patient's relationship to medications with decreased reliance on medication frequently occurring toward the end of a successful treatment.

Awareness of the transitional properties of pills may aid therapists in making sense of clinical phenomena and in developing effective treatment strategies. When medications are prescribed in an authoritarian manner or when the therapist is frustrated by the patient's lack of progress, it is not surprising that the introduction of medication often brings about an untimely termination. Borderline patients who experience untoward and unexpected drug side effects frequently swear off all future pharmacologic interventions. This may occur because the medication's ill effects, which might have been predicted by the therapist, violate the patient's illusions about the medication, and thereby preclude its use as a TO.

It has been my experience that by providing certain patients with p.r.n. sedatives, I have been able to overcome their reluctance to take antipsychotics, antidepressants, or lithium carbonate. Because of their pharmacologic effects, use at times of stress, and relative lack of side effects, the sedatives have the most transitional properties of all the psychotropics. The prescription of medication with lesser transitional properties may be linked to the prescription of sedatives. Some patients have responded impressively to one of the "less traditional" drugs, justifying the cautious use of p.r.n. anxiolytics. This somewhat unorthodox use of medication may be a form of corrective emotional experience for patients who did not benefit from "good enough mothering" in their early years.

Although most applicable to borderline personalities, the notion of "pills as transitional objects" can be usefully employed in understanding the psychopharmacotherapy of other patient groups. It should be emphasized that even for the borderline category, this concept is probably one of many that may ultimately prove useful in interpreting complex psychopharmacotherapeutic phenomena. In the context of psychotherapy, the patient–therapist interaction around pills may be understood in terms of transference, defensive style, psychosexual development, and so forth. The purpose of this paper is to demonstrate that the application of one psychoanalytic concept to a single patient group sheds light on a confusing area of clinical psychiatric practice. One can envision future investigations focusing on other dynamic concepts, different patient groups, and individual pharmacologic agents. Such studies will serve to widen the scope of the nascent "integrative model of psychopharmacotherapy for the 80s" envisioned by Karasu.

References

Arkema, P. (1981). The borderline personality and transitional relatedness. *American Journal of Psychiatry* 138:172–177.

Bellak, L. (1966). Effects of antidepressant drugs on psychodynamics. *Psychosomatics* 7:106–114.

Brody, S. (1980). Transitional objects: idealization of a phenomenon. *Psychoanalytic Quarterly* 561–605.

Cole, J., and Sunderland, P. (1982). The drug treatment of borderline patients. In *Psychiatry 1982 Annual Review*, ed. L. Grinspoon, pp. 456–470. Washington, DC: American Psychiatric Press.

Docherty, J., Marder, S. R., Van Kammen, D. P., and Siris, S. G. (1977). Psychotherapy and pharmacotherapy: conceptual issues. *American Journal of Psychiatry* 134:529–533.

Extein, I., and Bowers, M., Jr. (1979). State and trait in psychiatric practice. *American Journal of Psychiatry* 136:690–693.

Fintzy, R. (1971). Vicissitudes of the transitional object in a borderline child. *International Journal of Psycho-Analysis* 52:107–114.

Greenacre, P. (1977). *Emotional Growth*. Vol. 1. New York: International Universities Press.

Grolnick, S., Barkin, L., and Muensterberger, W., eds. (1978). *Between Fantasy and Reality: Transitional Objects and Phenomena*. New York: Jason Aronson.

Group for the Advancement of Psychiatry (1975). *Pharmacotherapy and Psychotherapy: Paradoxes, Problems, and Progress*. Vol. 9. Rep. no. 93. New York: Group for the Advancement of Psychiatry.

Gutheil, T. (1982). The psychology of psychopharmacology. *Bulletin of the Menninger Clinic* 41:321–330.

Havens, L. (1968). Some difficulties in giving schizophrenic and borderline patients medication. *Psychiatry* 31:44–50.

Irwin, S. (1974). How to prescribe psychoactive drugs. *Bulletin of the Menninger Clinic* 38:1–13.

Johansen, K. (1983). Transitional experience of a borderline patient. *Journal of Nervous and Mental Disease* 171:126–128.

Kafka, J. (1969). The body as transitional object: a psychoanalytic study of a self-mutilating patient. *British Journal of Medical Psychology* 42:207–212.

Kahne, M. (1967). On the persistence of transitional phenomena into adult life. *International Journal of Psycho-Analysis* 48:247–258.

Karasu, T. (1982). Psychotherapy and pharmacotherapy: toward an integrative model. *American Journal of Psychiatry* 139:1102–1113.

Klerman, G. (1975). Combining drugs and psychotherapy in the treatment of depression. In *Drugs in Combination with Other Therapies*, ed. M. Greenblatt. New York: Grune & Stratton.

Levy, S. (1977). Countertransference aspects of pharmacotherapy in the treatment of schizophrenia. *International Journal of Psychoanalytic Psychotherapy* 6:15–30.

Linn, L. (1964). The use of drugs in psychotherapy. *Psychiatric Quarterly* 38:138–148.

Luborsky, L., Singer, B., and Luborsky, L. (1976). Comparative studies of psychotherapies: is it true that everybody has won and all must have prizes? In *Evaluation of Psychological Therapies*, ed. R. L. Spitzer and D. F. Klein. Baltimore: Johns Hopkins University Press.

Modell, A. (1963). Primitive object relationships and the predisposition to schizophrenia. *International Journal of Psycho-Analysis* 44:282–292.

———— (1968). *Object Love and Reality*. New York: International Universities Press.

Ostow, M. (1962). *Drugs in Psychoanalysis and Psychotherapy*. New York: Basic Books.

Pope, H., Jonas, J. M., Hudson, J. I., Cohen, B. M., and Gunderson, J. G. (1983). The validity of *DSM-III* borderline personality disorder. *Archives of General Psychiatry* 40:23–30.

Rothschild, A. (1981). The combined use of psychotherapy and pharmacotherapy in a depressed outpatient. *McLean Hospital Journal* 6:75–85.

Sarwer-Foner, G., ed. (1960). *The Dynamics of Psychiatric Drug Therapy*. Springfield, IL: Charles C Thomas.

Savage, C. (1960). Transference and countertransference aspects of the tranquilizing drugs. In *The Dynamics of Psychiatric Drug Therapy*, ed. G. L. Sarwer-Foner, pp. 369–391. Springfield, IL: Charles C Thomas.

Schlierf, C. (1983). Transitional objects and object relationship in a case of anxiety neurosis. *International Review of Psycho-Analysis* 10:319–332.

Schoenberg, M., Miller, M., and Schoenberg, C. (1978). The mind-body dichotomy reified: an illustrative case. *American Journal of Psychiatry* 135:1224–1226.

Sheard, M. (1963). The influence of the doctor's attitude on the patient's response to anti-depressant medication. *Journal of Nervous and Mental Disease* 136:555–560.

Soloff, P. (1981). Pharmacology of borderline disorders. *Comprehensive Psychiatry* 22:535–543.

Stevenson, O. (1954). The first treasured possession. *Psychoanalytic Study of the Child* 9:199–217. New York: International Universities Press.

Van Praag, H. (1965). Tablets and talking: a spurious contrast in psychiatry. *Comprehensive Psychiatry* 6:255–264.

Winkleman, N. (1960). Chlorpromazine and prochlorperazine during psychoanalytic psychotherapy. In *The Dynamics of Psychiatric Drug Therapy*, ed. G. L. Sarwer-Foner, pp. 134–149. Springfield, IL: Charles C Thomas.

Winnicott, D. W. (1953). Transitional objects and transitional phenomena. *International Journal of Psycho-Analysis* 34:89–97.

8

How Does Psychiatric Drug Therapy Work?

MORTIMER OSTOW, M.D.

The author proposes that the conventional antipsychosis tranquilizers and antidepression energizers exert opposite effects upon a hypothetical clinical entity suggestive of an 'energy' function. The *sensitivity* of this function in the case of any given patient, its *resilience* and *reactivity* will all determine how the patient will respond to these medications. The various syndromes that respond to these medications may be imagined to lie along a spectrum of psychic states from 'low' to 'high', or to be elicited by movement from one point to the other. This theory permits the integration of clinical pharmacologic intervention with metapsychologic theory and thereby facilitates the coordination of drug therapy with psychodynamic psychotherapy.

This chapter suggests some answers to several questions that confront those who employ medications in the treatment of mental illness, and who simultaneously analyze illness on the principles of metapsychology. Given the limited categories of medication, how are they able to influence such a large number and variety of clinical states: mania, depression, schizophrenia, anxiety, phobia, borderline personality, and probably anorexia and bulimia? To ask the same question in a different way: Can we find within the theory of psychoanalytic metapsychology an individual parameter or a composite function that can be seen to be influenced by the medications that we use, and that can be seen to play a role in the genesis of the syndromes influenced? If that is so, then can we discern a linkage among the syndromes that we shall consider, by virtue of their common partial determination by this parameter?

First, I must express some caution about the acceptability of my observations, on which I base my theories. Judging from their reception, they are plainly ideas whose time has not yet come. They have been called "too dangerous," yet also obsolete. The problem will become evident very shortly, deriving from two sources. Although some psychoanalysts do use medication, very few of them have been willing to make way for it in their psychoanalytic thinking. Secondly, I shall fall back upon a parameter that Freud considered essential to psychoanalytic metapsychology, but that has been abandoned by the psychoanalysts of the last two generations as too mechanistic and as outdated—namely, psychic energy.

Clinical Observations

Let us look at an individual, susceptible patient under the influence of a relatively large dose of a true tranquilizer—one of the phenothiazines, thioxanthines, butyrophenones, or reserpine. I have not administered such a drug to a healthy individual, but from my experience with many patients, I'm able to construct a typical pattern that would obtain if the drug were administered to an individual without disease, but sensitive to its influence. The subject will convey the impression of age, harassment, a lack of erectness and vigor; he will display profound inertia or agitation, but little or no effective activity. Such a patient will be preoccupied with himself and show little interest in actual or potential love objects, or in activities, and will experience no ambition. He will focus and report on his inner sensations, his inner feelings, coenesthesia, rather than on any externally perceptible attribute of himself. These inner sensations will be perceived as distressing; in fact the individual will complain of misery and anguish. Often the distress will be attributed to specific organs or organ systems, felt to be diseased and threatening death.

The sensation of fault and defect will be generalized, so that we will hear complaints about the subject's age, competence, moral integrity, intelligence, wholesomeness, reputation, and economic status. Therefore feelings of guilt are commonly encountered, as well as the need for, and expectation of, punishment. Confidence, too, will be undermined, and give way not only to diffidence and a feeling of impotence but also to timidity and fearfulness. What anger exists will be expressed only toward the self. Others will seldom be criticized.

Sexual desire is lost, plus a certain capacity for sexual function: an impairment of sexual potency in men, and the diminution of lubrication in women. Appetite for food is diminished, and the subject loses weight, often rapidly. Sleep is impaired, the subject sometimes awakening after no more than a half-hour of sleep, and then lying in bed ruminating about his miserable and dangerous future.

The change effected by the drug influences not only the subject's inner feeling but his relations with others. In general he will efface and subordinate himself, submit to domination, avoid encounters, and surrender readily to the expectations of others. He will also surrender to reality, unable to mobilize any ingenuity, novelty, or creativeness. He sees himself limited and restricted by reality, defeated by the ordinary demands of daily life, unable to conceive of any solution to the simplest problem.

The subject also frequently exhibits some motor changes: initially there may be a dystonia affecting almost any of the motor groups; later, we may see the characteristic, distressing restlessness, akathisia; and finally, a fairly classical Parkinsonism with typically frozen face, tremors, motor inertia, bad posture, and salivation. Hormonal changes are reflected not only in the decrease in sexual desire and diminution in the readiness of the genitals to become sexually aroused: lactation and a loss of menses may occur in women.

It is not really relevant to discuss the pharmacology involved in the chemical action of the drugs on the central nervous system, nor in the elicitation of the specific changes I have described. We can make our clinical observations and utilize them without reference to the intermediate chemical and physiologic process involved. The pharmacology is complex, involving several different neurotransmitters that act on both pre- and postsynaptic neurons in ways, and at rates, that are influenced by other concurrent changes in the central nervous system. With our present knowledge, prediction is not possible. Therefore we shall leave what will ultimately be a most useful and interesting account—of the interaction of mental and physical effects—to some future date, and restrict ourselves here to the clinical data.

I have described the clinical syndrome of melancholic depression—except that the extrapyramidal syndromes, including the akathisia, are not ordinarily seen in depression. When the syndrome is induced chemically, these extrapyramidal syndromes can be selectively removed by the administration of an anticholinergic substance. In fact, because almost all of the true currently used tranquilizers possess a varying degree of anticholinergic action, the drugs themselves act to limit the extrapyramidal effects that their tranquilizing action tends to induce.

When the effective drug is removed, the syndrome does not always *relent* spontaneously: in the case of natural melancholia, the subject may display little, if any, *resilience*. It can be reversed by the administration of a substance that acts in the opposite direction.

Consider now the converse experiment: the administration of a drug that acts to undo the effects of tranquilizers, and, in susceptible individuals, to induce effects opposite to those mentioned. (The antidepression or energizing drugs do not resemble each other nearly as closely as the tranquilizers do: in the pattern of the response they elicit, the time course of the onset of these effects, side effects, and persistence of these influences. Nevertheless, a composite picture can be drawn that can reliably be used for clinical purposes.) Under the influence of such antidepression medication, we observe the following effects: the subject impresses the observer as erect, youthful, and vigorous. The subject will have little interest in examining himself, but will be occupied with actual and potential love objects, with activities, projects, and ambitions. To the extent that he must take account of himself, he will think of his visible and perceptible attributes—by which he is known to others—rather than his sensations, inner feelings, and sentiments. He will exhibit surprising amounts of energy in carrying out plans, and especially in embarking on new projects. His continual activity sometimes dazzles. The subject's affect can best be characterized not as cheerful, but as euphoric, though sometimes angry. The idea of illness does not occur to such an individual, and when actual symptoms occur, he will minimize and deny them, feeling literally invulnerable. The subject will admire himself and feel pride in his abilities, achievements, possessions, and status. He feels satisfied with himself and sees no fault in his conduct or personality; feeling confidence, he exhibits courage, and in fact, sometimes foolhardiness.

The patient desires, and actively pursues, sexual gratification. Sexual organs function effectively. Appetite for food is restored, but not necessarily in excessive degree. Weight is restored to normal, and may—but need not—exceed the patient's usual weight. As the subject recovers from his depressive state, sleep returns to normal; but as he passes from a state of euthymia into euphoria, morning awakening resumes, though now the patient awakens full of enthusiasm and vigor, and eager to get on with his planned activities, most of which he sees as succeeding and bringing him satisfaction.

In his relations with others the subject assumes a dominant role: challenging, competing, leading. Reality and its constraints do not impede him; he can devise plans to circumvent, overcome, and defeat it. He solves problems creatively, and his imagination makes him creative in all of his endeavors.

There are no visible motor or hormonal changes corresponding to those that occur in melancholia.

The state described corresponds to hypomania, a state of minor pathology. If carried further, it would become mania. The difference would involve intensifying all other qualities to a point where they would become dysfunctional. The patient becomes so active that he cannot complete any project; his energy and resources are wasted. His optimism, and sense of invulnerability and omnipotence, distort his judgment so that he undertakes foolish projects that are bound to fail. His ambition and his need to achieve make his object relations unsatisfactory to any actual or potential partner. His leadership becomes domination, eliciting resentment and rejection by others whose regard and cooperation he requires. The frustration that he no doubt encounters makes him irritable and very angry.

We have considered two syndromes: one is elicited by one set of chemical agents, and the other by a different set. (Some, but not all, of their pharmacologic properties oppose each other.) The two syndromes relate to each other almost as mirror images, with few exceptions. Although I have identified the first state with melancholic depression, melancholia usually displays abnormal behavior that modifies the basic state created by the chemical agent alone, so as to make it even more dysfunctional than it would otherwise be. For example, the state of misery gives rise to a wish to die, which may elicit anxiety and defensive activities, or may actually lead to suicide. The intrusion of others into the isolation that the subject desires may elicit inappropriate anger. Similarly, the second state, when carried beyond a certain point, becomes pathologic, and the pathology modifies what would otherwise be the pure syndrome. Although in any real situation, as the extreme of either position is approximated, defensive maneuvers and dysfunctional breakdowns modify the patterns described, it is still possible to imagine a hypothetical state in which the extreme syndrome is visualized, uncomplicated by these consequences and reactions.

How shall we designate these two polar states? It seems that the relevant parameter here could be called *psychic energy:* state *one* seems characterized by a dearth of psychic energy; and state *two* by a plethora. As late as 1940, in *Outline of Psychoanalysis,* Freud predicted that ultimately chemical agents usable for the treatment of mental illness would be discovered. He claimed they would work by altering the amounts of energy, and their distribution, in the mental apparatus. Nevertheless, whenever I propose this theory I encounter criticism regarding such things as reifying metaphors, resorting to nineteenth-century science, and mixing psychology and pharmacology. To avoid such useless controversy, let me suggest that the term psychic energy be treated as just a metaphor—albeit an intuitively relevant one—that can conveniently be used for purposes of labeling and designation, but not necessarily ultimate explanation.

Change of State

Having examined the two states of psychic energy—low and high—and having seen how each can be brought about by a type of medication, let us examine the clinical consequences of moving from one state to the other. If we administer an antidepression or energizing drug to a patient in a state of low energy, we shall encounter no surprises. Each of the qualities of that state listed above will gradually subside, giving way to its converse, and the complicating defenses, dysfunctions, and anger will disappear. This is indeed what we observe when we treat melancholic depression with antidepression drugs, though we aim to stop before a clinical state of mania is induced. However, we're not always able to avoid that—especially in bipolar patients—and frequently permit hypomania to develop, in which state the patient feels even better, and more appreciative, than if returned merely to normality.

When we have succeeded in overcoming a melancholic state through antidepression medication—so that the patient achieves a relative stability—we encounter a syndrome that I have called narcissistic tranquility (Ostow 1967). In fact, although it occurs most frequently in the patient protected by medication against depression, it can be encountered in any patient who has advanced from a state of major stress to a state of lesser—though not absent—stress. Consequently, it is frequently encountered among individuals without mental illness when they leave on vacation. The syndrome includes the following components: increased appetite; weight gain, even when food intake is controlled; somnolence, or even torpor, during the afternoon or evening; increased sexual desire; and the tendency to accumulate possessions. The syndrome contrasts with what

Selye has described as the general adaptation syndrome, and therefore invites correlation with glucocorticoid levels.

The *Physician's Desk Reference* attributes the unwanted property of inducing weight gain to most antidepression drugs. It has been my impression that the patient does not gain weight unless he is relieved of his depression. In other words, weight gain is induced, not directly by the drug, but by the psychophysiologic state that the drug brings about when it successfully combats depression, or when any psychiatric drug overcomes any stressful mental state.

When we try to bring a patient down from a high to a low energy state, we encounter some complications. We must consider three parameters of responsiveness to these drugs. The first parameter is simply *sensitivity:* some individuals respond sensitively to small amounts of medication, while others resist even large amounts. The second is *volatility:* some individuals tend to remain at a fixed energy level even under provocation, and to remain stably at another in response to medication. Others fluctuate in energy level—in response to external emotional and physical stresses, and to inner changes such as menstrual cyclicity. Medication may damp these fluctuations, but only partially.

The third parameter might be called *reactivity:* for many patients, the attempt, without medication, to change their energy level from high to low, encounters a reactive resistance. As tranquilizing drugs are administered in increasing doses, instead of becoming depressed the patient becomes more and more active in the manic pattern; the more medication given, the more paradoxically active he becomes. Reactivity also accounts for the paradoxical hypomanic or manic rebound often encountered when an antidepression drug is withdrawn.

It is actually a modified—and not the pure—manic syndrome that is elicited in reactive patients by tranquilizing drugs. When a small amount of a tranquilizing agent is given to a depressed patient who possesses the quality of reactivity, the depression may lift within 12 to 24 hours. This phenomenon can be used as the basis for treatment of depression, and it is likely to succeed in reactive patients. (I have stopped using it in recent years only for fear of triggering a tardive dyskinesia.) It can also be used to reinforce the therapeutic action of true antidepression drugs when they themselves fail, in moderate doses, to alleviate depression. When the energizing small dose is exceeded, the reactivity is overcome, and the tranquilizing medication then exerts its expected depressing effect. As the dose of tranquilizing medication is increased, other patients— especially the truly manic-depressive—display an increasing manic overactivity, accompanied not by euphoria, but rather by agitation and a sense of depression, irritability, anger, and even belligerence; the patient may even periodically weep. Sometimes, the coexistence of manic and depressive features creates the impression of a "mixed state."

The statement that a relatively small dose of a tranquilizer exerts a reactive energizing effect, and that a larger dose exerts the expected damping effect, is incomplete. In many patients one finds a range of doses—greater than the depressive range of doses—that again elicits reactive energizing, and above that a dose that depresses again. I cannot say how many sinusoidal oscillations of this dose-response curve can be observed within the range of clinically practical doses.

While the experiment of imposing a depressive pull on an individual—by administering a tranquilizing drug—gives us an explanation of some kinds of manic and mixed states, it also gives us a clue to the nature of another common, puzzling, and difficult problem: the *borderline personality disorder* (Ostow 1987). If the clinical literature on this condition, or the clinical state of a number of patients who properly deserve this designation, reviewed, we see that it is characterized not by a specific collection of findings—for a large number of disparate psychiatric phenomena can be found in such patients—but by the phenomenon of, primarily, *volatility;* and, secondarily, anger. I believe that a good case can be made for the argument that the borderline syndrome is simply the expression of excessive *volatility,* compounded by *reactivity,* of the psychic energy system. As a result, extremes of affect are experienced in rapid succession, together with the anger accompanying depressive influences in reactive patients, and a consequent inability to hold the object and self-images constant or coherent. Impulsiveness, destructiveness, and belligerence on the one hand; and euphoria, affection, and optimism on the other, succeed each other with surprising rapidity. If that argument is correct, then the syndrome should be alleviated by a drug that damps oscillation of psychic energy, such as lithium; or one that resists the activating depressive pull, such as an antidepression drug; or both—and in many cases it is.

In the case of those patients who exhibit *sensitivity* to the effects of tranquilizing drugs—but not necessarily volatility or reactivity—we encounter two other phenomena, each associated with a specific syndrome. When the depressive pull asserts itself in the sensitive patient as a result of the administration of a tranquilizing drug, or as a result of a psychogenic depressive influence, either of two familiar syndromes appears. The patient, unaware that he is reacting to an affective threat, tends to cling to familiar, protective love objects and situations, or both. He becomes accommodating, agreeable, and submissive. In this mood, a patient in analytic therapy will accept interpretations and other interventions fairly uncritically, giving the therapist the impression that insight is being attained and that rapid progress is being made. It is only when the clinging fails to protect against the ultimate lapse into depression, and the patient retreats within the depressive armor, that the therapist realizes that the patient's behavior was meant only to encourage support and that the progress was illusory. If, during the clinging phase, the patient is separated from the reassuring, protecting individual or situation, anxiety may set in—sometimes quite abruptly. We see, then, a kind of separation anxiety manifest as *phobia, panic reaction,* or simple, unconditional *anxiety.* Since the anxiety is induced ultimately by a depressive pull, it can be effectively combated by the administration of an antidepression drug.

For other individuals, protection against anxiety and depression is offered not merely by proximity to a protecting figure but by words and gestures of admiration and affection. When these are offered in adequate amount, they protect effectively. However, when they are withheld, we see reactive anxiety; protest; abandonment of the object for others; and similar petty, vindictive, or replacement maneuvers. Such patients exhibit what impresses one as narcissism—the need for unremitting adulation. We may infer that this phenomenon forms a basis for a predisposition to the *narcissistic personality*. In other words, the narcissistic personality is likely to be found in an individual who is sensitive to external or internal depressive influence, and who defends himself against it by demands upon others for a constant supply of admiration. Such narcissistic individuals usually respond to antidepression drugs with at least partial relenting of their characteristic need.

All of the above syndromes may be defined solely in terms of energy equilibrium; that is, with little regard for childhood experience or current psychodynamic interaction, and can be alleviated by medication. Other patients, however, exhibit what seem to be similar—if not identical—syndromes, but do not respond to antidepression medication. We must infer that the psychic energy parameter plays a part in the pathogenesis of the syndrome in the case of some patients but not others.

Schizophrenia

A surprisingly similar analysis applies to schizophrenia. Again, let us start with the facts. Given patients in a state of active schizophrenic psychosis, the conventional administration of antipsychosis tranquilizers will elicit any of four different responses: Some patients will recover promptly, and, continuing with the same dose of medication, will remain well; some will recover briefly and then relapse—psychotic but no longer agitated—even when the dose of medication is increased; others will become less agitated but no less psychotic, or more so; and finally, some patients will become more agitated, more psychotic, and more disturbed. These responses will be affected by the dose, but usually there is no essential difference between one tranquilizing agent and another.

The explanation for these discrepancies lies in the difference between one person and another with respect to the variables discussed: sensitivity, volatility, and reactivity of the psychic energy parameter. First we must ask why the chemical agents that produce changes on the manic-depressive spectrum—that I therefore designate as regulators of psychic energy—can influence schizophrenia. We must infer that schizophrenia—at least those forms of the illness that respond to medication—is a disorder that necessarily involves variation in the psychic energy parameter. Evidently, *both* a constitutional susceptibility to schizophrenic decompensation *and* a variation in psychic energy adequate to trigger that decompensation are required to elicit a schizophrenic reaction. (We must consider, though, that because all of these drugs exert influences in addition to the influence on psychic energy, a response to these, such as anticholinergic phenomena, does not necessarily imply that psychic energy is involved.)

We can now consider the possibility that the differences in response of the schizophrenic patient to tranquilizing medication reside in the differences in response to changes of the psychic energy parameter. Specifically, if an actively psychotic patient recovers in response to a moderate dose of an antipsychosis tranquilizer, then we may infer that the condition resembles simple mania, in that in both instances a deviation in the direction of energy excess is remedied by a drug that reduces that excess. A second group of schizophrenic patients will recover promptly with tranquilizing medication, but within days thereafter, as the medication continues, will become simply depressed, or psychotic again, with evidence of depression in the psychotic picture. These are patients who are particularly *sensitive* to the depressing effects of the drug, driven downward into depression once the pathogenic energy plethora has been resolved. In some, but not all, schizophrenic patients, a state of depletion of psychic energy—melancholic depression—will create a picture of psychosis. This syndrome, clearly psychotic, nevertheless includes telltale signs of the depleted, depressive state, such as hypochondria; expectation of death; and feelings of guilt, direct or projected. The high and low states of psychosis may not always be recognizable as such when seen alone, but when both are seen in the same patient, they differ clearly and leave little doubt as to which is which.

A third group of schizophrenic patients will respond to tranquilizing medication with aggravation of their illness, though the agitation may be alleviated. These patients resemble manic-depressives in a depressed state—tranquilizing medication only makes them psychotically depressed to a greater degree, though it subdues the accompanying anger that tends to make them agitated. A fourth group of schizophrenics becomes more psychotic, angry, and agitated; more homicidal, suicidal or self-mutilating, under the influence of tranquilizing medication. They can be compared to the "mixed," excessively reactive bipolar patients, those who resemble manics in their overactivity and feelings of omnipotence and omniscience but also exhibit depressive anticipation of defeat, punishment, loss, and frustration, and easily fluctuate from laughter to tears.

A fifth group of psychotic patients resembles those described as borderline. They exhibit relatively rapid oscillation between psychotic and nonpsychotic states; the former may include indications of being either high or low. In fact, the borderline rubric, as commonly used, includes patients who periodically slip briefly into states of psychosis. The factor that determines this characteristic I termed *volatility*. The coexistence of *reactivity* adds the components of anger and destructiveness to the syndrome.

The considerations to which I have drawn attention make it clear that a depressive pull is responsible for several of the separate schizophrenic syndromes. It follows, therefore, that antidepression medication can be useful in the treatment of these conditions. Antidepression drugs will counter the excessive sensitivity of those patients who lapse into a depressive psychotic state in response to tranquilizers. They will also prevent or repair the reactive syndromes. For borderline patients, antidepression drugs alone may suffice in providing some stability if the energy excursions tend primarily downward. Combining antidepression drugs with tranquilizers will offer even more stability, and lithium, too, may contribute. Paradoxically, small amounts of tranquilizers, by virtue of their ability to elicit reactively an increment of psychic energy, may suffice in resolving a psychotic state, when the latter is attributable to mild energy depletion.

Apocalyptic Dynamics

But the pathogenesis of schizophrenia involves more than just fluctuations in psychic energy. How does it differ from illnesses of the manic-depressive spectrum? We have known since the Schreber case (Freud 1911), that the mental change associated with psychosis could be described as a withdrawal of cathexis from reality. What happens during the definitive outbreak of the illness is that the patient mentally disengages from the real world, perceiving that disengagement as an awareness that the world is coming to an end. This awareness is immediately associated with acute anxiety, followed by the experience that the world is being reborn. The reborn world, as seen by the patient, is free of the humiliations, frustrations, and disappointments of the real world.

We encounter many variations on this theme. If there is a good deal of anger associated with the psychotic retreat, the end of the world is seen to come about through a violent struggle, a cataclysmic war, in which the patient's destructive and defensive impulses vie for control over his behavior and are seen as contending forces projected into the cosmos. If the destructive forces are ascendant, the patient may see himself as a diabolic destroyer and actually become murderous or suicidal, or both. On the other hand, if the defensive forces prevail, the patient may become a messianic deliverer, a new Moses or Jesus.

The classical apocalypses of religious scripture strikingly resemble these solipsistic apocalypses of the psychotic patient. We must infer, therefore, that this dynamic mechanism that achieves hallucinatory and delusional immediacy in psychosis is available far more prevalently as an unrealistic defense against pain that arises in the encounter of the inner with the outer world. Clinically, we also find it in the fantasies and dreams of borderline patients—even when they are not psychotic—and in patients who fall into other diagnostic categories, but who require devices to cope with rage. I suspect that faced with the prospect of loss, and especially death, the psyche almost automatically becomes involved in attempts at renewal, rebirth, and creation—often in a frankly erotic manner. An interesting project would be to trace the specific circumstances that encourage the appearance of the apocalyptic pattern, and what favors, or disfavors, each of its components.

The sequence of anger followed by rebirth suggests the *reactive* pattern of response to energy-depleting stress; whereas the reactive pattern may therefore underlie the full psychotic apocalypse, I suspect that there are far more complex relations to take into account.

Implications for Theory

What can we conclude from these considerations? These syndromes are elicited and shaped by the status, and its changes, of a parameter that functions on the border between physiology and psychology. For most patients this parameter responds only faintly, if at all, to interpretation, reconstruction, reassurance, education, or any other usual psychotherapeutic maneuvers. There are some patients, however, who exhibit a considerable *resilience*, responding to gratifying external changes—the return of a loved one, or alleviation of solitude—with restoration of the psychic energy parameter. Because borderline patients are inherently volatile, they are likely to show this resilience. It is true that the *specifics* of the *manifestations* of any of these syndromes, and the dreams and fantasies that accompany them, will be determined by the total experience of the individual patient. However, the *syndrome pattern* itself, which prevails at a given point in the case of patients dominated by psychic energy fluctuations, will be relatively fixed, uniform, and characteristic of the psychic energy status. In the same way, changes in symptomatology that are effected by *changes* of the psychic energy status will reflect the personal experience of the patient only in *content,* but will conform in *structure* to relatively fixed patterns of the type discussed.

To be sure, even in these fixed structures, we can discern psychodynamic mechanisms. Freud *did* perceive the world-destruction-and-rebirth dynamic in the case of schizophrenia, and he and Abraham *did* describe correctly the oral mechanisms, and the identification with the object, that regularly occur in melancholia. In the former case, this apocalyptic pattern is primary and essential, and other dynamics, such as homosexual inclinations and defenses against them, are secondary and nonessential. Analytic interpretation will affect neither helpfully. Similarly, in the case of melancholia, the essential dynamic is based upon the deficiency of psychic energy, and the low self-esteem, lack of interest and desire, hopelessness, and helplessness that flow from it. Analysis of these symptoms, or the mechanism of oral incorporation, or identification with the lost object, will do nothing to alleviate the patient's anguish.

It follows, therefore, that attempts to influence clinical states in these cases by psychotherapeutic methods are bound to be completely, or mostly, ineffective. Resilient patients may try, by seduction, manipulation, or threat, to engage the therapist in the kind of personal relationship that will supply their needs for love. A truly caring and devoted therapist can be helpful to such a patient through the personal concern and affection that he radiates, but it would be an error to infer that it is the interpretation to which the patient is responding, rather than the involvement that accompanies it. Some of the more dramatic displays of transference dependence, including the interminable analyses, are determined by the ability of the analysis to protect the patient against painful alterations in his psychic energy state.

The Recovered Patient

A priori, one would assume that when the deviation of energy state has been undone, or its volatility suppressed, we can focus on the more conventional psychodynamics with which, as psychoanalysts, we are familiar, and which we know how to influence usefully. We must attend to the personality changes upon which the psychic energy deviation has been superimposed, to the distortion of personality that ordinarily accompanies the schizophrenic or manic-depressive diathesis, and that caused by the experience of the disease. By and large, that is true, but there are some considerations we must keep in mind.

The restoration of the state of psychic energy equilibrium may well alleviate, or undo, the grossly pathologic behavior that brought the patient for treatment in the first place; but it also compels him, once again, to confront the frustration or disappointment that triggered the episode of illness. Frequently, anger is expressed toward the disappointing object, and hostile or even destructive solutions are undertaken. Obviously, an attempt to defuse such unfortunate projects must be made by the therapist.

Second, we must deal with residua of the psychic energy pathology, even when it has been brought under control by medication. Some patients who did not become depressed or manic until relatively late in life, had managed, nevertheless, in previous years to protect their equilibrium by establishing certain apotropaic maneuvers—those devoted wholly to providing magical protection—some of which are destructive and dysfunctional. Even when the medication provides a more reliable and realistic protection, the patient will tend to reestablish the unwholesome or exploitative type of behavior to which he has been accustomed.

Third, we must consider that for most patients who exhibit any unusual degree of psychic energy volatility, there is no normal, customary equilibrium point. Given the patient who has functioned fairly well for most of his life but becomes depressed for the first time in his fifties or sixties, when his depression is properly treated he will tend to slip back and remain in that state of psychic energy equilibrium that had been hitherto characteristic. However, when the patient has been plagued by destabilizing psychic energy volatility for most of his life—as is true of most borderline patients—there will be no stabilizing notch marking his equilibrium point; in that case, the therapist will have to choose, willy-nilly, that state of function he considers most helpful to the patient. This he does by regulating the dose of the tranquilizer, energizer, or both. He will obviously try to choose a state of mind that neither elevates the patient to an unrealistic state of self-confidence that impairs his judgment, nor fixes him into the rigid constraints of excessive realism that would stifle his imagination and motivation. What state the analyst chooses will determine primarily the patient's courage, enterprise, imagination, motivation, and whether he tends to dominate or submit, to lead or to follow; and secondarily, therefore, whether and whom he marries or stays married to; his vocation and success at it; his social life; relations with children, friends and community; and the quality of his life in general. The analyst, in other words, possesses a greater control over this patient's life and destiny than is usual, and that power imposes upon him a need for especial ethical concern, above and beyond ordinary clinical responsibility.

Conclusions and Summary

1. The classical theory of psychoanalytic psychodynamics that we have learned, taught, and employ in the treatment of patients is valid only within certain limits. It does not apply in the case of mental illness occasioned by deviation of a hypothetical quantity that I have been calling psychic energy, and it does not apply when illness has been caused by extraordinary external stress.

2. The treatment of patients for whom these two limits have been transgressed requires the use of modalities and theories other than classical.

3. The way in which certain illnesses respond to tranquilizing and antidepression medication reveals certain affinities among them and suggests that they are all evoked, influenced, and relieved in response to spontaneous or induced variations in one or, at most, a few common parameters. The most parsimonious hypothesis, and a serviceable one, is that a single function is involved. Different syndromes are induced in accordance with the *sensitivity* of this function to external or internal stress, or to the influence of medication, its *volatility,* and its readiness to respond *reactively* in the direction opposite to the one in which it is being displaced.

4. Schizophrenic patients respond to medication very much as patients on the manic-depressive spectrum do, and presumably are responding to the same variations in this function.

5. In schizophrenics, we often encounter a fantasy of world destruction, followed by rebirth, in a pattern that resembles that described in classical religious apocalypses. Probably this pattern is evoked, accented, and suppressed in susceptible patients by variations in the psychic energy function.

6. There are some patients on the manic-depressive spectrum, as among the schizophrenics, especially including borderline patients who, when the pathogenic deviations of the energy spectrum are corrected by medication, cannot revert to an established equilibrium position. For them the therapist can, and must, choose a particular position that he considers optimal for the patient, his quality of life, and destiny; and he must struggle to provide a wholesome stability for the patient in that position.

More generally, in the data provided to us as analysts, observing patients being treated with chemical agents more closely than any other psychiatrists, we can find answers to questions that were unavailable before. How do the various psychiatric syndromes, which we have been able to describe hitherto only phenomenologically, relate to each other? Are there fixed sequences in which the syndromes occur? Which syndromes will respond more readily than others to chemical agents? What kind of theory can we devise that will comprehend all of these phenomena, and provide at least a mnemonic device for predicting relations and sequences? How will such a theory articulate with classical psychoanalytic theory, or with variants? I have attempted to formulate a tentative, initial statement of description, relationships and theory; much more work has to be done.

Finally, reverting to the issue of psychoanalytic resistance to psychiatric drug therapy, at a time when psychoanalysis is being challenged as never before by alternative therapies and pseudotherapies, by the need for increased efficiency and decreased cost, we find in its literature a proliferation of theories, mostly unsubstantiated by data or evidence of therapeutic efficacy, while the wealth of information offered by the data of psychiatric drug therapy is disdained, and the inferences that can be drawn from it ignored.

Is it not clear that for us (and probably for members of all scholarly disciplines) a theory serves primarily to comfort and strengthen us in times of stress and uncertainty; that when we need the theory, we ignore its deficiencies, or we struggle to patch them up or mask them, rather than make the radical changes that reality requires? We can do that only when we have confidence in our observations, and in our ability to make sense of them and to use them helpfully.

Many questions remain unanswered about the use of psychiatric drug therapy during psychoanalysis, and about the meaning of the data that we collect, when the two procedures are combined. But we need the courage to do the combined procedure, to collect the data, to draw reasonable inferences therefrom, and to test the resulting hypotheses in clinical practice.

References

Freud, S. (1911). Psychoanalytic notes on an autobiographical account of a case of paranoia. *Standard Edition* 12:69–71.

_____ (1940). An outline of psychoanalysis. *Standard Edition* 23:182.

Ostow, M. (1967). The syndrome of narcissistic tranquility. *International Journal of Psycho-Analysis* 48:573–583.

_____ (1987). Comments on the pathogenesis of the borderline disorder. In *The Borderline Patient: Emerging Concepts in Diagnosis, Psychodynamics, and Treatment,* ed. J. S. Grotstein, M. F. Solomon, and J. A. Lang, pp. 289–315. Hillsdale, NJ: Analytic Press.

9

The Borderline Disorder

MORTIMER OSTOW, M.D.

The borderline disorder is characterized by volatility, overlaps with major mental illness, and tends to be familial. Psychic energy fluctuates consistently with change in status on the manic-depressive axis, which can in turn be influenced by chemical agents. As energy levels change, symptoms occur in characteristic patterns, whether the cause for the change is chemical or experiential. An effort is made to develop a model relating these changes to a physiologic substrate "virtual motivation" system. The concept of psychogenicity is not challenged by the assumption that physiologic changes accompany changes in manifest psychic energy level.

It is postulated that the striking lability of the borderline disorder is the result of commensurate lability of the psychic energy parameters. As the energy level rises and falls it triggers one syndrome after the other of those to which the patient is vulnerable. Thus the pattern of rapid variability by which these patients are so well known. Indeed, some patients do dramatically well when stabilized with lithium. Further comments are made on the complexity of integrating medication and management with dynamic psychotherapy in these difficult patients.

From the proliferation of books and essays on the subject of the borderline disorder, it seems evident that there is a need to define a diagnostic entity to accommodate a large, important, and otherwise unclassified group of patients. The group demands notice because it constitutes a significant portion of current psychiatric inpatients and outpatients. These patients usually demand a good deal of care and attention, often tend to injure themselves, and resist the establishment of a comfortable doctor–patient relation.

Conceptually this disorder differs from the other major categories of psychiatric illness in that it is characterized by no unique pathognomonic manifestations. Rather, it may exhibit signs and symptoms of such other conditions as neurosis, affective disorder, and episodes of psychosis. What seems to be especially characteristic is the mixture of manifestations of other disorders, the rapid fluctuations in the presenting signs and symptoms, and the stormy relation with the therapist. In other words, it is not the specific group of signs and symptoms that is definitive, but the pattern in which they occur.

It is not even clear that the borderline disorder represents a separate pathologic entity, rather than the pathologic extreme of a parameter whose less extreme values prevail in the normal population. The view currently accepted by many psychiatrists is that the disorder, if it is to be regarded as a parametric variant, occupies the interval between neurosis and psychosis.

One of the difficulties encountered in the attempts to delineate this condition arises from the fact that each of the observers deals with a somewhat different population. Most of the patients studied and reported have been selected from a hospitalized population and therefore differ, in at least their capacity for self-control, from patients seen in private practice. Among the samples reported, there are differences too in social and economic class, cultural background, and educational level of the source populations. As a result, the by now well-known and often-quoted study by Perry and Klerman (1978) determined that among four of the best known sets of diagnostic criteria, about half the items are each found in no more than one of the four sets. Perry and Klerman concluded, not that the syndrome as defined by the proponents of each was invalid, but that each of the reporters may have been dealing with a different population and that they might therefore have been describing variants or subgroups of the same condition.

Clues

If one looks beyond the visible manifestations for the underlying mechanism, one may discern what is common to and characteristic of most of the syndromes that have been described in the literature. These characteristics apply as well to those of my own patients who seem to me to belong to this real, though ill-defined, group. To that end, let us consider the following items as clues.

1. I referred earlier to the fact that it is not individual signs and symptoms that characterize the borderline disorder but rather the pattern that they display. This pattern consists of two elements. First, there is the surprising mixture of signs and symptoms of other, discrete disorders. The second element is simply the frequent, rapid, and pronounced fluctuations of their visible manifestations. Usually these fluctuations can each be seen to have been precipitated by some significant impinging event, a gratification or a disappointment, praise or blame, affection or rejection. The response is usually abrupt, incommensurate in degree with the precipitating incident, an overreaction of major

proportions. What is missing is perspective, proportion, equanimity, and serenity. In another generation, and in another context, Goldstein (1940) called this phenomenon "abnormal stimulus bondage," or "forced responsiveness to stimuli."

Cohen and his associates (1983) comment on difficulties in "modulation of activity and attention" in young adult patients with borderline personality disorder. Donald Klein (1977) observes that lability is "a central pathological trait."

Perhaps it is the difficulty of *modulation* that most characterizes this condition—modulation of activity and attention, as Cohen and associates suggest, but also modulation of affect (especially anxiety and depression), modulation of desire, approach and withdrawal, optimism and pessimism, idealization and disparagement, friendliness and hostility, self-aggrandizement, self-degradation, and self-injury.

2. The borderline disorder, as it is now understood, bears some intimate relationship with depressive illness. Two of the four sets of criteria examined by Perry and Klerman (1978) mention depression specifically. Many other observers and commentators note the unusually frequent occurrence of manic-depressive illness in the families of the designated borderline patients (Andrulonis et al. 1982, Stone 1980).

The specific kind of depressive illness that one encounters in the borderline patient and in his relatives is not always spelled out. Among my own patients I have observed melancholic depression; perhaps more often, severe but nonmelancholic unhappiness; and sometimes a mixture of the two. (I distinguish the former from the latter by the presence in the former of the usual vegetative signs—guilt, a feeling of having aged, withdrawal, and poor resilience. Nonmelancholic unhappiness conversely shows little if any of the vegetative phenomena—no guilt, persistent though often angry attachment to the love object, and ready remission. The ready remission is consistent with the lability discussed earlier.)

Confirmation of the participation of the manic-depressive mechanism in the borderline syndrome may be inferred from the response of the patients to antidepressive medication. Sarwer-Foner (1977), though he questioned their usefulness for long-term treatment, did report that many features of the borderline syndrome responded to antidepressive drugs. Klein (1977) distinguishes among several types of borderline patients but found that some responded to lithium and others to monoamine oxidase (MAO) inhibitors. Petti and Unis (1981) reported substantial "improvement" in the behavior of three borderline children treated with imipramine in usual doses (5/mg/kg per day). (I assume that borderline children share more with borderline adults than the adjective.)

3. The relation between the borderline state and schizophrenia is at present not clearly definable. Some of the earliest descriptions of the borderline state, although designated by other names (see Stone 1980, ch. 2, for a history of the concept), assumed that the border demarcated between schizophrenia, or psy-

chosis in general, and its absence. Even now Kernberg (1975) uses the term *borderline* to designate patients who "occupy a borderline area between neurosis and psychosis."

The borderline patient does at times regress to psychotic states. These differ from schizophrenia in that they are usually circumscribed. They may be brief, lasting hours, days, or weeks—that is, circumscribed in time. They may be limited to the transference relation—that is, circumscribed with respect to object. Yet the distinction is thought to be so sharp that one can reliably distinguish between borderline and truly schizophrenic patients (Andrulonis et al. 1982, Gunderson 1977).

4. The borderline patient in many instances gives evidence of organic brain disease. Cohen and his colleagues (1983) list five sectors of development in which the borderline child manifests disturbance. The fourth of these is "neuromaturation: unevenness in fine and gross motor development; odd posturing and gait; hyper- or hypotonia; atypicalities on neurologic examination, with disturbance in body image, sequencing and coordination (p. 200). (Cohen et al. do not assume that the borderline child grows up to become a borderline adult, but rather that he may pursue an even more pathologic career—namely, that he may become psychotic or regress to a more severely pathologic type of personality disorder.)

Andrulonis and his group (1982) distinguish three subcategories of borderline personality disorder: one with no evidence of organicity; a second with a history of trauma, encephalitis, or epilepsy; and a third with a history of childhood attention deficit disorder (ADD), learning disability, or both.

That borderline disorder and attention deficit disorder (ADD) overlap has been observed in recent years by a number of students of the subject. Hartocollis (1975), writing in Bellak's collection of essays on minimal brain dysfunction (MBD) in adults, lists a number of features shared by MBD and borderline patients: labile affective disposition, including a readiness for anger and temper tantrums, based on low frustration tolerance; low self-esteem; defective sense of identity; loneliness and emptiness; inclination toward impulsive self-destructive action; and a tendency to project blame. Cohen and associates (1983) note the "remarkable overlaps" of the characteristics of children with borderline syndrome and attention deficit disorder. "Thus it seems conceivable," they write, "that the ADD and borderline syndrome might represent at least in part, similar clinical entities of some common underlying biological dysfunctions" (p. 202). Similarly, the borderline disorder often overlaps with what *DSM-III* calls antisocial personality disorders, and the latter is often associated with subtle and sometimes even gross evidence of brain dysfunction (Elliot 1978).

5. Finally, there seems to be little question that heredity plays an important role in the etiology of borderline disorder. Stone (1980) reports that about one quarter of both psychotic and borderline patients in the hospital have first-degree relatives with serious psychiatric disorders. For ambulatory patients the incidence of psychiatric disorders in first-degree relatives was again about 25

percent among borderlines, but only about 6 percent among neurotic patients. Wender (1979), reporting on a group of patients defined by the Hoch and Polatin criteria for pseudoneurotic schizophrenia, ascertained that 44 percent of these borderline schizophrenic adoptees were born of parents who satisfied criteria for the same diagnosis. Andrulonis and colleagues (1982) reported that about one third of both borderlines and schizophrenics had family histories of depression and the same proportion of relatives who abused alcohol or other drugs. Only 4 percent of their borderline patients had schizophrenic relatives; in contrast, about one fifth of their schizophrenic patients had such relatives. They observed too that about 40 percent of female borderline patients had depressed relatives, but male borderline patients had only half that number of depressed relatives.

Even more interesting was that one eighth of their borderline patients, but none of their fifty-five-member control group, were adopted. One might infer from this observation that absence of a natural and loving parent contributed to the pathogenesis of the condition. Since most adoptive children are born of unplanned pregnancies, I think it is fair to infer that the parents of borderline children in many instances are as impulsive and irresponsible as their children; that is, they too may be borderline.

In summary, it seems fair to say of the borderline disorder that it is characterized by pronounced volatility and poor modulation of many parameters of psychic function; that it overlaps with major mental illnesses, including manic-depressive disease, schizophrenia, and organic brain disease; and that it is especially likely to occur in families that carry mental illness of one type of another. Our problem, then, is to try to understand what kind of basic dysfunction could create such a condition.

Hypothesis

To introduce the hypothesis I propose, let me review another hypothesis that I have suggested on several occasions in the past in order to provide a rationale for psychiatric drug therapy (Ostow 1962, 1970, 1979). If we omit from consideration the modern sedatives (such as members of the benzodiazepine series), lithium, and carbamazepine, then the other therapeutic medications we possess can do only one of two things to a manic-depressive patient. Some of the medications will move a depressed patient out of depression and towards or into mania. These we call antidepressive agents (or, less elegantly, antidepressants) or energizers (Ostow and Kline 1957). The other group of substances, tranquilizers or neuroleptics, may move the patient downward from mania or hypomania toward normality and, further, toward or into depression.

Since the state of depression is characterized by mental and physical inertia (or impotent agitation) and a disinclination to initiate action and change, and since the state of mania is characterized by an eagerness to act and to do, to move and to change, I have associated the state of depression with a dearth of "psychic energy" and the state of mania with a plethora of "psychic energy." Freud (1911) anticipated that chemical agents would be found that would alleviate mental illness. The new agents, he said, would influence "the amounts of energy and their distribution in the apparatus of the mind."

That a change of position on the manic-depressive axis is subjectively and intuitively perceived as a change in the availability of "energy" is suggested by the following observation. A depressed patient was treated with isocarboxazid (Marplan), 40 mg per day. Because his response seemed excessive with respect to activity, planning, and extravagance, and because of insomnia, he was told to decrease the dose to 30 mg per day. Within the next week there were dreams about deficit and disease, though there was no conscious sense of impairment. Two weeks after the reduction of dose, the patient reported the following dream: "Someone was driving a boat that was completely filled with coal, which was needed for energy, to sell it and make a lot of money." He awoke that morning, depressed and exhausted for the first time since his recovery began, and could not mobilize himself to go to work.

The patient was a technically trained professional who was familiar with the meaning of the word "energy" in scientific disciplines. Referring to coal as a source of "energy" is technically correct. He invoked the concept here when he was compelled in the dream to deal with the feeling of enervation that characterized the depressive relapse, a feeling that many people experience as "impoverishment" in its broadest sense.

Obviously the term does not denote energy in its physical sense, or even the chemical potential for the liberation of energy. It does denote motivational impetus, a psychological parameter. Klein (1977), dealing with the same clinical phenomenon, suggests that psychotropic agents work through modification of "activation-affective dysregulation." His term implies that affect and activation are influenced together, and it probably refers to the parameter that Kline and I have designated as psychic energy (Ostow and Kline 1957).

The function that I am here designating "psychic energy" does fluctuate consistently with change in status on the manic-depressive axis. Also, position on the manic-depressive axis varies monotonically with estimated "psychic energy" level, except that the antidepressive defensive maneuvers that I describe later often alter the manifest, as distinguished from true, "energy" level. That manifest and essential levels may differ, one from the other, is demonstrated in the case just described. There, for 2 weeks following the reduction of dose, the patient dreamed of defect and deficiency, but continued consciously to feel well. Only after 2 weeks did the defensive denial break down. Then the patient abruptly found himself depressed and lacking in "energy."

Position on the manic-depressive axis can be influenced by chemical agents, the antimanic and antipsychotic drugs exerting a downward pull toward depression, and the antidepressive drugs an upward push toward mania, in either case approaching or passing a normal midpoint. Since "psychic energy" as I have defined it, and status on the manic-depressive axis, both clinical parameters, correlated with each other, are also powerfully and consistently influenced by drug therapy, one may reasonably infer that whatever the drug therapy does in the central nervous system, it alters those functional systems that bring about the clinical changes that we are discussing. That we do not know exactly what chemical and physical changes are involved—in spite of the mass of data that have been assembled and the plethora of hypotheses that have been proposed—is essentially irrelevant to the argument. Apparently it is a multitude of processes that the drugs initiate—chemical, electrical, and structural. Nor do all the drugs act in a similar way, or operate by the same mechanism. Antipsychotic and antimanic effects can be obtained not only with the phenothiazine, thioxanthine, butyrophenone, and reserpine type agents; beta-adrenergic blockers, alpha agonists, and calcium ion blockers produce cardiac and autonomic, but also antipsychotic and antimanic, effects. One may infer that the complex process that results in those alterations of behavior that I consider expressions of psychic energy level can be influenced at a number of points in the physiologic process and in a number of ways.

In 1962 I tried to adduce evidence in support of the following three propositions:

1. The basal ganglia are concerned with the generation or distribution of instinctual energy.

2. Tranquilizing and energizing drugs act upon the basal ganglia.

3. Tranquilizing drugs act to decrease the amount of instinctual energy available to the ego; energizing drugs act to increase it.[1]

If we observe patients closely as they move from one point on the manic-depressive axis to another, we find that toward the depressive end patients tend to be self-effacing and submissive, whereas toward the manic end they tend to be controlling and domineering. Also, the depressed patient tends to exaggerate the limitations and restrictions of reality, being able to find no way to overcome obstacles. While in a manic state, however, this same patient is able to mobilize ingenuity and imagination so as to circumvent or override the obstacles presented by reality.

The contribution of the psychic energy entity and its neurophysiologic correlates to the pathogenesis of manic-depressive illness is duplicated in the case of schizophrenia, but there is an additional element. In the case of a patient with a schizophrenic diathesis, as the psychic energy level rises and exceeds a certain threshold, which differs from patient to patient, a fairly abrupt change takes place: the classical psychotic retreat from reality occurs, together with its usual concomitants, panic and subsequently restitutive delusion. The administration of an antipsychotic agent (tranquilizer) will undo the energy deviation and its consequent psychosis. When, conversely, the psychic energy level falls, the patient vulnerable to schizophrenia declines into a melancholic depression.

---

[1]The term *instinctual energy* here is used in its metapsychological sense.

In some instances the depressive syndrome may be classical and unremarkable. In others, sometimes on different occasions in the same patient, the depression elicits a psychotic detachment from reality. Although I have observed this sequence on many occasions, I do not know what determines whether or not the depression will trigger psychosis. In either instance, the administration of an antidepressive agent (energizer) will undo the energy deficiency and the accompanying depression or depressive psychosis.

Observing the patient who is undergoing the changes that terminate in the energy plethora breakdown, I have regularly encountered the following phenomenon. The increment in energy level is, as usual, accompanied by a tendency toward grandiosity, to dominate, and to challenge authority. However, the about-to-become schizophrenic patient cannot tolerate his improvement in status, and the ensuing psychotic break is accompanied by delusions of inferiority and worthlessness. I shall not take our argument even further afield than I already have by discussing the delusional defenses against this conviction of inferiority. For example, the male patient who under ordinary circumstances is timid about asserting his masculinity, under the influence of a rising energy level will find sexual desire and urge for sexual domination increasing beyond the point that he can tolerate. When that happens, the psychotic detachment begins, accompanied by feelings of having been castrated or being now female (compare, for example, Freud's [1911] Schreber case). He may then defend himself against this delusion by obvious efforts to deny it and to assert visible masculinity once more. Usually this whole sequence can be clearly seen if the patient is observed daily, as he is in psychoanalytic treatment.

It is relevant to our argument to record here another phenomenon that accompanies the incipient schizophrenic, energy plethora (high) breakdown. As the energy increases, the patient becomes more and more anxious, agitated, and angry. Beyond a certain level, anxiety and anger become intolerable and are then projected out into some person or object of the environment, or onto one's own body. The environment, or some designated enemy, becomes delusionally endowed with dangerous potential, or one's body seems to be disintegrating, as if diseased. As the energy level continues to rise, the definitive psychotic break ensues.

What triggers these changes in psychic energy level? We do know chemical triggers. They include the tranquilizing and energizing drugs that we use therapeutically. In susceptible individuals, cocaine and in some instances even marijuana will elicit an energizing effect. On the other hand, some drugs used in internal medicine, such as beta-blockers and calcium blockers, may in susceptible patients elicit an energy-depleting effect, thereby inducing depression or depressive schizophrenia. Some humoral energy-altering influences arise internally, for example, those responsible for the premenstrual and postpartum psychic changes, both of which tend, in predisposed individuals, to deplete energy and elicit states of depression.

Experiential factors obviously account for most of the incidents of pathogenic energy changes. Serious loss is generally recognized as an adequate precipitant of depression. Frustration and a need to achieve control over a painful situation often elicit an energy-elevating alteration. In many cases, especially in patients who possess susceptibility to movement in both directions, the initial response to a frustration or disappointment may be elevation of mood, followed, after a shorter or longer interval, by depression.

Age, too, plays a role. Most borderline patients, and probably psychopaths too, tend to experience a subsidence of turmoil and agitation once past the age of 30 or 35. I suspect this "burning-out" effect corresponds to a diminution in lability as well as level of the psychic energy parameter, doubtless as an expression of a concomitant decrease in lability and resilience of neurohumoral regulation and a decrease in the level of activating neurohumors. The same factor probably accounts for the increased frequency of melancholic depression with age. However, true manic-depressives may continue to experience manic episodes, and even an enduring hypomanic disposition indefinitely.

It would be helpful to have some model relating these various inputs to each other and to the physiologic substrate that underlies the behavioral complex whose manifestations I have called *psychic energy*. Let me suggest the following as consistent with the clinical facts.

Let us assume that the nervous system of vertebrates includes a phylogenetically archaic mechanism that controls a fundamental parameter of behavior that corresponds to what in humans we call motivation. (In my 1962 book, I argue that the basal ganglia complex is the likeliest candidate for the locus and regulation of that function.) Even in the lowest vertebrates, this parameter will be influenced by internal and external inputs. Some inputs will elicit adaptive responses—for example, the circadian and seasonal rhythms, the sequence of secular maturation, and climate and availability of food sources. Some will elicit maladaptive responses—for example, aging and disease. These factors certainly influence psychic energy in humans, some more significantly and others less significantly than they influence virtual motivation in lower vertebrates. Of course, chemical agents that bind to receptors on the neurons in any portion of this "virtual motivation" system will influence its level and responsiveness.

In addition to these general and universal determinants of motivational level, we must anticipate individual differences in base level and responsiveness to these determinants. Heredity will make some contributions to these differences and fortuitous influences, others. In some cases the base level or responsiveness to external influence will deviate so far from an average normal that pathologic behavior will ensue no matter what inputs are provided.

At some point in the evolution of complex mental function, extremes of experience begin to play a significant role in setting the level of virtual motivation. Syndromes similar to human melancholia can be observed in mammals under such circumstances as separation of young from mother and isolation from the group. One could say that these experiential influences modulate the level established by the physiologic determinants.

If this model applies to humans, then it can help to organize the way we visualize the mutual interplay of the various determining inputs to the motivational or psychic energy system. There is an archaic motivational system, which, by virtue of heredity or fortuitous incident events, may be set to provide levels of energy either too high or too low for optimal function, or it may be too unstable to provide a consistent energy level. The system is subject to influence by circadian and seasonal cycles directly and also indirectly, that is, in response to hormonal changes. It is also influenced by growth and maturational pressure. It can be maladaptively altered by illness and trauma. It will respond to the introduction of chemical agents that bind to any of the components of the system. Frustration and disappointment will elicit changes in the level of energy provided. Because, in the human, behavior is to such a great extent liberated from rigid, instinctual control and governed by psychic experiences and processes, it is reasonable to expect that these too will strongly influence the psychic energy level. And the influence would be exaggerated in those individuals whose motivational apparatus is constitutionally set either unusually high or low, or is inherently unstable.

The purpose of this extensive excursion is to make clear that the concept of psychogenicity is not challenged by the assumption that physiologic changes accompany changes in manifest psychic energy level, and that once triggered by psychogenic influences or by more material biologic alterations, these physiologic changes acquire, so to speak, a life of their own. They may not remit when the experiential influences is withdrawn, but have to be corrected by countervailing agents.

Let me make the argument somewhat more concrete by giving a specific clinical example.

A successful 65-year-old businessman became depressed after he was confronted by a serious financial loss caused by a strike of his workers, which he could not have prevented. The stress was purely external and experiential. However, there was an inherited vulnerability: there had been manic-depressive illness and hypomanic personality in his family. Yet his individual vulnerability was sufficiently mild that he was able to withstand the usual frustrations and disappointments that life brings without breaking down until now, that is, until the process of aging had reinforced the vulnerability, or decreased his resistance. Once the melancholic depression set in, the syndrome that appeared resembled the typical syndrome of melancholic depression, namely, inertia, guilt, self-criticism, a wish to die, pessimism, withdrawal, anorexia, weight loss, morning insomnia, and loss of sexual desire. Although the way in which these signs and symptoms were expressed and reported was influenced by the patient's personality and style, the syndrome itself was independent of his experience. It was a manifestation of the psychic energy depletion and its underlying physiologic changes. After the strike was settled, not too much damage having been done, the illness did not remit. However, it was easily dissipated by antidepressive drug therapy.

The illness had been elicited by a stressful experience impinging upon a mild, inherited vulnerability in an aging individual. The resulting clinical picture was independent of current or past traumas, and relatively uninfluenced by his personality. It was a manifestation of a specific dysfunction of the central nervous system. This dysfunction, once initiated, was not undone by alleviation of the stress, but was undone by a chemical agent that corrected the dysfunction on a physiologic level.

Lability

I regret that we have had to detour so far from our principal interest, the borderline disorder, but we can now return to it. If we address ourselves to the borderline patient's pronounced lability and ask what is the basic parameter that fluctuates so rapidly and so widely, one may consider the possibility that it is the parameter of psychic energy, or at least that the volatility of psychic energy accounts for a large part of the volatility of the borderline patient.[2] Corresponding to this psychological volatility, we must assume an underlying instability of the neurohumoral equilibrium (a simplistic term designating a complex and poorly understood set of processes, intracellular and intercellular, secretory and electrical and possibly structural, that determine the behaviors we are considering).

In previous writings, I have described clinical states that I have observed appear as a patient begins to sink toward a state of energy deficiency or melancholia. I have interpreted these states as expressions of an effort to defend against the impending melancholic state. The first response may be a manic hyperactivity—not an unproductive agitation but a true manic busyness, characterized by attitudes, each the opposite of a corresponding dimension of depression (i.e., optimism, grandiosity, ambition, enthusiasm, joy). The syndrome may include immoderate degrees of counterproductive self-indulgence, such as sexual athletics of one type or other, indulging in alcohol or one or more drugs of abuse, and gambling.

If this paradoxical hyperactivity cannot be maintained, or if it fails to arrest

---

[2]Because psychic energy is not an objective entity but a hypothetical construct devised to provide a theoretical correlate to "energetic" behavior, this statement sounds circular. The statement relates the source of this lability to psychic energy as it is applied elsewhere, for example, to an "explanation" or systematic ordering of various psychic states on the manic-depressive axis such as those described immediately below; and to a systematic description and approach to the prediction of the effect of the various pharmaceutic agents used in the treatment of mental illness. Psychic energy is a *virtual* entity.

the downward slide, the patient's mood changes more or less abruptly. Now, instead of overriding the needs and sensitivities of others, the patient looks to them for support, clinging by making himself subservient, trying to please and ingratiate himself. The abrupt shift from self-indulgence to self-denial may sometimes present as an unexpected religious conversion and may be encouraged by the seductive recruiting activities of a cult group. When the patient is separated from the object for whom he has developed this anaclitic need, he becomes anxious. As a result we may observe a phobic aversion to separation, or a panic disorder.

When the clinging fails to protect against further depressive decline, or if the patient should experience it as a threat, the patient may enter into the phase that I have called angry withdrawal. He turns angrily and sometimes violently against the object who has failed to protect him. We may see a detachment disorder of neurotic quality, such as hysteria, or of psychotic quality, such as catatonic or paranoid forms of schizophrenia. If the patient is in psychotherapy at the time, he may turn angrily against the therapist and leave treatment. If some degree of psychotic diathesis exists, we may see a transference psychosis.

Finally, if the attempt to deter depression by angry withdrawal fails, the patient may lapse into definitive melancholic depression, which may or may not exhibit a psychotic flavor.

By virtue of this mechanism of defense against depression, the manic-depressive patient may come to exhibit any of a number of clinical syndromes in addition to clear-cut mania or clear-cut melancholic depression, including phobias, panic attacks, dissociative phenomena, or ego-syntonic destructiveness toward others or oneself. Whether the syndromes include psychotic features depends on whether the disturbance on the manic-depressive axis is accompanied by a schizophrenic diathesis. If the syndrome is elicited by this antidepressive mechanism rather than by some other neurosogenic or psychotogenic mechanism, it will be alleviated by the administration of an antidepressive drug. (Some colleagues will not accept the argument that syndromes that respond to the same drug are likely to be caused by the same mechanism, preferring the less parsimonious hypothesis that the same drug may influence various disorders by different mechanisms. To be sure, the inference is not a necessary one, but it should be seriously examined before it is rejected.)

Now the ordinary phobic, hysteric, or depressed patient will, if untreated, remain in the same state of mind steadily over a reasonable time. When, however, the patient moves up and down quickly from one of these manic, depressive, or antidepressive syndromes to another, when happiness and unhappiness alternate rapidly, and when one neurotic or psychotic syndrome follows another, the clinical picture approximates that associated with the borderline disorder.

In short, I am suggesting that the striking lability of the borderline disorder is brought about by a commensurate lability of the psychic energy parameters (and an underlying lability of neurohumoral regulation) associated with or triggered by profound overreactions to experience. As the energy level rises and falls, it triggers one syndrome after another of those to which the patient exhibits inherent vulnerability. That is why borderline patients may differ from one another with respect to which symptoms they exhibit, while they resemble each other in the fact that one state of mind succeeds another in relatively rapid sequence.

To support my argument, I can adduce the following facts. My suggestion accounts for the observation that some borderline patients respond to drugs used for the treatment of depression, specifically, tricyclic or MAO inhibitor antidepressive agents, and lithium. (I discuss the specific response to medication below.) What gives the patient most relief is stabilization of mood, which can sometimes be achieved with lithium alone. Sometimes the results are dramatic. My suggestion accounts for the fact that some borderline patients exhibit brief episodes of psychosis, including transference psychosis. Since it has been established that vulnerability on the manic-depressive axis is inherited, my suggestion accounts for the fact that the borderline disorder is often accompanied by a family history of manic-depressive disorders, borderline disorder, or both.

If the borderline patient is indeed subject to vigorous fluctuations of psychic energy, then one would expect that there will be occasions when he is precipitated into melancholic depression or true schizophrenic episodes. The fact is that I have encountered several characteristic borderline syndromes among patients who first presented for treatment of manic-depressive illness or schizophrenia. After these presenting conditions were alleviated by appropriate drug therapy, the underlying borderline disorder was disclosed. It follows that attempting to define borderline disorder by excluding manic-depressives or psychotics from the sample will necessarily yield a skewed composite profile.

Poor Object Relations

Most criteria for the borderline disorder specify, in one language or another, impairment of object relations. All the patients I have seen whom I would include in the group of borderlines could not sustain an amicable relation with anyone. That is not to say that they were indifferent, remote, or detached, like the deteriorated schizophrenic. On the contrary, they were intensely object oriented and eager for a close relation. They knocked loudly and persistently on the doors of parents, siblings, spouses, children, and friends and would display appreciation when admitted. However, within days or weeks usually, sometimes months, the relation lost its charm and instead became a source of intolerable unhappiness. They seldom recognized that the discontent arose within their own psychic economy, and they exhibited considerable ingenuity in justifying the attribution of fault to the partner in the relation. What we see therefore is object pursuit, object abandonment or alienation, regret, grief, perhaps depression with or without contrition, all leading to a great deal of family and social turmoil, as well as misery for the patient and for all those involved with him. These vicissitudes in object relations induce in the psychic energy parameter vigorous changes, which, in turn, are accompanied by the volatile shifts in symptoms and further vigorous shifts in object relations, often leading to vicious cycles.

Because my argument involves both psychogenic and physiologic elements, it may seemed confused to readers who ordinarily think in only one of these frames of reference. I contend that psychic energy is a psychological metaphor that can be used to order clinical observations of individual pathologic states of mind and other relations among them. It also helps to predict the effects of the major psychiatric medications on these states of mind. I assume therefore that is not merely a metaphor but the expression of the function of a true neurophysiologic entity, a virtual source of motivation. This function responds to experience, and, therefore, alterations in psychic energy and the clinical effects that flow therefrom may be considered psychogenic. On the other hand, once the alteration has taken place in vulnerable individuals, it does not recover promptly with the alleviation of the stress, or it may correct or overcorrect, so that the clinical picture then comes to be determined by the physiologic events, which, once initiated, are no longer controlled by the external stress. Also, given an inherited or acquired hypersensitivity, the psychic energy function may be caused to deviate from a normal level by ordinary impinging stimuli such as seasonal cyclicity impinging from the outside, or by stimuli impinging from the inside, such as hormonal changes. Annual recurrence of mania or depression at the same season each year would be an example of the former, and postpartum mental illness would illustrate the latter. In such cases, psychogenicity, though not absent, plays a minor role.

The recurrent rejection of the object is usually followed by serious unhappiness, sometimes by suicide or by attempts at self-mutilation. If the disappointment is followed by a withdrawal of psychic energy of major magnitude (read: impairment of neurohumoral transmission in the critical brain structures, brought about by whatever mechanism), then we see a true melancholic depression. If, on the other hand, the energy supply is not depleted, the so-called depressive state may assume quite a different form, exhibiting object orientation, resilience, and absence of guilt. Attempts at self-injury may follow either of these states.

How do we explain this object intolerance? The mechanisms proposed to explain it—for example, infantile trauma or disturbance of the mother–infant relation—do not compel conviction in all cases. Certainly many of these patients experienced inadequate, incompetent, or frankly hostile handling by their mothers or mother surrogates. In fact, the dynamic interplay with the object who is the target of the adult ambivalence usually seems to reproduce fairly accurately the patient's ambivalent relation with his mother, especially as he remembers it from childhood. Therefore, it is reasonable to suspect that a pathologic deformation of this prototypic relation underlies and causes the pathology of the successor relations of the adult world. Other patients, on the other hand, seem to be solitary ugly ducklings in otherwise healthy families, and the fixating effects of unwholesome parent–child relations are far from evident.

We could invoke the concept of bonding and suggest that borderline patients cannot sustain object relations because they were not properly bonded to the early objects of infancy, either because of an inherent incapacity for bonding, or because the opportunity for wholesome bonding was not available. Some of Harlow's (1964) experiments with mechanical mother surrogates for monkeys seem to have produced monkey infants that could not subsequently bond to parents, siblings, peers, or offspring. When the females who had sustained this trauma were impregnated, their maternal behavior was completely abnormal, ranging from indifference to outright abuse of their infants. Harlow observed that the second generation, born of "motherless mothers," were more precocious than their peers in sexual activity and, "have exhibited more aggression and day to day variability in their behavior than have the members of other playpen groups. The two male offspring of the most abusive mothers have become disinterested in the female and occupy the subordinate position in all activity" (p. 64). He continues, "The extreme of sexuality and aggressiveness observed in their behavior evoke all too vivid parallels in the behavior of disturbed human children and adolescents in psychiatric clinics and institutions for delinquents." Obviously the behavior that Harlow described reminds one of the borderline disorder. If we take this experiment as an etiologic paradigm, we are encouraged to credit the hypothesis that the disorder is the result of the influence of a hostile mother.

On the other hand, we hear often enough of infants who fail to mold to the mother's body when held almost immediately after birth, who can tolerate no body contact, and this in families in which all other children responded normally to the same mother. We are led to infer that some infants just cannot bond satisfactorily in their earliest days and never subsequently develop the capacity to sustain a love relation. Are we dealing then with prenatal or perinatal trauma, or with inherited deficiencies? Perhaps either can serve as a sufficient cause in some cases, and perhaps both are involved in others.

One may consider the possibility that inherited volatility of the psychic energy parameter that I am suggesting may itself prevent adequate bonding; it may fail to adjust the level of tension of the infant so as to permit bonding to the mother. Such infants are usually described as "very tense." That possibility cannot be rejected, but we need more evidence to consider it seriously.

Status Pathology

The final component of the borderline syndrome that I shall consider concerns the parameter of status within the individual's family and society. I refer here to the observation that in a society that permits vertical mobility by its citizens, some struggle to rise to the top and remain there; others sink from a high position to a low one; still others remain at the same status as the families into which they were born. In our mobile society we assume that the tendency to climb is the norm. When we speak of an individual's fulfilling his potential, we generally mean not only that he does as well as he can at whatever it is that he can do, but also that his success brings him some recognition that confers a commensurate improvement in status. A failure to seize opportunities to rise in status, or a tendency to let oneself sink, earns a mental health demerit.

An increase in psychic energy provides a sense of confidence, a motivation to overcome obstacles, to assume leadership and control. Such activities bring with them an elevation in status. Conversely, depletion of psychic energy is associated with a loss of confidence, low self-esteem, relinquishment of leadership and control, and therefore a decline in status.

Among borderline patients, we encounter alternating struggles upward and declines. To some extent these fluctuations in status seeking are to be attributed to the fluctuation in psychic energy. However, in some borderline patients, we can detect another factor at work. We see the same kind of mechanism that Freud (1916) called attention to in his essay on "Those Wrecked by Success," namely, an intolerance for success and achievement. We have already described this mechanism in considering the pathogenesis of the acute schizophrenic breakdown—having achieved a state of being highly energized, the vulnerable patient retreats from it by a lapse into psychosis in which he delusionally sees himself as defective. Similarly, as his energy level rises and he finds opportunity for success, if he does not become acutely psychotic, the borderline patient may engage in some direct or indirect self-injury: he may mutilate himself or attempt suicide; or he may do something calculated to discredit himself or disrupt whatever family or vocational life he has established. It is important to emphasize that this self-imposed deprivation of success is seen in many, but not all, borderline patients. Some do indeed allow themselves success for relatively long periods of time.

What is the mechanism that limits success and improvement in status? In some instances we can discern the oedipal conflict that Freud described. In others one detects a fear of growing up and a fear of assuming responsibility, a lack of courage. One is almost tempted to infer that for whatever inherited or fortuitous reason, some individuals are endowed with or acquire the disposition to rise in social status or to leadership, while others seek a lower level. When individuals of the latter type are pressed by family or social pressure to strive upward or are placed in a leadership position, we can expect some negative consequence such as anxiety, depression, or some disengagement maneuver.

In those borderline patients who exhibit this status infirmity and in other, nonborderline personality disorder patients who share it, we can often detect a specific set of behavior patterns. There are those patients who completely lack the courage and the will to achieve any kind of independence and the responsibilities appropriate to their age. These are the helpless, dependent patients. Second, there are those patients who make their way painfully out of the nursery and into the adult world, but who engage in an unceasing struggle with their mothers, or with whoever comes to replace the mother in their psychic economy. These are patients in constant turmoil, struggling to contain their agitated hostility. Third, there are those patients who do achieve a reasonable degree of success but live in dread of the time when it will all be taken away from them. They seem to believe that they didn't deserve the success, that they are living on borrowed time, and that ultimately they will pay a devastating price. One may think of this as a Faust or Cinderella complex. These are individuals who fear being "wrecked by success." Many patients will shift from one of these positions to another as time goes on, or may exhibit all of these at different times.

Let me be clear about my suggestion. I believe that lability of psychic energy and impaired or absent ability to form affectionate bonds are to be found among all borderline patients (at least all borderline patients in the group with which I am familiar). Many, but not all, also exhibit an inhibition of the tendency to rise in status and to succeed. Lability of psychic energy is, I believe, specific to and pathognomonic of the borderline syndrome. The other two phenomena can be found also in potential schizophrenics and in patients with other personality disorders.

Borderline Disorder and Attention Deficit Disorder

I have already called attention to a generally acknowledged overlap between borderline disorder and attention deficit disorder syndromes. I referred to the observation of Cohen et al. (1983) of the overlap among children and to Hartocollis's (1975) similar comments about adults. Both adults and children share impulsiveness, turmoil, agitation, incapacity for object relations and proclivity for self-injuring behavior.

It would be helpful to say also how they differ. Because I do not see children, I have no contribution to offer to the distinction in early years. Hyperactivity, inability to attend, dyslexia, and learning disorders are the distinctive qualities cited most frequently. I have observed that older adolescents and adults for whom there is reason to suspect attention deficit disorder display, in addition to the qualities mentioned above, a sense of incompetence, inferiority, defeat, and an accompanying feeling of resignation. These patients are more likely to become depressed on that account, to limit their expectations of themselves and of life, and, reluctantly, to withdraw from competition and isolate themselves from their fellows. There are others, however, who manage to deny their inadequacies and to exploit their talents. Some of these, in an effort to reinforce the denial, pursue an exhibitionistic and narcissistic lifestyle. I suspect that the latter type, if not too disabled by borderline disabilities, may never come to the attention of psychiatrists and may never, therefore, acquire a diagnosis.

That leaves us with the question of the pathologic mechanism common to the two disorders. I have proposed that lability of psychic energy contributes strongly to the borderline disorder. The lability is a psychological quality that probably expresses a pathologic lability of the function of the basal ganglia centers of motivation.

The term *minimal brain dysfunction* (which has been replaced by attention deficit disorder) points to an organic basis for the syndrome. However, neither the pathologic nature nor the principal locus of the disorder, if there is one, has been clearly established. Focusing on the problem of difficulty in attending or the problem of hyperactivity as a characteristic disability, several investigators have attempted to single out one or more structures or systems as the site of the controlling disturbance (see Bloomingdale 1984). No clear-cut pathologic change has been demonstrated, however, and we are left with only many different educated guesses. Because the manifestations of the disorder are so varied, it is likely that the structural pathology is not confined to any one system, but rather that the lesions are diffuse or that the repercussions of the principal dysfunction interfere with brain function fairly diffusely.

Nevertheless, Cohen and his associates (1983) call attention to the literature commenting on the resemblance between the postencephalitic syndrome in children and the syndrome of attention deficit disorder (ADD). The postence-phalitic syndrome typically expresses dysfunction that is fairly diffusely distrib-uted in the brain but derives principally from dysfunction of the basal ganglia, specifically, disturbances of motility and motivation. ADD patients, or at least one group of them, exhibit the motility problem of hyperactivity. The charac-teristic inattention and impulsivity of the ADD patient reflect disturbance of motivation. Whereas the quality of the motility and motivation disturbance in the postencephalitic differs from that in ADD patients and while their histories are different, the functional systems that seem to be involved coincide.

Both Cohen and colleagues (1983) and Wender (1979) are impressed by the effects of stimulants on ADD children, interpreting them as evidence that brain catecholamines play a role in the etiology of the disorder. According to current theory, the catecholamines, and especially dopamine, also play a major role in the manic-depressive set of disorders and schizophrenia. Dopamine function seems to be concentrated in the basal ganglia, specifically in the striatonigral system. The stimulants amphetamine and methylphenidate both make dopa-mine more available; therefore the therapeutic efficacy of these substances seems to support the hypothesis that basal ganglia dysfunction is involved in the ADD syndrome.

Recent work by others supports this suggestion, providing a mechanism relating imperfect cerebral dominance, often associated with dyslexia, to neu-rohumoral dysfunction. Glick (1983), at a conference on the biological founda-tions of cerebral dominance, reported that dopamine asymmetries in the nigro-striatal pathways of rats account for turning preferences, which he relates to cerebral dominance. Among humans, too, he finds concentrations of dopamine in the nigrostriatal pathways correlated with laterality. At the same conference, Denenberg (1983) reported that whereas rats that had not been handled during their first 21 days after birth displayed no turning preference, male rats that had been handled, displayed, as adults, a marked preference for turning left and also a reduction in the tendency to kill mice. The brain changes that were responsible for these alterations in behavior were localized in the right hemisphere. It is a fair guess, then, that neurohumoral dysfunction of the basal ganglia underlies some aspects of both ADD and borderline disorder, and that this dysfunction alters the normal balance between aggressiveness and tameness, creates problems of lateral dominance such as those that are usually associated with impaired reading and learning, causes disturbance of motility and motivation, and makes some attention deficit disorder and some borderline patients therapeutically responsive to stimulants and other antidepressive agents.

Psychodynamics of the Borderline State

Kernberg (1975) offers an approach to the borderline disorder based upon dynamic considerations alone. He describes signs of ego weakness: lack of anxiety tolerance, lack of impulse control, and deficiency in capacity to sublimate. He observes a tendency toward primary-process thinking. He specifies a number of fairly primitive "defensive operations"—splitting, primitive idealization, primitive projection, projective identification, denial, omnipotence and devaluation—and he associates all these with a pathology of internalized object relations. He has little to offer about etiology, considering as possibilities traumatic experience with the mother and constitutional deficiencies. However, whatever its origins, it is the infant's disturbed relation with the mother that is considered responsible for establishing the paradigmatic, paranoid distortion of early parental images.

I have no dispute with Kernberg's description. Certainly one can readily confirm the presence of the phenomena he describes in borderline patients. Lability of psychic energy does relate fairly closely to the anxiety intolerance, poor impulse control, and poor capacity to sublimate that Kernberg describes; and lack of capacity for object relations can subsume and account for the "pathologically internalized" object images and the "primitive defensive operations" that accompany them. On the other hand, it is conceivable that whatever the deficiency is that creates the three components of the borderline syndrome I have described, it can also create the characteristic failure of the synthetic function of the ego ("splitting"), rejection of reality, and inconsistency of attitude. In short, I am proposing a set of biologic impairments that achieve expression in the specific clinical findings described by Kernberg. The impairments as a group may represent a nonspecific resultant of very early trauma of whatever nature, organic or psychogenic, prenatal, perinatal or postnatal, fortuitous or inherited.

"Splitting" of the ego, that is, assigning contrasting and inconsistent qualities to the "internal object," manifested by the alternating exhibition of similarly inconsistent attitudes to the corresponding real object, has been promoted by Kernberg (1975), by Masterson (1975), Rinsley (1977), and others as the most common and characteristic property of the borderline disorder. So avidly has this formulation been accepted by analytic students of the borderline problem that the term has become a virtual shibboleth distinguishing between the analytic and the nonanalytic scholars.

Kernberg maintains that this phenomenon originates as a defect in the integration of ego images but that the defect is subsequently used for defensive purposes. The view that I am proposing here accounts for the same clinical phenomena without requiring the complex apparatus of object relations theory. When the patient is depressed, "low," his view of the object of his affection differs from his view of the same object that accompanies his "high" state. Similarly, each of the various defensive maneuvers elicited by the descent toward depression possesses its own view of the object, so that the borderline patient, his energy level fluctuating, finds himself confronted with an ever-changing set of attitudes toward the same individual. Further, as every psycho-pharmacologist knows, there is usually a latency of days to weeks between the time that the abnormal energy level (designated by whatever term the psycho-pharmacologist prefers) is restored to normal in response to remedial medica-tion and the time the ego regains its equilibrium and reconstitutes its equilibrium views. One observes a similar lag in deviating toward abnormality. Accordingly, the affective volatility of the borderline patient prevents him from consolidating his attitudes toward an individual who is important to him, so that his attitude at any given moment is determined by the then-prevailing affect. One might say that he has no "object constancy" (that is, no constant, coherent view of the object) because he has no "subject constancy."

Inconsistency is favored not only by energy volatility but also by the patient's inability to sustain affectionate relations. Affectionate closeness is regularly and inexplicably succeeded by rejection and hatred, and these then by reconciliation. This purely dynamic, as distinguished from energetic, fluctuation also contributes to the prevention of the consolidation of ego attitudes.

It is not only that the patient cannot experience ambivalence, as Akhtar and Byrne (1983) suggest. He cannot tolerate it. At any given moment, the object is either-or; he cannot be both.

It would be a mistake to fail to take notice of the effect on the patient of the defects of mental function that impair him. In most patients I have found that the disabilities, and the disappointments and frustrations that they necessarily incur, powerfully reinforce whatever tendencies exist to devalue oneself, and ulti-mately lead to a depressive sense of demoralization and defeat. This develop-ment is itself reinforced after the third decade, when the upward thrusts of psychic energy subside and leave the patient with little relief from discourage-ment.

Treatment

A theory that has implications for therapy seems to me both more persua-sive and more useful than a theory that has none.

Since volatility is one of the most disturbing and distressing of the symptoms of the borderline patient, an attempt to overcome its effects should be a primary goal of treatment. If I am correct in suggesting that a large proportion of the volatility is contributed by the specific volatility of the psychic energy parameters, then drug therapy might be employed to stabilize the latter. My suggestion that the psychic energy parameter is involved in the pathology is based partly on the observations noted earlier (where I reviewed some of the recommendations made by others regarding drug therapy for borderline patients) to the effect that borderline disorder does respond to the administration of drugs used for the treatment of other disorders in the manic-depressive group. Antidepressive medication is indicated when the patient is seen in a depressed state. I refer here to true melancholic depression, for which antidepressive medication can be considered specific. When the patient is unhappy because of frustration or disappointment but does not show the classical signs of melancholia, antidepressive drugs may alleviate his unhappiness by inducing an inappropriate euphoria. On the other hand, they may precipitate self-destructive behavior, or even psychosis.

Given the lability of the psychic energy mechanism in these patients, the primary goal must be not simply to protect the patient against depression, but to establish some degree of stability. That is, doubtless, why lithium is reported to be effective in some patients. It stabilizes the borderline just as it deters excursion into either manic or depressive territory.

If the patient responds to lithium, what does that response consist of? My own experience with lithium in borderline cases is too limited to permit me to generalize, but a priori I would assume that it can only damp down the affective swings and thereby deter the appearance of those syndromes elicited by them, such as manic, depressive, and psychotic episodes; phobias and panics; symptoms of detachment; and bouts of intemperate anger. In the cases with which I am familiar, that is exactly what happened. On the other hand, the difficulty in object relations, with its consequent frequent disappointment and loneliness, and the self-defeating tendency cannot be undone by a drug that influences only the neurohumoral substrate of the affective regulatory system.

Lithium does not help every borderline patient, even when the affective excursions play an important role. In some instances, therefore, one attempts to achieve affective equilibrium, just as one does in some schizophrenic individuals, by combining antidepressive and tranquilizing drugs in a carefully titrated ratio. In most schizophrenia cases, that is not difficult to accomplish. When it is done successfully, it can keep a schizophrenic patient symptom-free for years. My experience with borderline patients, however, has been more problematic. Often I have found that the most precise titration fails to establish a satisfactory equilibrium. What usually happens is that one can achieve a balance of antidepressive and tranquilizing influences, but the equilibrium is so unstable that the smallest practical dosage change elicits an excessive behavioral change. If more tranquilizer is added, the patient becomes depressed and may even become so depressed, discouraged, and demoralized as to contemplate suicide. If more energizer is added, the patient experiences invigoration and renewal but cannot make peace with love objects to whom he is attached or with the vocational obligations he has accepted. Whereas in the schizophrenic patient behavior equilibrium can be achieved in a narrow but workable range of ratios, in some borderline patients the range has been almost infinitesimal; the patient is either on one side or the other of the equilibrium point but is never stabilized at it. This therapeutic problem can be attributed to the properties of borderline patients: lability of their affective regulation system and their incapacity for sustained object relations. Intolerance for success, when it too is present, contributes to the defeat of the technique.

Of the twenty-eight patients whom I have treated in recent years, almost half required drug therapy for alleviation of some acute, current turmoil. In each instance, the medication succeeded in alleviating the turmoil for which it was introduced, but because of the considerations I have just mentioned it did not alleviate the continuing personality disorder. I anticipate that with newer agents and better understanding future efforts may be more successful. In another six instances I introduced medication in an attempt to overcome the paralyzing lack of courage or a stubborn dependence. Again, because of the pronounced lability of these patients, or their persistent incapacity for object relations, or paralyzing fear, although the medication was able to influence their behavior, it could not budge them off the pathologic track.

I believe that for some of these patients drug therapy is necessary and for others it may very well be helpful. We require reports of experience with the combination of antidepressive and antipsychotic drugs with stabilizing drugs, such as lithium and possibly carbamazepine, and with sedative drugs given in regular daily dose.

The patient's reactivity to stimuli, his low stimulus barrier, which contributes to a lack of stability in psychic economy, requires an attempt to protect himself against unexpected and extreme impressions and demands. We can attempt to help him create a structure that will regularize and limit his exposure to such impingements. The structure may include recommending living arrangements that will remove him from a source of contention. For example, the adolescent may be encouraged to leave his parents' home, or quarreling spouses may be encouraged to separate temporarily until they acquire some perspective. The comfort of living in a consistent, constant, and reliable universe is unavailable to these patients. One of the attractions of the religious cult for the adolescent is that it provides him with a firm, utterly predictable, and protective surround that will buffer him against surprises and prescribe a daily ritual that contributes to the impression of constancy.

The structure should encourage assumption of full-time engagement in a group of activities. Full-time employment, even if it is volunteer and unpaid, or full-time education will protect the patient against the embarrassment and demoralization of visible idleness and against the seduction of troubled and troublesome companions.

Frequent visits to the psychiatrist provide both the structure of regular appointments and a reliable, protective, affective relation that, to some extent, dilutes the impact of conflict with love objects. Obviously, hospitalization, when it is available and acceptable, offers the most effective protection against random input on the patient's delicate sensibilities.

The absence of equanimity and perspective leaves the patient open to overinvolvement in the vicissitudes of his affective swings and limits his capacity to test reality, to observe and criticize himself realistically, and to maintain stable goals and attachments. Therefore, it would be helpful in psychotherapy to reinforce these functions: reality testing, self-observation, and steadiness in maintaining goals and object relations. Similarly, it will be helpful to undermine the ego syntonicity of the patient's self-injurious behavior, and to expose it as such, challenging the rationalizations usually adduced to defend it.

For many borderline patients, and especially those who suffer a residue of childhood ADD disability, low self-esteem creates endless misery and depression. The best way I know to deal with these feelings is to help the patient who does not have one to undertake some occupation that he can perform competently, and that will earn for him some appreciation, provide him some status within his own social group, and augment the internal structure of his life. I have found embarking on a career especially helpful to many self-deprecating borderline individuals.

Of course, the therapist's influence in doing this work depends on how well the positive transference is maintained. The therapist must thus deal promptly and effectively with negative transference and attempt to anticipate it by questioning and challenging those aspects of positive transference that are obviously defensive denials and idealizations, as well as those that implicitly express expectations of the fulfillment of unrealistic demands.

I find that in general the noninterpretive techniques are even more helpful than interpretations with these patients. I refer here to education; encouragement; serving as a model for rationality, equanimity, and self-possession; and even making practical suggestions. I find it frequently useful to be far more encouraging and directive than one would be in the analysis of a neurotic patient.

I also find that the discussion of death wishes and fantasies is useful. This discussion includes not only death wishes toward others but also wishes for one's own death as a means of uniting with mother. It is also useful to discuss defenses against the wish for one's own death.

What can be achieved with these patients in treatment varies greatly from one patient to the next. At one extreme are those who lack the courage and will to advance beyond the position of helplessness and so either resign themselves to a life without achievement or devote all of their energies to squeezing as much sustenance, emotional and material, from parents and others as they can. These patients are the most resistant to treatment and use the therapy only as an auxiliary source of protection and love. At the other extreme are those who do achieve but who fear retribution. They can be protected against their fears and helped to find a modus vivendi that is restricted much less by the protective shield with which they tend to circumscribe their lives. A great deal can be done for those whose chief manifestation of illness includes continuing ambivalent conflict with parents and spouse. The amount of energy invested in these conflicts can be reduced and liberated for some self-fulfilling activity. A peaceful home environment can be promoted for the benefit of the patient, the spouse, and the children.

By whatever means, the analyst should attempt to replace turmoil with equanimity, timidity with courage, and bravado with realism.

Prognosis

How effective is psychotherapy for borderline patients? The results of psychotherapy with borderline patients are no easier to evaluate than the results of psychotherapy with any other kind of patient. One finds in the literature recommendations for techniques of treatment but little about results. One is led to infer that although not all patients recover, many do. I don't know whether that inference is correct.

In my own practice, more than half of the last twenty-eight borderline patients left treatment abruptly in a pique of negative transference, something no other patients in my practice have done. Some had been with me for years, others for weeks. In each case, it was after disappointment with respect to one or another demand to which I had refused to accede.

Eight of those twenty-eight patients continued in treatment for months or years and demonstrated unequivocal improvement in stabilization of life pattern, partial reconciliation in object relations, and more realistic views of themselves and their capacities. Of two of these eight cases, the results can be said to be very good.

It is also relevant that more than half had been treated previously by others and had been referred to me only after other therapists had failed. Some of my successes were in this group and some in the group that had had no previous treatment. It is interesting, too, that during some phases of their treatment, some of these patients felt warm and close to me, indulging in a good deal of unrealistic idealizing. Those periods were characterized by the syndrome of clinging dependence that I previously described as a defense against depression. I infer that in office practice, that is, with borderline patients who are free to come and go, nobody has any impressive success. Some patients make a number of attempts at therapy, usually starting each enthusiastically and abruptly leaving in disappointment, as they do in all other object relations.

Considering the degree of overt pathology with which unimproved patients leave, it is surprising that one sees so few borderline patients during and especially after middle age. I suspect that as the turmoil subsides, beginning in the early thirties, these patients find some sort of niche of minimum discomfort in which they suffer a muted pain. I have encountered a number of these "burned-out" borderlines among older patients who have come to nonmedical counseling centers for assistance. Almost all continue to project blame on to others. They come only after some relatively stable supportive equilibrium has been disrupted, typically after divorce or the death of a spouse, a parent, or some other supporting relative. I am impressed that in the literature most of the discussion of therapy speaks of years of treatment. I suspect that at least some of the implied improvement is attributable to aging and the burning-out process rather than to true achievement of self-control by way of insight.

References

Akhtar, S., and Byrne, J. P. (1983). The concept of splitting and its clinical relevance. *American Journal of Psychiatry* 140:1013–1016.

Andrulonis, P. A., Glueck, B. C., Stroebel, C. F., and Vogel, N. G. (1982). Borderline personality subcategories. *Journal of Nervous and Mental Disease* 170:670–679.

Bloomingdale, L. M. (1984). *Attention Deficit Disorder.* New York: Spectrum.

Cohen, D. J., Shaywitz, S. E., Young, G. J., and Shaywitz, B. A. (1983). Borderline syndromes and attention deficit disorders of childhood: clinical and neurochemical perspectives. In *The Borderline Child,* ed. K. S. Robeson, pp. 197–221. New York: McGraw-Hill.

Denenberg, V. (1983). As reported in *Science* 220:488–490.

Elliot, S. A. (1978). Neurological aspects of antisocial behavior. In *The Psychopath,* ed. W. H. Reed, pp. 146–189. New York: Brunner/Mazel.

Freud, S. (1911). Psychoanalytic notes on an autobiographical account of paranoia (dementia paranoides). *Standard Edition* 12:3–84.

——— (1916). Some character types met with in psychoanalytic work, II (those wrecked by success). *Standard Edition* 14:309–336.

Glick, S. (1983). As reported in *Science* 220:488–490.

Goldstein, K. (1940). *Human Nature in the Light of Psychopathology.* Cambridge, MA: Harvard University Press.

Gunderson, J. G. (1977). Characteristics of borderlines. In *Borderline Personality Disorders,* ed. P. Hartocollis, pp. 173–192. New York: International Universities Press.

Harlow, H. F. (1964). Social deprivation in monkeys. In *Vistas in Neuropsychiatry,* ed. Y. D. Koskoff and R. J. Shoemaker, pp. 51–67. Pittsburgh: University of Pittsburgh Press.

Hartocollis, P. (1975). Minimal brain dysfunction in young adults. In *Psychiatric Aspects of Minimal Brain Dysfunction in Adults,* ed. L. Bellak, pp. 103–112. New York: Grune & Stratton.

Kernberg, O. (1975). *Borderline Conditions and Pathological Narcissism.* New York: Jason Aronson.

Klein, D. S. (1977). Psychopharmacological treatment and delineation of borderline disorders. In *Borderline Personality Disorders,* ed. P. Hartocollis, pp. 365–384. New York: International Universities Press.

Masterson, J. F. (1975). The splitting defensive mechanism of the borderline adolescent: development and clinical aspects. In *Borderline States in Psychiatry,* ed. J. E. Mack, pp. 93–102. New York: Grune & Stratton.

Ostow, M. (1962). *Drugs in Psychoanalysis and Psychotherapy.* New York: Basic Books.

——— (1970). *The Psychology of Melancholy.* New York: Harper & Row.

———, ed. (1979). *The Psychodynamic Approach to Drug Therapy.* Psychoanalytic Research and Development Fund.

Ostow, M. and Kline, N. S. (1957). The psychic action of reserpine and chlorpromazine. In *Psychopharmacological Frontiers*, ed. N. S. Kline, pp. 481–513. Boston: Little, Brown.

Perry, J. C., and Klerman, G. L. (1978). The borderline patient: a comparative analysis of four sets of diagnostic criteria. *Archives of General Psychiatry* 35:141–150.

Petti, T. A., and Unis, A. (1981). Imipramine treatment of borderline children: case reports with a controlled study. *American Journal of Psychiatry* 138:515–518.

Rinsley, D. B. (1977). An object-relations view of borderline personality. In *Borderline Personality Disorders*, ed. P. Hartocollis, pp. 47–70. New York: International Universities Press.

Sarwer-Foner, G. L. (1977). An approach to the global treatment of the borderline patient: psychoanalytic, psychotherapeutic, and psychopharmacological considerations. In *Borderline Personality Disorders*, ed. P. Hartocollis, pp. 345–364. New York: International Universities Press.

Stone, M. H. (1980). *The Borderline Syndromes.* New York: McGraw-Hill.

Wender, P. H. (1977). The contribution of the adoption studies to the understanding of the phenomenology and etiology of borderline schizophrenics. In *Borderline Personality Disorders*, ed. P. Hartocollis, pp. 255–270. New York: International Universities Press.

_____ (1979). The concept of adult minimal brain dysfunction. In *Psychiatric Aspects of Minimal Brain Dysfunction in Adults*, ed. L. Bellak, pp. 1–15. New York: Grune & Stratton.

10

On Beginning with Patients Who Require Medication

Combined treatment literally widens the scope of analysis to include sicker patients whose suffering can be reduced rapidly. In addition, masochistic character, anxiety, and panic may respond dramatically to antidepressants. Patients who will profit from combined treatment are distinguished from those who will profit optimally from either one alone. The author strongly urges that the analyst do the actual prescribing, because of the analyst's access to unconscious material. Techniques of analyzing the transference and resistance to medication are described, as are the procedures for starting treatment with medication or introducing medication into an existing analysis. The concept of psychic energy is used to organize observations relating behavior to drug therapy. Techniques of ascertaining a patient's position on the high–low spectrum are outlined, including specific analysis of dreams to determine the required direction of the medication.

After years of rejecting the possibility of combining psychiatric drug therapy with psychoanalysis, our profession is becoming reconciled to its necessity. To a certain extent this reconciliation has been forced by the current dearth of patients considered appropriate candidates for psychoanalysis. By starting with a course of drug therapy, one can alleviate depression or even psychosis within a relatively short period of time and bring a patient to a state of mind that will permit a normal psychoanalytic procedure.

Complementary use of medication literally widens the scope of psychoanalysis. The combined procedure implies that we acknowledge that for the treatment of psychosis, mania, and melancholic depression, psychoanalysis is an inefficient tool if it is effective at all. We are learning to face the fact that these conditions should not be treated with psychoanalysis, because even if it could be demonstrated in any given case that the analytic treatment resulted in the patient's recovery, it has become evident to everyone that drug treatment can produce the same relief in a much shorter period of time, not only saving the patient time and money, but sparing him months or years of unnecessary suffering.

What has not become well known yet is the fact that many conditions that we do not recognize as depression, and that seem to be the neurotic or character disorders that we consider appropriate for classical analysis, for example, masochistic character, or anxiety or panic disorder, may also respond dramatically to antidepression drug treatment. In many such instances, psychoanalysis becomes unnecessary, and in others it can be curtailed. It follows that although psychiatric drug treatment makes some patients available for psychoanalysis who would not otherwise be available, in other cases it makes psychoanalysis superfluous. We must conclude that there are common pathogenic processes that respond poorly, if at all, to insight treatment. Some of these respond easily to psychiatric drug therapy.

The profession's resistance to acknowledging the power of medication and its potential for complementing the analytic procedure in the treatment of some patients was based, it seems to me, on two considerations. Psychodynamic drug therapy seemed, at first glance, to be another method for devaluing psychoanalysis and the unique contribution that it makes. Although every psychoanalyst knows that Freud anticipated the availability of psychiatric drug therapy and correctly related it to the humoral messenger system (Freud 1933, 1940), nevertheless, most psychoanalysts have seemed to believe that if one took the possibility of psychoanalytic drug therapy seriously, one was betraying the psychoanalytic profession. I learned from Dr. Herman Nunberg that Freud spoke of anticipating a time when it would be possible to use chemical substances during a therapeutic analysis in order to direct the analysis into the most fruitful channels.

Second, the technique of psychoanalysis is carefully structured so as to minimize all influences upon the patient other than insight derived from his own free associations. The analyst is not to influence him by revealing to the patient more than a minimum amount of his own personal life, nor by making decisions for him, nor by advising him, nor by communicating with members of his family. By prescribing drug therapy, the psychoanalyst seems to violate this basic principle of treatment: he advises the patient, makes decisions for him, he steps inside his arm's length distance from the patient, and if he is a good physician, he encourages, instructs, and attempts to mobilize and motivate. All of this seems to threaten the "purity" of the analytic procedure itself, and to contaminate the transference irreparably.

The title of this chapter, "On Beginning with Patients Who Require Medication," requires some discussion. One may begin a psychoanalytic procedure with a patient already being treated with medication. One may commence a treatment with a patient who requires medication at first, with the intention of initiating a psychoanalytic procedure as soon as the patient is ready for it. One may introduce medication in the course of an existing psychoanalytic procedure. The principles involved in all three situations are the same: one responds appropriately to the clinical state of the patient, but tries to avoid maneuvers that will irreversibly compromise analytic technique. One introduces each departure from classical analytic technique with a clear explanation of why it seems to be indicated at this point, what one hopes to accomplish, what are the prospects for its success, and, if the patient can tolerate such a discussion, what undesirable complications might ensue. If the clinical situation is not too urgent, one asks the patient to consider the recommendation and to bring back his views, which one then responds to, first on the basis of manifest content, and then where possible, on the basis of unconscious meaning. Ultimately, one attempts to analyze the meaning of the extra-analytic intervention to the patient.

The Indications for Combined Treatment

The specific population of those who will profit from combined treatment must be distinguished from those who will profit optimally from either treatment alone. Patients who will profit from psychoanalysis but not from drug therapy include those with classical transference neuroses, and patients with personality disorders, except for borderline personality and various forms of depressive personality. Patients who will profit from drug therapy include those with conditions that appear on the manic-depressive spectrum, that is, melancholic depression, mania and hypomania, also panic disorder and nonspecific anxiety, and other syndromes when they are based upon a depressive diathesis. They include also schizophrenia, some but not all borderline patients, and according to some recent claims, some obsessive-compulsive patients.

Not all patients who profit from drug therapy are suitable candidates for psychoanalysis. Many patients are just not interested in anything but immediate relief of their most distressing symptoms, depression, or anxiety. Others really don't require any further treatment. Especially after the fifth decade, the successful treatment of a discrete episode of depression that is not based upon a personality disorder or an ongoing neurosis leaves the patient without evidence of any important neurotic disability and therefore no indication for analysis. Some patients with manic-depressive disease, when their excursions into illness have been controlled with lithium, exhibit neither indication nor desire for psychotherapy of any type.

Many patients who recover with proper drug therapy are poor candidates for psychoanalysis. For example, in the case of young schizophrenics, even the most skillful treatment with medication alleviates only the gross psychotic symptoms, but leaves the underlying personality disorder, the intense timidity, the paranoid attitude toward the world, untouched. For such patients, an insight-oriented therapy is a remote, if at all achievable, goal. Many borderline patients, especially the most primitive among them, are too preoccupied with dealing with their frequent and painful mood swings to be able to take interest in underlying dynamic states. Although they may accept the format of an analysis, that is, treatment frequency of three to five times a week, lying on the couch, and free association, no psychoanalytic process appears.

The indications for analysis in patients whose symptoms can be controlled with drug therapy include the following: a continuing personality disorder; neurotic symptoms that derive from early trauma rather than from constitutionally poor regulation of affective excursion; object relations and self-image that are impaired by the recurrent disruption of continuity in mood and affect caused by rapid or slow cycling manic-depressive excursions.

After my very first experiences with psychiatric drug therapy, it seemed to me interesting that those conditions that responded to medication were conditions that responded poorly, if at all, to any psychotherapy, and similarly, those that responded to psychotherapy were not likely to respond to psychiatric drug therapy. For example, an acute episode of schizophrenia will ordinarily be resolved easily with medication, but psychotherapy is relatively ineffectual and psychoanalysis is inappropriate. On the other hand, a patient with a neurotic problem with object relations will not be helped by medication, only by an intensive psychotherapy.

By and large, I consider that conclusion still valid. But then why do we consider treating any given patient with both modalities simultaneously? There are some patients who suffer acute breakdowns, most commonly depression, as episodes imposed upon a continuing personality disorder. One ascertains from the history that before the onset of the presenting bout of depression, the patient exhibited difficulty in his relations with others—parents, spouse, business associates. Before one can commence a definitive psychotherapy or psychoanalytic treatment of this latter continuing problem, one must overcome the depression. For that drug therapy is initiated, and psychoanalysis as soon thereafter as the patient becomes available for it. Combined treatment is also indicated for those patients whose lives are seriously disrupted, whose object relations and identity are distorted by the affective fluctuations, by the conflicts between impulse and inhibition that constitute the primary illness. The most common of such patients are the relatively high-level borderline patients that we encounter in our practice, the narcissistic personalities, the rapid-cycling manic-depressives, and the adult attention deficit disorder patients.

When medication first appeared, I hoped and expected that it would restore the equanimity necessary for analysis and that the analysis would eliminate the need for the medication (Ostow 1960). Thirty years later, that prediction seems to have been woefully incorrect. It seems to me that no psychotherapy can overcome the pathologic instability or impaired regulation of psychic "energies" that I believe to be the basis of the drug-responsive mental illness. It is always striking to see rapid loss of insight, perspective, and objectivity when medication is abruptly withdrawn. I have seen a few patients who require medication only during the course of one or a few relatively brief episodes of depression or of schizophrenia, and I like to think that the psychotherapy or analysis that they had during the intervals contributed to the long periods of remission, but I cannot be sure that it did.

One does have the satisfaction of seeing patients whose neurotic needs seriously impair interpersonal relations and work improve in these areas, clearly in response to analytic therapy. But the analysis itself and the improvement in performance are contingent upon the concurrent control of mood with medication when a mood disorder or psychosis would have prevented analysis. Although there are exceptions, I find that many patients who require medication exhibit a surprising rigidity in analysis. They may follow the rules properly—although some have difficulty doing so—but the analytic process that we are able to cultivate in responsive patients fails to appear. Nevertheless the procedure has some value. For such patients the analyst functions as a guide, a teacher, a constant parental object in an otherwise remote and impersonal universe. Over a period of years, the analyst walks the patient through the crucial periods of his life, the challenges that he encounters, and tries to compensate for the absence of courage and self-esteem.

Technique of Drug Therapy

In the title of this chapter, who prescribes the medication is not specified. All nonmedical analysts who believe that a patient requires medication will refer the patient to a psychopharmacologist and leave the decision of whether to prescribe and what to prescribe and how much to the latter. Most will deal analytically with everything that the patient brings into the analysis that relates to the drug treatment. The nonmedical analyst has no choice. However, many medical analysts, too, prefer to refer their patients out for psychopharmacologic intervention; they do not wish to become involved in the treatment. Those analysts who do this do not know how to prescribe, but that is because they have not learned how to use medication, and they have not learned because, in most instances, they consider prescribing medication inappropriate for a psychoanalyst while conducting an analysis.

I should like to take a strong stand here in urging the analyst to prescribe the medication himself. I recall a conversation I had with Herman Nunberg in the 1950s, when the first psychiatric medications appeared, about the ultimate effect of such agents on the practice of psychoanalysis. No matter how effective medication might be, he argued, one would still need analysts to select medication and to regulate dose and combination. Although analysts are not really necessary for this task, by virtue of their command of psychodynamics they can do it better than others once they have acquired mastery of psychopharmacology.

Medication cannot just be prescribed. For the medications that we currently possess it is important to select, to monitor, to titrate, and to combine. The psychopharmacologist does these things on the basis of the clinical evidence that he accumulates during a 15- or 30-minute conversation with the patient (after the initial workup examination), once a week initially, and then once a month or once every several months after a while. The psychoanalyst, on the other hand, is in a much better position to select, monitor, titrate, and combine, because he has access daily or almost daily to what is going on in the patient's mind. It is not uncommon, for example, to hear the patient report at the beginning of the session that he is feeling fine, but then to hear the recitation of a dream that discloses a worsening depressive state. The psychopharmacologist will hear only the conscious report; the psychoanalyst has the truly revealing data.

Splitting the treatment between a psychopharmacologist and a psychoanalyst can be compared to driving a car with one person steering and the other controlling the throttle, with little if any communication between them. It can be done, but badly. The psychopharmacologist has little access to the truly important clinical data, and the psychoanalyst never knows whether he is hearing the patient speak or the medication. It follows that even when the treatment is split, a psychopharmacologist who is psychoanalytically knowledgeable will do considerably better than one trained purely as a nondynamic, biological psychiatrist.

Of course, psychoanalysts who have not prescribed medication are concerned that doing so violates the classical arm's-length position of the psychoanalyst vis-à-vis the patient. He is trying to influence the patient extra-analytically. I can only say that in 35 years of combining drug therapy with psychoanalysis, I have never encountered a situation in which I felt that the one treatment interfered with the other. Neither writing the prescription; asking about drug response, whether therapeutic or toxic; nor even occasionally checking blood pressure; recommending laboratory testing; or examining the patient for tremor, ataxia, or nystagmus, has evoked analytic fantasy or activity that could not be analyzed in session, frequently with profit. (Touching the patient is not required for any of these procedures except for placing a blood pressure cuff.)

As in unmodified analysis, the analyst must focus clearly on the transference, especially at the beginning of a drug therapy. A., a 56-year-old man who came to me in a state of fairly pronounced melancholic depression, was treated with a monoamine oxidase inhibitor and daily psychoanalytic sessions on the couch. Twelve days after starting treatment (monoamine oxidase inhibitor treatment usually requires about 4 weeks before an adequate dose becomes effective) he reported:

> I got through okay. I'm about the same, but at moments I feel better. I may as well confess that I'm figuring out how to get out of New York. I am claustrophobic. New York frightens me. I keep wanting my brother-in-law to help me, to give me a job. I see my mother reaching out her hand to help me. I see my mother's face and she wants to help me. Sometimes I see a child's face near hers, like the infant Jesus. One time I had a vision of my mother and Jesus Christ both reaching out their hands to help me. The only

happy time in my whole day is when I get into bed. It's killing me to pay that much money, but I have to do it. I think I am better in some ways; the panic is less. The thought I choke back is, "Thank God I've got you to come to." At least you gave me the medication, in which I have great hopes. I would like to go out and screw someone else's wife, someone nice. Too many people, fire engines, noise; it terrifies me. Christmas terrifies me. I have just gotten to be a big fat slob. I worry about cancer all the time. I have been making up lists for my wife, my safe deposit keys, etc. I suppose I have a fear of homosexuality. I used to sit in the office with my factory manager, and I would get a pain in my balls as I spoke to him. I'm in a state of fury that this should happen to me. I have lived a fairly decent life, except that I screwed a few women and evaded the draft.

Here it was clear that my providing medication was interpreted as being fed by mother. The infant is being rescued magically. However, that very anaclitic dependence invokes a fear of homosexual attack. That had to be interpreted to him to prevent his flight from treatment, which he was already considering.

The patient's response to the medication will strongly influence the transference. If the medication alleviates his distress, he will be grateful to the analyst and see him as a loving and protective parent. It is also frequently interpreted as impregnation in preparation for rebirth. At the end of the fourth week of treatment of this same patient, in order to encourage him, as he left, I said, "Maybe you'll have a surprise for me on Monday." He replied without hesitation, "A baby."

Again, B., a borderline young woman, was referred to me after her discharge from a psychiatric hospital on a large dose of antipsychosis tranquilizer. She seemed to me depressed and so I replaced the latter with an antidepression drug. As her depression lifted, she dreamed that her father was giving her pills that had holes in them. When I asked what kind of pills had holes in them she replied, "Life Savers." Associated with the pills in the dream was a white, jellylike material, which clearly symbolized semen. Evidently the treatment had fulfilled her fantasy that an experience of fellatio with her father had effected rebirth by oral impregnation.

If the medication fails to alleviate the distress for which it was intended, or if it produces distressing side effects, as some medications do, the patient may come to feel that he is being poisoned by the analyst. If the patient is impulsive, he may on such occasion abruptly leave treatment, even if he had been warned that the procedure of selecting medication is one of systematic trial and error. Usually when the transference becomes negative as a result of untoward drug response, analyzing will have little therapeutic effect. The reality of the physiologic toxic change makes interpretation unconvincing. However, the situation and its analysis can be recalled on some subsequent occasion when they are relevant, and when the patient is capable of greater insight. The converse is also true; the transference will influence the patient's attitude toward the medication.

If the transference is positive, the patient will report a positive response to the medication and minimize its side effects. When, on the other hand, the transference is negative, the patient will minimize the therapeutic effect of the medication and complain about side effects. The perception of medication and the effect of the medication make a reality contribution to the transference fantasy comparable to what day residue does in dreams. (I owe this formulation to Joseph Sandler.) When the drug has been effective, the transference is influenced to become more positive and to remain positive longer than otherwise. The patient becomes more forgiving toward the analyst. However, I have seen no evidence that the prescription of medication per se alters the transference or any other aspect of the psychoanalysis permanently and significantly.

While some patients will welcome the idea of medication readily, others will resist it. Resistance to medication is something that all psychopharmacologists encounter, but they have no real understanding of its nature, and no means of contending with it. The psychoanalyst may be able to deal with it analytically.

Some patients fear, as retribution for what they consider inappropriate oral-aggressive wishes, that they will be poisoned. Such a fear engenders a paranoid attitude, which can cause the patient to resist taking the prescribed medication. Occasionally, such patients, while resisting therapeutic medication for fear of being poisoned, will at the same time use marijuana or alcohol or other dangerous drugs, thereby revealing their own tendency to poison themselves while projecting the wish onto those who are trying to rescue them.

Resistance is sometimes created by the patient's fear for his own physical integrity. We encounter this issue among those who are subject to recurrent attacks of panic and anxiety. They, like all phobic patients, fear that they will literally fall apart during an anxiety attack, and so they tend to avoid any experience over which they do not possess full control, or at least the illusion of full control. Medication represents to them an influence that is beyond their control, and therefore they resist it. Interestingly enough, these patients respond to doses of medication considerably lower than the doses ordinarily required. It is as if their lower threshold for anxiety is related to or caused by a low threshold for response to chemical agents.

Among those patients who resist psychiatric drug treatment, one finds those who come for help, but who nevertheless resist it out of a neurotic need to suffer. This need does not necessarily lead to seeking pain, but may easily create resistance against opportunities to be relieved from current distress. They seem to fear the rapid therapeutic power of medication more than the slow influence of a psychotherapy.

Some patients seem to recognize in themselves a tendency to become excessively dependent, and they react by resisting close relations that might become dependent relations. They seem to try to dilute the attractiveness of the analysis by keeping the frequency of visits as low as possible, and by looking for opportunities to discontinue treatment. These patients frequently displace their fear of dependency from the analyst to the drug that he prescribes, or that he arranges for someone else to prescribe.

In the minds of many patients, an illness that can be treated by psychologic means is less threatening and less shameful than one that must be treated with an organic modality. Drug treatment means brain dysfunction or permanent defect, while psychotherapy merely means temporary and reversible psychic perturbation. If the patient avoids the drug, he loses less self-esteem. A related resistance appears when a member of the family or close friend has been treated with medication either unsuccessfully or partially successfully. The patient feels that accepting drug therapy, especially if the same drug is prescribed, means that he is just as unfortunate as the other.

Patients whose illness creates euphoria, such as hypomanic, manic, or "high" borderline characters, or certain incipient schizophrenics, enjoy their "high" and resist any procedure that threatens it. If their behavior becomes dangerous, medication may have to be administered against their wishes.

It is difficult to recommend a specific procedure since cases differ so much from one to the other, just as it is difficult to specify procedure for analysis in general. In what is perhaps the most common situation, the patient applies for treatment in a state of clear-cut, melancholic depression. From the history the analyst infers that the depression can be understood as an incident in the course of and prepared for by a continuing neurosis or personality disorder. He conveys this conclusion to the patient, and recommends that treatment start with an attempt at chemotherapy for the depressive episode, and that it continue, as the depression subsides, with analysis, giving the reasons for his proposal. If the patient concurs, the analyst opens the first phase of treatment by prescribing a specific medication and explaining why he has chosen that medication, what effect is desired, how soon it might come about, and what toxic side effects might be encountered on the way. It is important to reassure the patient that if this drug must be abandoned, prescribing it represents merely the first phase of what could be a systematic program for achieving relief. (I shall not here discuss the pharmacologic aspects of choice of medication, dosage, monitoring and titration, nor of combining medications, since these issues alone would require book length treatment. However, the psychoanalyst, whether or not he has prescribed the drug, should have this information because it enters into the day residue, not only of dreams, but of conscious fantasy and thought.) In most instances, during the first phase of treatment, only the most superficial psychotherapeutic maneuvers are appropriate—reassurance, comfort, support, offering hope and advice. Therefore, initially the patient need be seen less frequently than he might be seen later. There is little process in the presence of depression, and the sessions soon become dull and boring, and discouraging for the patient, except for those who need continuing contact.

The analyst must then look for responses to the medication, both desired therapeutic responses and undesired side effects. If the patient resists the medication, he will complain noisily about side effects and minimize evidence of improvement. If he welcomes the intervention, the opposite may occur; that is, he will minimize or fail to report side effects and exaggerate indications of improvement. In order to assess what is really happening, the therapist must evaluate all of the patient's statements in the light of his knowledge of the expected course of recovery and the common side effects of the medication being used, as well as their time course. Even if the analyst is not himself prescribing the medication, he must still evaluate the reports of the patient. For example, if the patient reports clear-cut improvement within a day or two after starting medication, the analyst must know how likely it is that improvement will be felt so soon. Is this a true drug effect, or a placebo effect? If it is the latter, then the patient must be protected against the disappointment that will follow when it disappears.

When the recovery that is hoped for actually starts, the patient is helped to recognize the specific changes in psychic function that have occurred. Recognizing the difference between the parameters of psychic function in recovery contrasted with depression is a form of superficial insight that gives the patient a sense of some mastery of his illness. When we are dealing with psychosis, but even to a certain extent in the case of depression, after recovery, the episode of illness appears as a gap in the patient's psychic function, and he appreciates the analyst's assistance in filling in that gap, in being helped to understand why the psychic continuity was disrupted, and what was the content of his thought during the interruption.

In only a very few cases will the first drug and first dose serve to achieve the desired results. In most cases the dose will have to be increased gradually and one drug may have to be replaced by or combined with another, or the principal drug or drugs might require reinforcement by adjuvants. (These procedures require a sound knowledge of psychopharmacology and should be pursued with a light and sensitive touch. I say this not to discourage the analyst from prescribing medication but to encourage him to inform himself really well before doing it, initially perhaps by consulting with competent psychopharmacologists when a difficult problem arises.) As each of these changes is made, the patient must be prevented from becoming disappointed and discouraged. The reason for each change should be explained clearly, and he should be reminded on each occasion that a systematic program is being followed—that the procedure is not random guesswork.

In most cases, sooner or later, a desired, or at least acceptable, result is obtained. It will be a few days or weeks before the extent of the recovery and its stability can be ascertained. During this period, the patient will be celebrating the improvement, and the transference will become quite positive. During the period when the medication starts to become effective, but before a true stabilization has occurred, the patient will present with varying degrees of comfort or distress, with fluctuating symptoms and mental states. In unmodified psychoanalysis, the psychoanalyst is constantly challenged by such fluctuations to try to ascertain whether they are the result of spontaneous intrapsychic processes, whether they are responses to the analysis or the transference, or whether they have been elicited by external events, or whether two or three of these influences are simultaneously active. If a varying drug therapy is going on, the additional variable makes the assignment even more complicated. How much of this process of assessment and its results should be communicated to the patient is a matter of analytic judgment.

As the desired mental state and the medication regimen that has established it becomes stabilized, the true psychoanalytic process begins to develop. Now the psychoanalyst can address himself primarily to that, and to encourage free association, and the reporting of fantasies, dreams, and behavior. He becomes able to intervene and interpret in exactly the way that he would in an uncomplicated analysis. When he judges that the time has come, he may readjust the frequency of sessions and suggest the use of the couch. From the point of view of the analysis, the procedures of the drug therapy, and the various mental responses that it elicits, are all proper subjects for analytic scrutiny.

While many patients will do well on an appropriate dose and combination of medication for years, others exhibit mood swings and symptom fluctuations at intervals of days, weeks, or months. In that case, the analyst may have to vary the medication from time to time. In some such cases, lithium may induce some stabilization.

Not infrequently, a patient already in a conventional analysis for what has seemed to be a simple neurotic state or personality disorder becomes depressed or, less often, even psychotic. If this supervening state is not overcome by appropriate analytic work within a reasonable time, and especially if the condition precludes analytic work or threatens the life of the patient or those about him, then medication should be introduced. I usually introduce the idea of medication by citing the indications for it, describe what I expect it to do, what is the likelihood of its success, and what are the drawbacks. If the situation is not acute, I generally wait for a few sessions while the patient digests and accommodates to my recommendations and I try to analyze his response to it. The patient generally likes to be assured that the analysis will not thereby become jeopardized, and he can be assured that it will not. If the patient is frightened by what has happened to him, he may welcome this extra-analytic intervention, and it will help him to overcome his resentment toward the analyst for permitting the deterioration to occur. When the medication is prescribed, and as its effects are developing, the sessions may become concerned with it, especially because the clinical state that has required the medication will usually prevent much analysis from taking place. As in the case of the new patient, with the attainment of a stable state of remission of the complicating episode, the analysis can resume its normal course. In most cases, neither the frequency of visits nor the use of the couch need be affected by the interruption.

Theoretically, we should also consider the case of the patient, already on drug therapy, who then applies for psychoanalytic treatment. I can imagine, for example, that a manic-depressive patient or a borderline patient, already stabilized on lithium, may wish to overcome problems with object relations and then seek analysis. In fact, however, I have never been approached by such a patient. On the contrary, I have seen patients, after obtaining satisfactory results with drug therapy that was initiated only after a long and unsuccessful analysis, then leave the analysis that had failed over a period of years to bring the relief desired.

Because the psychoanalyst has immediate access to both the conscious and unconscious processes of the patient, he is in a much better position to monitor the parameters of manic-depressive disease and psychosis as well as other drug-susceptible conditions, and the effect of medication upon them, than the psychopharmacologist who can assess, in a brief period of time or limited by the constraints of a fixed questionnaire, the conscious reports of the patient.

I accept Freud's suggestion (1933, 1940) that psychopharmacologic agents—which he merely anticipated—act to influence the psychic energy available to mental functions, because it seems clear to me that what these drugs change is motivation, specifically libidinal motivation, as distinguished from aggressive motivation. (Aggressive energies are elicited by distressing perturbations in the supply of libidinal energies, as well as by actual external danger.) Under the influence of antidepression agents, subjects exhibit increased motivation, increased interest in seeking and exploiting opportunities for gratification, optimism, self-confidence, and enthusiasm. Contrariwise, under the influence of antipsychosis tranquilizers, subjects will display inertia, lack of interest, pessimism, diffidence, and discouragement. (Psychiatrically normal individuals respond to these chemical influences as well as to spontaneous internal changes with corrective maneuvers so that the drug effect is muted or suppressed. The drug effect becomes visible especially easily among those individuals who cannot correct for energy deviations spontaneously, and who are therefore easily driven to manic or depressive extremes by these chemical agents.)

My formulations are based purely upon clinical observation, but deal with fluctuation of clinically visible behavioral parameters. The term *psychic energy*, as I use it, is not identical with, and may not even correlate directly with, physiologic energies. The complexities of drug effect upon neural transmission within the brain, which fill the literature of psychopharmacology and the biochemistry of the brain, cannot yet be translated into clinically visible processes and cannot yet be used to make clinically useful predictions. The behavioral parameters that they affect and the effect that they have upon them are visible clinically, and certain patterns and sequences can be distinguished and used to prescribe and to monitor.

The chief advantage of this concept of psychic energy is that it links metapsychologic thinking to the kind of behavioral change that responds to medication and that is induced by medication. It makes it possible to organize one's thoughts and observations in relating behavior to drug therapy. The energy concept is out of favor nowadays among psychoanalytic theoreticians, but I anticipate that it will be resuscitated as psychoanalysts become more familiar with the action of psychopharmacologic agents (Loeb and Loeb 1987).

Simply put, those conditions that respond to antipsychosis tranquilizers or antidepression energizers can be thought of as caused by excessive excursions of the energy level from a midpoint of a spectrum. One end of the spectrum is the position that induces a manic state, and the other end, a state of depression. A movement toward either end in the individual without disease will induce a corrective tendency. Those individuals whose ability to correct deviations is impaired will suffer from manic, depressive, or schizophrenic illness. When the failure to regulate level is compounded by an instability of the system, we have conditions that favor borderline personality.

For example, conventional psychopharmacologic wisdom has it that the proper treatment for mania is lithium combined with an antipsychosis tranquilizer. But there is a problem: many manics treated that way will become more agitated before they are overwhelmed by large doses of medication, while others will recover with relatively small doses of medication. Again, those in the first group will improve with an antidepression drug—paradoxically and against the rules—whereas those in the second group will become worse with an antidepression drug. The psychopharmacologist has no explanation for this paradox. I have seen no discussion of it in the literature. The dynamic psychiatrist on the other hand, familiar with psychic mechanisms of primary tendencies and secondary corrections, will infer that the mania of the second type is a primary mania, while that of the first type is a reactive mania, a secondary attempt to resist a threatening depressive state. Although it may be difficult to distinguish between these two states before they have both been seen in the same patient, one will suspect a corrective rather than a primary manic state if the patient is more volatile, exhibits paradoxical weeping, expresses more anger than expected, and especially if he reports depressive dreams. In other words, the corrective manic state is more likely to resemble what *DSM-III-R* (1987) calls Bipolar Disorder, Mixed. However in many instances, the depressive component of the mixture may be all but invisible to any but the psychoanalyst.

Similarly, the proper drug formula for treating an acute episode of schizophrenia, or schizoaffective disease, is not immediately self-evident. Some patients respond to antipsychosis tranquilizers alone, and others require the concurrent administration of an antidepression drug. A schizophrenic patient may exhibit a psychotic state under any of three circumstances: when he is at the "high" end of the spectrum, as the primary manic is; when he is at the "low" end of the spectrum, as a depressed patient is; or when he is trying to struggle against being overwhelmed by depression, as the secondary manic does. It follows that those patients who belong in the first category will, like the primary manic, respond well to treatment with an antipsychosis tranquilizer, whereas those in both the second and third categories should be treated with an antidepression energizer, usually together with the tranquilizer. Those in the first and third categories resemble each other in the same way that primary and secondary manics do.

For the purposes of monitoring, I have found the following parameters useful. The primary indicator of status is the patient's mood. A good mood indicates a high position on the manic-depression spectrum, and a low mood, a low position. In other words, a good mood, if it is associated with a pathologic condition that requires treatment, indicates the use of an antipsychosis tranquilizer, and a bad mood, though somewhat less reliably, an antidepression energizer.

The patient's self-observation tells us about his status fairly sensitively. If the patient speaks ill of himself, he reveals that he is descending toward or is at lower levels of the manic-depressive spectrum, or a homologous "high-low" schizophrenic spectrum. One must allow, however, for defensive denial of a true depressive state. Again, if the patient reports on subjective feelings (primary self-observation) rather than reporting accounts of his activities (secondary self-observation), I infer that he approaches the lower end of this spectrum. Self-criticism, especially the expression of feelings of guilt, also suggests a low position.

A tendency to become involved with love objects and others suggests a "high" state, which I interpret as the consequence of a profusion of libidinal energy; conversely, a tendency to withdraw to solitude suggests a "low" state.

The patient's outlook, whether optimistic or pessimistic, is usually consonant with his mood, and may reveal his status fairly transparently.

The degree of objectivity that the patient is able to maintain tells us how close to the midrange of the spectrum he can remain. Toward either end he tends to lose objectivity, perspective, and insight.

The problem of monitoring and assessing the patient's "energy" status is complicated by the fact that people do not move or drift directly toward either end of the spectrum without a struggle. Usually as extreme positions are approached, we see counteractive, corrective tendencies that create the impression of turmoil and struggle.

Most manics of the primary type seem to become euphoric without evidence of any corrective tendency. However, the schizophrenic differs from the manic in that as he becomes higher and higher, a corrective tendency is invoked which he interprets and projects out as a destructive force. The corrective tendency may express itself in attempts at self-destruction, self-mutilation, and/or rejection of the world of reality. When it is projected out, it becomes the basis of paranoid delusions and/or the perception that the world is being destroyed, a projection of his rejection of it. An antipsychosis tranquilizer suppresses the excess "energy" and thereby makes the pathogenic corrective tendency unnecessary. The hypochondria and narcissism of the schizophrenic may suggest a depressionlike, low-"energy" syndrome. However, they may be phenomena created in reaction against the "high" state that instituted the pathogenic process.

As the patient descends toward the depressive position, we observe a number of maneuvers that seem intended to arrest the descent. (All of these changes, primary and corrective, can be observed not only when they occur naturally, but also, almost experimentally, when they are induced by the administration of one or the other of the medications that we have been discussing.)

Frequently, the earliest evidence of the struggle against depression is a paradoxical overactivity, which, when sufficiently intense, may become the secondary hypomania or mania that we discussed above. An early corrective maneuver is clinging to a protective love object. When that love object is lost, or threatens to become unavailable, anxiety may appear. I infer that in such cases the anxiety signals a loss of support against depression. The syndrome suggests separation anxiety or agoraphobia. As the patient descends further toward depression, he becomes angrier and angrier. Although some anger can be seen in the secondary manic and in the phobic, it becomes the primary presenting manifestation of illness when the descent to depression is not arrested. In many instances, the anger itself seems to be able to induce an organized campaign that aims to overcome what is thought to be the depressing influence, so that some paranoid characteristics might appear. If any one of these syndromes becomes symptomatically overwhelming so as to require drug therapy, the proper drug in each of these cases is an antidepression energizer. Sometimes, if the system is labile, it may swing too far to the up side, so that ultimately a combination of antidepression energizer and antipsychosis tranquilizer may be necessary. Lithium too may contribute to stabilizing this "psychic energy" system. My purpose in spelling out these corrective maneuvers here is to make it clear that it is not always easy to ascertain what the "energy" status is at the moment, and therefore which drugs are appropriate. The distinction between primary tendencies and secondary corrective phenomena is essential.

I have observed that the manifest content of dreams can frequently be used to monitor the patient's "energy" changes and therefore to guide one in drug selection and titration. Patients who require drug therapy for control are likely to report apocalyptic dreams, namely, dreams that portray, in manifest content, widespread destruction and/or death followed by a rebirth indicated by a reunion with mother. In my 1962 book, *Drugs in Psychoanalysis and Psychotherapy*, I reported in some detail the analysis of two patients who were receiving medication, one a patient with conversion and anxiety hysteria, and the second with paranoid schizophrenia. The latter patient, C., during her second visit, volunteered two dreams from the previous week:

Dream 1: One was a painting of a city that seemed dead—a "ghost city." It was painted in black and white and no human or animal figures appeared. All at once the doors of the houses opened and gaily dressed people came out, including my husband and me.

Dream 2: The patient was driving very fast in an automobile with her husband. She was afraid of a crash. Suddenly she was resting on a peaceful green meadow.

Sometimes the union with mother precedes the destruction. A schizophrenic young man, D., who maintained fairly comfortably on a combination of antidepression energizer and antipsychosis tranquilizer, one night omitted his medication and reported the following dream:

I had a nightmare. I found myself in bed with my mother. We had no clothes on. She was insisting that I start sexual advances. I touch her breasts. I don't know whether she had anything on the lower part of her body.

I watched a movie that became real life. Grand Central Station was about to explode and kill everyone inside. A great ball of fire. It would pass from that building onto Park Avenue. I ran for my life.

I watched it again. People were being led into a theater innocently, without knowledge of what's to come. They would die. I watch from the second level. Chaos. No one had the authority to call the police. I ran out to 39th Street. Swimming for my life. As fast as possible. Tough enemies with machine guns were firing indiscriminately.

You appeared in the station. I was assured that chaos wouldn't break out again.

I recognize in these dreams the conflict between primary and secondary movements. In dream 1 of patient C., the image of the world has been destroyed. Then a corrective rebirth occurs spontaneously. The depressing influence has been overcome by the rebirth influence. It is the latter that creates the psychosis and the delusional fantasy. Therefore an antipsychosis tranquilizer was indicated. After the psychosis subsided, the patient became depressed, since the depressing influence was now unopposed. Accordingly, an antidepression drug was added. The combination has kept the patient stable for 30 years now.

Dream 2 starts with the union of the patient with her caretaking spouse in a vehicle, which we commonly encounter in apocalyptic fantasies and dreams. Then the destruction occurs and it is followed by a rebirth. The destructive phase did not succeed in overcoming the pathogenic upward striving. The second dream then confirms the picture in the first dream, namely, that the upward movement must be suppressed.

D.'s dream starts with an oedipal approach to mother, impelled by the imbalance of medication caused by the omission of the scheduled dose of medication that evening. Note that there was no alteration of behavior and no new symptoms appeared. The effect of the omission of the medication appeared only in the dream. The inappropriate oedipal striving was promptly subdued, overwhelmed by an apocalyptic destruction. The upward and downward impulses are evenly matched here and, in the end, tranquility is restored by the analyst, a messianic rescuer. (I have discussed the apocalyptic characteristics of all of these dreams elsewhere [Ostow 1986].) The omission of the medication released both upward and downward tendencies and created a potential for instability, rather than for relapse into their "high" or "low" pathologic states. What was indicated here was the resumption of both medications in order to restore mental stability.

Not uncommonly a patient will report that he is feeling well; he will deny depression. However, he may, during the same session, report a dream like this (patient E.):

> He saw someone suffering wounds all over his body. Then he saw and was impressed by a large house, but once inside, he discovered that it was supported by only very thin and insubstantial uprights. It could easily topple.

Here we find an unopposed depressive tendency, the falling of the house because the uprights are too fragile. (That detail suggests a problem with potency. All of these dreams can, and in an analysis, should, be interpreted in the usual way, using associations, memories, fantasies, and day residue to uncover the meaning of the details of the dream for the individual. In this discussion I am focusing only on the manifest dream, demonstrating how it can be used for the purpose of assessing "psychic energy" status and conflicts without the personal associations.)

A borderline, but now chronically depressed man (patient F.) who was taking large doses of antidepression medication, reported one day that his mother had returned home from visiting him, and that whenever she left, he would become more depressed. A few days later he reported the following dream:

> I was in Brooklyn on Eastern Parkway driving past the headquarters of the Lubavitch Rebbe. I was sitting in a room with Hasidim. They said, "This time it really happened.—No, it couldn't." What were they talking about? I walked out. They were all talking. It turned out that the Rebbe had died and these people believed that he was directly related to God. A number of times he'd been sick, but hadn't died. Now he had died. If he had had divine protection he should not have died. They paraded him around on a chair. He would ascend to heaven in a fire. They put me in the chair, which I thought was strange. They were rocking me back and forth. I fell off the chair. There was a fire. I fell into it.

The patient associated falling into the fire with going to hell, and being carried around on a chair to a common practice at Jewish weddings of elevating the bride and groom on chairs to be carried around on the shoulders of their friends. The man said, "After I awoke I thought, 'There's a depressive dream, death and rebirth.' "

In the dream, the patient invokes religious sentiments, which he never does in conscious life. We see evidence of a struggle upwards, in fact literally upwards, but a struggle that involves usurping the role of father. (The chair represents mother.) However, instead of the ascent, that is, the rebirth that he hopes for, he is cast down into the fires of hell. Clearly the depressive forces prevail.

This type of dream analysis can assist in following the progress of the patient's treatment. Before he came to treatment and while visiting his parents, a seriously depressed borderline young man, G., dreamed: He was on a roof eating a hot dog. As he finished it, he noticed a building nearby. There were some fire escapes crisscrossing, leading down from the roof. A young man was being restrained by some uniformed men. He was able to get away from them and jump. Here the patient attempts to find comfort in oral gratification with his parents. An oral aggressive tendency accompanies that effort. But the downward pull asserts itself, literally represented as a compulsion to jump off the roof.

When he started to recover as a result of both antidepression medication and psychotherapy, the quality of his dreams changed. He had started treatment on January 4th and on the 15th he reported: "I was floating down a river, away. My mother saved me, pulled me out." The following day he dreamed:

> I was with my two sisters. We were walking over a walkway over a highway to get to some sporting event. We went over a bridge. There were three: one, another, and then a third. We went over it. We would come back. The third one was only a plank of wood. Going back I go first. I had trouble. I was scared I would fall. My sisters went over it. Then I was able to. One of them showed me how to do it.

The water and the bridges represent separation anxiety and death. The fear of falling off the bridge reproduces the pretreatment fear of jumping off the building. However, now he is rescued by his mother or his sisters. As a result of treatment, the rebirth tendency is powerful enough to counteract the destructive tendency. It was almost a week later before the patient was able to acknowledge that he actually did feel better.

Examination of apocalyptic death and rebirth tendencies that appear in dreams and fantasies can reveal the dynamics of the conflicting forces and their relative strength at each point in the treatment.

Potential and Limitations of Combined Treatment

Although we are focusing on the opening phases of analysis when it is combined with psychiatric medication, let us glance at the outcome of the procedure. The methods that I have described and the approach apply to the combined procedure in general, but the results depend to a large extent upon the patient and on his clinical problem.

First let us note that while we would expect the concurrent use of psycho-analysis and psychopharmaceutical modalities to permit a greater degree of success than we obtain with either alone, it seems to me that many patients who require medication to permit analysis to proceed exhibit a surprising rigidity, a greater resistance to the offering of free associations and to the incorporation of insights offered. While they seem to make a genuine effort to comply with instructions and they dutifully accept and repeat interpretive interventions, nevertheless the enlightenment is accepted only superficially and influences behavior only to a relatively small degree.

Patient G., the suicidally depressed young man, started psychotherapy on a three-times-a-week schedule. He accepted medication, though reluctantly. I tried to engage him in an analytic procedure but obtained only rigidly limited reports. At first I attributed his lack of interest in psychodynamic formulations and understanding to his depressive pain. However as he improved and over-came his depression and engaged joyously and hopefully in many activities, his interest in treatment dropped even further. These activities themselves revealed serious inhibition in selecting and pursuing age-adequate goals. Nevertheless he produced almost no analytic material, restricting his reports to poor descriptions of daily events in a stereotyped way, unaccompanied by reflections, thoughts, fantasies, or dreams. He insisted on reducing the frequency of sessions to twice a week and then once a week. (He had left a number of previous psychothera-pists completely, after brief attempts at psychotherapy.) Within a few months he discontinued the medication without telling me, certain that he had no need for it. Over the course of the next several months his depression returned insidi-ously and he gave up one activity after another. He acquiesced to resuming medication only after it became obvious that he was deteriorating rapidly and that he had no control over the situation. He was no more amenable to an analytic procedure when he recovered again.

Yet the treatment is indeed very helpful to such patients to the extent that it offers them guidance in the sense of instructing them in appropriate responses to social situations that they seem incapable of coping with on their own, and support against the frequent occurrences of despair that they incur by virtue of their illness, and to which they are so sensitive. The analyst functions as a companion and guide and the patient regards him as a kind of messianic rescuer with whom he ultimately identifies as he gradually begins to look after himself. Profound insight into unconscious dynamics and the reconstruction of childhood experience seem to play little role in the improvement that is obtained. One may with some justice conclude that what has started out as an analytic procedure becomes a supportive psychotherapy.

I find it surprising that the patient who, with proper medication control, becomes so self-possessed, so self-critical, and so insightful, nevertheless when the medication is inappropriately altered, quite abruptly loses his objectivity and insight and relapses into profound neurosis or psychosis. One is impressed to a greater degree than one is in the case of unmodified psychoanalysis, with the fragility of the normal mental state and its dependence upon fairly precise regulation of affects and "energies."

Let us look at the individual syndromes. The situation of the patient who presents in a state of depression that is superimposed upon a personality disorder, someone whose difficulty with object relations creates distress for others and defeat for himself, is probably least complicated. Overcoming the depression permits the conduct of a psychoanalytic procedure that is not remarkable in any way other than its being accompanied by a fairly constant regimen of drug therapy. The analysis can be quite successful by both internal criteria of a satisfactory analytic process and external criteria of improved functioning. Yet the susceptibility to recurrent depression may be unaffected.

The manic-depressive patient whose illness is controlled by lithium or other medication or both may be able to participate in an analytic procedure in a quite unexceptional way. In the course of the treatment it will be useful to discuss previous manic and depressive episodes, how they have influenced the patient's life, how they were perceived by others and by himself, and what effect they might have had on his self-esteem. But the psychoanalyst should not expect that the analysis will prevent subsequent episodes of illness. In most instances one will have to rely on the medication for that.

A group of patients exhibits rapid, successive, or alternating manic-depressive attacks, or at least highs and lows. Psychopharmacologists speak of them as "rapid cyclers." When this rapid cycling is accompanied by an unusual degree of aggressiveness, of overt hostility, whether directed inward as suicidal or self-mutilating behavior, or whether directed outward toward others and when it is accompanied by impulsiveness and an inconstant sense of personal identity, we speak of borderline personality disorder. However, I'm not sure how often rapid cycling occurs without the other qualities of the borderline personality. I attribute the volatility of the borderline, the poor sense of identity, and perhaps some of the anger to the "energy" instability. However, my experience with drug therapy suggests that there may indeed be two different syndromes. It is simply that some borderline patients respond with impressive improvement to the administration of lithium, whereas others do not. It may be that the latter are just nonresponders to the drug, as some manic-depressives are. On the other hand, it may be that an additional factor may be at work. I was impressed by one borderline patient who failed to respond at all to medication or whose responses were short-lived. However medication affected her when it did, it did nothing to deter her insistent self-destructive drive, which ultimately succeeded. The rapid cyclers who respond well to medication lend themselves to concurrent analysis. Those who do not respond can scarcely be engaged in a true analytic procedure.

Schizophrenics, of course, cannot be considered a homogeneous group. There are those whose psychosis can easily be contained with relatively small doses of medication and who can then engage in a psychotherapeutic procedure. Perhaps these should be considered instances of schizoaffective disorder. Some can participate genuinely in a true analytic exploration, in search of insight that they can utilize for therapeutic purposes. Others, on the other hand, find it difficult to comply with the formal requirements of psychoanalysis, that is, to give free associations and even to report accurately their mental state and recent experiences. Therapy serves the purpose merely of guiding them, encouraging them to continue with medication which they may resist, and being alert for changes in mental state that would require changes in the medication regimen.

One encounters also schizophrenics, many of whom are no less involved affectively, who respond only incompletely to medication despite one's best efforts to titrate dosages carefully and to seek optimal combinations. Although the most prominent signs of illness, for example, hallucinations, may be suppressed, the patient may remain quite paranoid and therefore difficult to deal with psychotherapeutically. Obviously an analytic process is impossible. In these patients one must infer pathogenic processes other than the spectrum shift that I described above. Here the primary tendencies and corrective processes are determined dynamically rather than "energetically." For these the outlook must be considerably more unfavorable than for the group that responds well to medication.

Conclusions

The possibility of combining psychiatric drug therapy with psychoanalysis opens the opportunity to treat patients otherwise inaccessible to psychoanalysis, and to continue psychoanalytic treatment despite intercurrent episodes of depression or even psychosis.

Experience demonstrates that the departure from what has become "classical," abstinent psychoanalytic technique need not affect the analysis adversely. Responses to accepting medication and experiencing its various desired and undesired effects must be treated as "day residue" in the analytic material, especially in assessing the transference.

When a new patient requires drug therapy before he becomes ready for analysis, the analytic procedure can be begun gradually as the patient's mental state stabilizes and he acquires sufficient self-control and perspective to participate.

Though the combined treatment opens doors hitherto closed to many patients, a good number of them demonstrate a surprising rigidity that makes their compliance with instructions only nominal, insight only superficial, and true behavior change limited.

In my opinion the drug therapy should be administered by the same person who does the analysis, and it should be informed by true psychopharmacologic sophistication.

References

Diagnostic and Statistical Manual of Mental Disorders (1987). 3rd. ed., rev. Washington, DC: American Psychiatric Association.

Freud, S. (1933). New introductory lectures on psychoanalysis. *Standard Edition* 22:5–182.

——— (1940). An outline of psychoanalysis. *Standard Edition* 23:144–207.

Loeb, F. F., and Loeb, L. R. (1987). Psychoanalytic observations on the effect of lithium on manic attacks. *Journal of the American Psychoanalytic Association* 35:877–902.

Ostow, M. (1960). The effects of the newer neuroleptic and stimulation drugs on psychic function. In *The Dynamics of Psychiatric Drug Therapy,* ed. G. Sarwer-Foner, pp. 172–191. Springfield, IL: Charles C Thomas.

——— (1962). *Drugs in Psychoanalysis and Psychotherapy.* New York: Basic Books.

——— (1986). Archetypes of apocalypse in dreams and in religious scripture. *Israel Journal of Psychiatry and Related Sciences.* 2:107–122.

PART III
Integration in Clinical Practice

11

Treatment of Depression

GERALD L. KLERMAN, M.D.

The data available from controlled studies demonstrate no negative interactions between drugs and psychotherapy for major depression. On the contrary, there are probably synergistic effects due to the different processes that influence the two treatments. Psychotherapy seems to influence interpersonal relations and social performance, while drug therapy reduces symptom formation and affective distress. The hypothesis that drugs render the patient more accessible to psychotherapy is most clearly supported by the data. There is relatively good evidence for the rejection of the hypotheses that postulate either a positive or negative placebo effect. There is also not much evidence in support of the hypothesis that patients experiencing symptom relief will be undesirous of exploring their interpersonal relations, social functioning, and psychological distress. The data from the Boston-–New Haven Collaborative Depression Study present no evidence for the hypothesis that drug-induced reductions of anxiety and symptoms are motives for discontinuing psychotherapy, that pharmacotherapy undercuts defenses, that there is possible deleterious effect of pharmacotherapy upon psychotherapy expectation, that drugs have an abreactive effect on the patient, or that psychotherapy may be symptomatically disruptive.

In the treatment of depression, drugs are frequently combined with individual, family, or group psychotherapy. This combination is probably the most commonly prescribed regimen for depression in current clinical practice. However, the theoretical rationale and empirical research supporting this treatment combination are limited in two ways: first, in regard to the modes of actions related to pathogenesis of depression; second, in regard to the empirical justification for its therapeutic efficacy and safety.

This situation is not unique to the treatment of depression. In fact, most treatments in clinical psychiatry are pragmatically rather than scientifically based. Clinical practices in the treatment of depression have been markedly altered in the past decade by the introduction of new antidepressant drugs; yet basic concepts underlying the treatment of depression have remained relatively unchanged. The efficacy of the monoamine oxidase (MAO) inhibitors and the tricyclic antidepressants and lithium has generated the monoamine theory of depression, which constitutes a major contribution to research in neurochemistry and psychobiology of depressive states. However, relatively few attempts have been made to integrate the available pharmacologic findings into currently accepted clinical views as to the psychogenesis and psychotherapy of depression to provide an internally consistent and scientifically supportable rationale for combined treatments.

The Psychiatrist's Dilemma

Ideally, in prescribing combined treatment the psychiatrist should have available three types of evidence: (1) evidence for the efficacy of each of the treatments, (2) understanding of their respective modes of action, and (3) verified concepts that bridge the two treatments and provide a reasonable and understandable basis for the combination. It must be acknowledged that in the use of drugs and psychotherapy for depression we are far from having these three types of information. On the one hand we have excellent research evidence for the efficacy of the drugs and partially verified hypotheses as to their mode of action. On the other hand there are very few controlled studies supporting the efficacy of psychotherapy in depression, although there is a well-developed and highly elaborated theory of the psychodynamics of depression. Bridging concepts between pharmacology and psychodynamics are relatively few, and empirical research as to the value and limitation of combined therapy is limited, albeit supportive.

Faced with this situation, the psychiatrist empirically has devised various programs for treatment of depression, the most common being the combination of drugs and psychotherapy. In doing so, most American clinicians act in conflict with their stated theoretical persuasions and therapeutic preferences. In practice, drug therapy is widely prescribed even though it may conflict with the value system of the psychiatrist. Almost all studies of the attitudes and values of American psychiatrists have found that they give greatest primacy and value to individual psychotherapy and hold drug therapy in low esteem and value, while acknowledging its efficacy for symptom reduction.

The psychiatrist's behavior in this situation can be understood, in part, as an example of "cognitive dissonance," the concept developed by Festinger (1957). Applied to psychiatric practitioners, "cognitive dissonance" describes the situation where, faced with a lack of congruence between their clinical practices and theoretical rationales, psychiatrists will adopt partial theories that are incompletely justified by the available data.

The psychiatrist's preference for drugs and/or psychotherapy is usually determined more by his training, his therapeutic orientation, and his pragmatic goals than by reference to a well-defined body of theory and empirical research. The psychiatrist cannot avoid this dilemma, since he must act on the basis of the balance of available information and ignorance, usually tempered by his own therapeutic orientation and theoretical persuasion. If the psychiatrist were to be guided by the research evidence, he should give highest value to drug therapy rather than psychotherapy. Yet in actuality the order of preference is reversed. Research data and theoretical views are seldom explicit in the psychiatrist's thinking when he is faced with therapeutic decision making. Vague concepts, incomplete formulations, and ideological commitments are to varying degrees explicit in this decision-making process. His stated treatment rationale is usually the manifest expression of partial theoretical models often based on his ideological beliefs and professional group membership.

For example, when we ask psychiatrists to explain their rationales for prescribing various therapies for depression, we can readily identify conflicting views. If we ask a psychotherapeutically oriented psychiatrist why he uses a particular psychotherapeutic technique, he will almost always answer in concepts and terms derived from psychodynamic theory, for example, resolution of conflict, change of personality structure, and reduction of depression. If, however, we ask a psychotherapist why he prescribes drugs, he will seldom answer in psychodynamic terms; rather, he will refer to the patient's need for reduction of symptoms and occasionally mention that drugs facilitate psychotherapy, but he will probably be vague about either the psychodynamic or pharmacologic processes whereby this facilitation occurs.

Although a drug-oriented psychiatrist's rationale in prescribing drugs is similar in some respects to the psychotherapist's in that he expects drugs to reduce target symptoms and ultimately reduce the patient's subjective distress, his long-term aims are usually different. Whereas the psychotherapist views the reduction of distress as facilitating constructive learning engendered by the psychotherapeutic process, the drug-prescribing psychiatrist tends to see symptom reduction as primarily facilitating the patient's social adjustment and accelerating spontaneous remission. The goals of drug therapy are usually more modest than those of psychotherapy. If pressed further, the pharmacotherapist may shift from this aspect of his rationale to more complex formulations of the mode of action of the antidepressant drugs in pharmacologic and neurochemical terms, citing, for example, the recent studies on catecholamines and indoleamines.

The preceding examples illustrate the partially supported theories and rationales that underlie and justify (perhaps better stated, rationalize) the therapeutic decisions made by psychiatrists. These views are ultimately subject to scientific discussion and research verification, but are perhaps better understood

realistically as the cognitive mode by which psychiatrists "explain" their treatment decisions to themselves, to their clients, to psychiatric colleagues, and to
the larger public.

Unfortunately, in the development of a scientific basis for psychiatry,
clinical practices are usually ahead of empirical research. In most therapeutic
decisions, pragmatic experience more often guides the psychiatrist than does
evidence from systematic clinical trials, experimental studies on animals, or
basic laboratory findings.

Depression serves as only one example of a compartmentalized and fragmented state of contemporary theory and practice in building a scientific
psychiatry. The issues raised in the treatment of depression apply equally to
treatment of other clinical psychiatric states, and most of the problems described
in this paper are only specific illustrations of general problems in psychiatric
therapeutics.

Hopefully, the psychiatrist will attempt to attain integration of empirical
research findings into his clinical practice and begin to modify his theoretical
basis to be congruent with his revised treatment practices.

Therapeutic Issues

Available Evidence for Therapeutic Efficacy

As stated previously, the ideal situation in assessing the theoretical and
therapeutic aspects of combined psychotherapy and drug therapy would be to
possess empirical evidence about the efficacy and safety of each of these
therapies. With respect to the efficacy and safety of antidepressant drug therapy,
the evidence is very favorable. Since the mid-1950s there have been a large
number of controlled clinical trials that have demonstrated the efficacy of the
phenothiazines, lithium, tricyclic antidepressants, and MAO inhibitors, as compared to placebo or other control group. For symptom relief and resolution of
the acute depressive episode drug therapy has demonstrated efficacy. Moreover, there is now substantial evidence for the value of two classes of drugs for
maintenance therapy to prevent relapse and recurrence: lithium for both bipolar
and unipolar depressions and the tricyclics for unipolar recurrent depressions
and various forms of neurotic depressions characterized by relapse and fluctuation (Klerman et al. 1974).

However, when we review the psychotherapy of depression, the evidence
for efficacy is more limited. There are almost no controlled studies of psychotherapy for depression, and the efficacy of psychotherapy is itself a subject of
continual controversy (Luborsky et al. 1971). Interestingly enough, the few
controlled studies have only recently been reported and were initiated by
research groups primarily experienced in the evaluation of drug therapy. The
three controlled clinical trials that have been reported were interested in

assessing combinations of drugs and psychotherapy. The outcomes of these studies from groups in Baltimore, Philadelphia, and Boston and New Haven provide important information about the relative efficacies of these two treatment approaches and their interactions (Friedman et al. 1972, Covi et al. 1974, Klerman et al. 1974). Aside from these controlled clinical trials there is a lack of evidence as to the efficacy of psychotherapy and its range of suitable patients, expected areas of change, and maximal duration of effect, which renders full assessment of the value of combined treatment difficult.

Practical and Therapeutic Issues in Combining Treatments

Drugs and psychotherapy derive from different theoretical realms and should be neutral toward each other, but ideologically they are competitive. Linkages and bridges between the theories supporting these treatments are few and weak in their empirical support. Although considerable psychophysiologic research has been undertaken in animals and humans to document the possible mechanisms by which conflict and stress influence brain function (particularly via pituitary, hypothalamic, and subcortical mechanisms), endocrine activity, and amine metabolism, experimentally based formulations for the use of psychotherapy combined with drug therapy are rare. In clinical practice, however, these approaches are used simultaneously, usually in an eclectic, pragmatic, and inconsistent manner.

Little attention has been given to the possible interactions between these two therapeutic approaches. A number of questions should be asked: What are the effects (positive and negative) on the psychotherapeutic process and outcome of the introduction of drug therapy? And conversely: What are the effects on drug treatment of the addition of psychotherapy? Are there negative interactions between drugs and psychotherapy? Under what conditions do drugs facilitate or retard psychotherapeutic communication? Will too rapid reduction of symptoms remove the patient's motivation for insight? These and similar questions require careful theoretical analysis and controlled empirical investigation. Although the effects of drugs and psychotherapy upon each other will be discussed for depression, it should become apparent that similar considerations may arise for combined treatments of other disorders.

Effects of Drug Therapy on Psychodynamic Processes

In prescribing drugs as adjuncts to the psychotherapy of depression, psychiatrists expect that the drugs will reduce manifest symptoms and lower the subjective distress of the patients. Prominent symptoms such as anxiety, insomnia, tension, and autonomic manifestations become the target symptoms for drug prescription. The psychiatrist attempts to reduce the patient's subjective distress and hopes thereby to facilitate communication, to reduce resistance to therapeutic insight, and to accelerate psychotherapeutic progress.

Drug therapy produces significant changes, not only in target symptoms, but also in psychodynamic functioning. Theoretically, studies of the actions of antidepressant drugs involve the possible relationship of Central Nervous System (CNS) substrates to affect, ego functions, and symptom formation. Ostow (1962) has interpreted drug effects in terms of psychoanalytic libidinal theory. Sarwer-Foner (1960), Azima (1961), Bellak and Rosenberg (1966), and other psychoanalysts have emphasized drug effects on various ego functions. Changes in sleep mechanisms and patterns as a result of drugs have also undergone psychodynamic study. Kramer and colleagues (1968) in Cincinnati have placed emphasis on drug-induced changes in dream content. In addition, there have been studies of drug effects on hostility, anxiety, and other affects (Gottschalk 1965, Klerman and Gershon 1970). Further studies in this area offer promise of elucidating psychodynamic mechanisms involved in antidepressant drug actions; conversely, experimental alterations of CNS amines by pharmacologic means could clarify the role of neurochemical substrates in the psychodynamics of affect regulation.

Possible Negative Effects of Drug Therapy on Psychotherapy

Interestingly, most attention has been paid to the possible negative effects on psychotherapy of introducing drug therapy. Although relatively little empirical research has been done on this problem, it is possible to identify a number of proposed hypotheses.

Hypothesis 1: The negative placebo effect. Much of the criticism of drug therapy enunciated by psychotherapists in the 1950s implied a negative placebo effect—that pill taking had harmful effects on psychotherapy. It was hypothesized that the prescription of any drug had deleterious effects upon the psychotherapeutic relationship and upon the attitudes and behavior of both patients and therapist—effects independent of the specific pharmacologic actions of the drug. Moreover, it was hypothesized that the prescription of medication promoted an authoritarian attitude on the part of the psychiatrist and enhanced his belief in his biological-medical heritage. At the same time, the patient would become more dependent, place greater reliance on magical thinking, and assume a more passive, compliant role, as is expected in the conventional doctor–patient relationship in fields of medicine other than psychiatry. Thus the introduction of medication into the psychotherapeutic process is hypothesized as initiating and/or augmenting countertransference and transference processes that run counter to the development of insight and the uncovering of defenses.

Hypothesis 2: Drug-induced reduction of anxiety and symptoms as motives for discontinuing psychotherapy. In contrast to the negative-placebo-effect hypothesis above, which deals only with the symbolic and psychological meaning of drug administration, another hypothesis acknowledges the pharmacologic and therapeutic actions of drugs, but expresses concern lest the resultant decrease of the patient's anxiety and tension reduces motivation for continued active psychotherapeutic participation. The hypothesis predicts that too effective a drug will initiate psychodynamic forces operating counter to progress in psychotherapy. Thus if a psychoactive drug, such as a phenothiazine or diazepoxide derivative, is highly effective in reducing psychotic turmoil, neurotic anxiety, or other symptoms, the patient's motivation for reflection, insight, and psychotherapeutic work will be lessened (Meerloo 1955, Szasz 1957). According to this hypothesis, it is predicted that if drug therapy is too effective, patients will no longer seek psychotherapy because they will be satisfied with symptom reduction and therefore cease working toward deeper personality and characterologic changes.

Hypothesis 3: Pharmacotherapy undercuts defenses. This hypothesis predicts that if the pharmacologic effect of a drug prematurely undercuts some important defense, symptom substitution or other compensatory mechanisms of symptom formation will ensue. For example, in psychotherapeutic practice, Seitz (1953) has reported instances of new symptom formation following hypnosis, and Weiss (1944) has cautioned against an overly rapid relief of the anxiety of the agoraphobic—if such anxiety is reduced too rapidly, before new defenses are developed, other symptoms may occur. This hypothesis assumes that symptoms maintain a balance between conflict and defenses, and that the precipitous reduction of anxiety, depression or tension may upset this equilibrium and release deeper conflicts. If so, this disequilibrium would obviously generate new symptoms for the depressive patient; but systematic research data and replications germane to this specific hypothesis are few and inconclusive.

Hypothesis 4: Possible deleterious effects of pharmacotherapy upon psychotherapy expectation. This hypothesis predicts that there may be a negative reaction when the patient is prescribed drug therapy instead of psychotherapy, if he expected the latter. The patient may feel that the prescription of a drug defines him as "less interesting," not a candidate for insight. Thus the use of drugs may initiate a loss of self-esteem on the part of the patient, especially if he belongs to a cultural subgroup whose values emphasize insight, psychotherapeutic understanding, and self-actualization. This expectation varies with the social class and subculture in which the patient participates. Within groups that value psychotherapy, the use of drugs is often regarded as a failure or a crutch.

Possible Positive Effects of Drug Therapy on Psychotherapy

The four aforementioned hypotheses predict negative influences of drugs on the psychotherapeutic process. Although these possible negative influences have been given the most attention by clinicians, in a comprehensive analysis equal consideration must be given to the possible positive effects by which drug therapy may facilitate, augment, and interact in a synergistic manner with psychotherapy and other therapies. At least four such hypotheses may be identified.

Hypothesis 5: Drugs facilitate psychotherapeutic accessibility. This hypothesis is embodied in the most commonly stated rationales for the use of combined therapies, and it supports prevailing clinical practice in psychiatry. Advertisements and other promotional materials of many pharmaceutical firms propose that the introduction of their drug facilitates psychotherapy by making the patient "more accessible." The proposed mechanism for this effect is readily specified—the pharmacologic action of the drug ameliorates the presumed CNS dysfunction underlying symptom formation, resulting in reduction of the patient's symptomatology, psychopathology, and/or affective discomfort. Drug-induced reduction in discomfort renders the patient better able to communicate in and benefit from psychotherapy. Whereas some level of anxiety, dysphoria, or symptomatology is believed necessary to provide the "drive" or "motivation" for participation in psychotherapy, on the other hand this hypothesis presumes that excessive levels of tension, anxiety, or symptom intensity result in a decrease in the patient's capacity to participate effectively in psychotherapy. Research evidence that will be presented later in this chapter supports this hypothesis that drugs facilitate accessibility.

Hypothesis 6: Drugs influence the ego psychological functions required for participation in psychotherapy. Another hypothesis predicts that drugs may positively influence the psychotherapeutic process through their pharmacologic action on neurophysiologic substrates for the ego functions necessary for psychotherapeutic participation. Some drugs may influence verbal skills, improve cognitive functioning, improve memory, reduce distraction, and promote attention and concentration. Since it is widely accepted that adequate ego functioning is a prerequisite for psychotherapeutic participation, these psychological functions and abilities are components of the large domain of ego function and enhance the patient's benefit from participation in psychotherapy.

Hypothesis 7: Abreactive effects of drugs. Abreaction is one of the earliest psychotherapeutic techniques. Breuer and Freud (1950) in their studies of hysteria described the use of hypnosis to promote catharsis or abreaction. A number of drugs, especially intravenous barbiturates and amphetamines, have been used to promote this effect. Wikler (1957), in his monograph on the pharmacologic basis of psychiatric therapy, referred to such methods as "psychoexploratory" techniques. These drugs help to uncover memory, break down defenses, and bring into consciousness material against which the person otherwise defends. A variant of this practice is the recent use of LSD, mescaline, and psilocybin to promote "peak experiences" in which the heightened sense of self-awareness and emotional, affective, and bodily experiences that occur under these psychedelic drugs are advocated as facilitating the psychotherapeutic process.

Hypothesis 8: Positive placebo effect of drug therapy. In addition to the short-term symptomatic relief of drug therapy, a positive placebo effect may often contribute to a general attitude of optimism and confidence on the part of the patient. The advocates of publicly congenial biologic methods, such as the megavitamin treatment of schizophrenia, are, in effect, removing some of the stigma from psychiatric illness and are in some instances making it easier for the patient to accept the definition of himself as mentally ill. Thus the request for drug therapy may itself be a vehicle through which the patient can seek psychotherapeutic help and counseling. In this sense, the skillful psychiatrist often uses the patient's initial request for drug therapy as a starting point for initiating a psychotherapeutic process.

Effects of Psychotherapy on Pharmacotherapy

Most of the discussion in the literature has focused on possible effects of drug therapy upon psychotherapy. Relatively little attention has been paid to the other side of the process, namely, the impact of psychotherapy upon the patient receiving pharmacotherapy. It is interesting to note how seldom this problem is discussed or even mentioned.

Perhaps considering the demonstrated efficacy of drugs for the treatment of depression and the relative absence of evidence for the efficacy of psychotherapy, the question should be stated: What benefit accrues to the patient to have psychotherapy added upon drug therapy? Although during the discussions in the 1950s and 1960s the psychotherapists were the more assertive members of the dialogue, and the drug therapists were on the defensive, one can discern a subtle but significant shift in recent years with the impact of evidence from controlled studies. Nevertheless, it is important to analyze the possible theoretical interactions. At least three further proposed hypotheses can be identified.

Hypothesis 9: Biochemical replacement effect of drugs. Some pharmacotherapists compare psychotropic drug treatment to the conventional nonpsychiatric use of drugs in medicine, especially endocrine agents such as insulin for diabetes. For those who hold this view, the rectification of the presumed neurophysiologic dysfunction or deficiency is the critical factor, and psychotherapy is considered unnecessary and irrelevant, or at best neutral. A variation of this single-factor reductionist hypothesis is expressed by some proponents of lithium treatment of mania. The most extreme version is proposed by those who advocate megavitamin therapy for schizophrenia. Those holding such views feel that drugs alone are both necessary and sufficient.

Hypothesis 10: Psychotherapy may be symptomatically disruptive. Furthermore, some pharmacotherapists hypothesize that psychotherapy may be deleterious to the pharmacologic treatment, since symptoms may be aggravated by excessive probing and uncovering defenses. Some psychiatrists who have worked with depressives and schizophrenics feel that harm is done to the patient by psychotherapeutic intervention, particularly during the acute stage, and that during the early recovery process the patient is best left alone to "heal over" and to reconstitute his defenses. There is a clear conflict between psychiatrists who advocate working through underlying conflicts in depression and others who support healing over or sealing over by promoting denial, repression, and other defenses. The fear hypothesized by many pharmacotherapists is that psycho-therapy, by uncovering areas of conflict, will increase the levels of tension. Implicit in this controversy over the validity of this hypothesis may be the variable of timing: What are the appropriate points in the process of therapeutic planning at which primarily supportive psychotherapy should be pursued, and when is it appropriate to use uncovering, probing insight techniques?

Hypothesis 11: Psychotherapy as rehabilitation. Many drug therapists hy-pothesize a value for psychotherapy, but in a secondary and ameliorative way. They propose that psychotherapy operates not upon ideologic mechanisms or upon the core of the depressive process, per se, but to correct secondary difficulties in interpersonal relations and in self-esteem and psychological func-tions that follow upon the impact of depressive symptoms. In this hypothesis, psychotherapy is seen as rehabilitative rather than as therapeutic in the classical medical model. As such, it would be purely elective rather than a necessary component of the treatment program.

The Boston–New Haven Depression Project

Thus far we have analyzed the various theoretical positions and identified at least eleven hypotheses specifying various interactive effects between psy-chotherapy and drug therapy. Let us now look at the empirical evidence. As stated previously, there have been only a few controlled studies of drugs and psychotherapy. Of the studies that have been reported, only the results from the Boston–New Haven Collaborative Depression Study (Klerman et al. 1974) have thus far been described in sufficient detail to allow analysis of the "goodness of fit" between the empirical data and the various hypotheses identified earlier in this paper.

The Boston–New Haven Collaborative Depression Project studied a large sample ($n = 150$) of depressed female outpatients treated with drugs, individual psychotherapy, or a combination of the two. The overall goal of the study was to evaluate maintenance treatment of depression, including its feasibility, efficacy, and safety. We developed this study in the mid-1960s as a collaboration between research groups at the Connecticut Mental Health Center in New Haven, Con-necticut (affiliated with Yale Medical School), and the Boston State Hospital in Boston, Massachusetts (affiliated with Tufts Medical School).

At that time we were convinced of the value of treatment for hospitalized depressed patients, and we decided to focus our research upon outpatients, who comprise the predominant proportion of depressed patients found in community and epidemiologic surveys (Paykel et al. 1970). We were convinced that drug therapy had established its efficacy for the symptomatic resolution of acute depressive episodes and believed that the more pressing research problem was to assess maintenance treatments, where the major goals are prevention of relapse and recurrence and maintenance of social performance. Moreover, we decided to study individual psychotherapy because in clinical practice this modality, together with drugs, has been and probably will continue to be the most common mode of treatment for depressed patients in outpatient settings.

The design of the maintenance treatment phase, which constituted the main experimental treatment phase of the total project, called for a sample of 150 patients to complete 8 months of treatment; these 150 patients were assigned randomly to a six-cell design. In order to develop this sample it was necessary first to treat a larger number of patients in a preliminary treatment phase to yield the group of 150 patients who had been symptomatically responsive to amitriptyline. Accordingly, the study was divided into a preliminary treatment phase and a maintenance treatment phase.

The preliminary treatment phase was an open trial of amitriptyline therapy for neurotic depressed patients. A total of 278 depressed outpatients were treated for 4 to 6 weeks with moderate dosages of amitriptyline (100 to 200 mg). Following this preliminary phase, 175 patients who had shown significant clinical improvement were assigned to the experimental treatment design. In the maintenance phase of our project, patients were assigned to treatment in a six-cell design in a double-blind controlled manner and were maintained for 8 months while they were being treated with drugs or psychotherapy or both.

The drug did produce significant reduction in the relapse rate. Amitriptyline, the active drug, clearly demonstrated its reduction of relapse rate using the strictest criterion of the 0.05 level of significance. There was no difference between tricyclic therapy alone and in combination with psychotherapy. Psychotherapy did not offer any additional therapeutic benefit over maintenance drug therapy in the prevention of relapse. Significant psychotherapy effects were shown on measures of social adjustment and interpersonal relations. The Social Adjustment Scale was the main outcome measure showing these psychotherapy effects. Previous factor analysis of the items on the scale had identified six factors: work performance; anxious rumination; interpersonal friction, which principally reflects hostility in the marital situation; inhibition of communication and reticence; submissive dependence, a factor that seems to be characteristic of acutely depressed women; and family attachment, which is a pattern of social adjustment in which social involvement is almost exclusively limited to those within the primary family group. The psychotherapeutically treated group did show statistically significant improvement in most of these components of social adjustment (Weissman et al. 1974).

Moreover, a differential time course was observed. Amitriptyline had immediate effects on symptoms and prevention of relapse; the effects of psychotherapy did not fully appear until the eighth month of treatment, and they became maximum later on. The effectiveness of psychotherapy took a longer time to build up, and when it did appear it showed mainly in interpersonal relations and social adjustment.

Relatively few, if any, systematic attempts have been made to study psychotherapy in depressed patients. In planning for this study we were not able to find a single systematic published report of the psychotherapy of depression that included more than twelve reported cases or described any attempt at a quantitative measure of outcome. In our experience, psychotherapy of the type described in our study (a once-a-week interview focusing on interpersonal, transactional relations of the patients) is effective in improving the patient's social adjustment and family relations.

We did not find any negative interactions between psychotherapy and drug, although many psychotherapists have argued that taking pills may impede or interfere with the psychotherapeutic process (Hypothesis 1 above). Our data indicate that medication had no negative effects on the content or the nature of the psychotherapeutic interaction. Our interpretation of the effects of psychotherapy in our study follows the point of view proposed by Frank (1965) and his associates at Johns Hopkins University. The main impact of individual psychotherapy is on patients' interpersonal relations and social effectiveness, whereas the main effect of drug therapy is on symptom reduction and prevention of relapse.

The design of this study permitted the testing of interactions between drugs and psychotherapy, and none was found. Psychotherapy is not an alternative to antidepressant treatment and does not prevent relapse or the recurrence of symptoms. Maintenance amitriptyline has little effect on social adjustment and is no better or worse than a placebo or no pill. The effects were largely independent, operating on different outcome measures. Drugs did not have a negative effect on psychotherapy, and psychotherapy did not have an adverse effect on symptom reduction achieved by drugs (Hypothesis 10). This finding is contrary to clinical speculations about combined treatments.

There were no beneficial psychotherapy effects for patients who were terminated early from the study owing to symptomatic worsening or relapse. Moreover, the psychotherapy effects were greatest for patients remaining symptomatically well. We know that drugs help to prevent relapse (Weissman et al. 1974) and to maintain patients in a symptomatically well state. The result was a kind of synergistic effect of the two treatments (drug and psychotherapy) that did not produce any formal interactions, since they affected different areas at different times. These findings are a strong argument for combined treatments.

This study supports the value of drugs and psychotherapy over a period of months in enhancing the social adjustment of recovering depressed female outpatients.

Conclusions

The combination of drugs and psychotherapy in psychiatric treatment is widely used but little understood. Ultimately, data from controlled trials will be necessary to clarify the therapeutic issues. These issues are currently evident in the treatment of depression where drugs and psychotherapy, the most frequently prescribed therapeutic modalities, can be related to relatively well-specified, although only partially validated, theoretical models—the neurochemical models that explain and justify drug treatment, and the psychodynamic models that underlie psychotherapeutic methods. Depression, therefore, presents one area of psychiatry that is theoretically active and therapeutically successful and where linkages between theory, experiment, and practice are emerging.

The data available from controlled studies demonstrate no negative interactions between drugs and psychotherapy for depression. On the contrary, there are probably synergistic effects due to the different processes that influence the two treatments. Psychotherapy seems to influence interpersonal relations and social performance, while drug therapy reduces symptom formation and affective distress. There are, moreover, sequential interactions such that sustained symptom reduction seems a necessary condition for the efficacy of psychotherapy. Of all the various hypotheses, the one that postulates that drugs render the patient more accessible to psychotherapy (Hypothesis 5) is most clearly supported by the data. There is relatively good evidence for the rejection of the hypotheses that postulate either a positive or negative placebo effect (Hypothesis 1 and Hypothesis 8). There is also not much evidence in support of the hypothesis that patients experiencing symptom relief will be undesirous of exploring their interpersonal relations, social functioning, and psychological distress (Hypothesis 2).

The data from the studies reviewed in this paper support the hypotheses that drugs facilitate psychotherapeutic accessibility (Hypothesis 5). There is a positive effect of drug therapy in contributing to a general attitude of optimism and confidence on the part of the therapist and patient. This stems from the fact that with drug therapy symptom control is feasible and the fear of the emergence of a relapse is reduced. The drug effect on symptom reduction can be considered consistent with the fact that there is a biochemical replacement effect of drugs that rectifies some sort of neurophysiologic dysfunction or deficiency in the patient (Hypothesis 9) or that there is a reduction of stress that renders the patient more accessible to therapeutic intervention.

Furthermore, the data from the Boston–New Haven Collaborative Depression Study present no evidence for the hypothesis that drug-induced reductions of anxiety and symptoms are motives for discontinuing psychotherapy (Hypothesis 2), that pharmacotherapy undercuts defenses (Hypothesis 3), that there is a possible deleterious effect of pharmacotherapy upon psychotherapy expectation (Hypothesis 4), that drugs have an abreactive effect on the patient (Hypothesis 7), or that psychotherapy may be symptomatically disruptive (Hypothesis 10). The hypothesis that psychotherapy is rehabilitative cannot be either supported or denied by the present evidence (Hypothesis 11), and there is insufficient evidence either way for the hypothesis that drugs influence the ego psychological functions required for participation in psychotherapy (Hypothesis 6).

Ultimately, further studies are needed, not only upon the type of supportive or situationally directed psychotherapy studied thus far, but enlarged studies to include other aspects of psychotherapy, particularly those forms of psychotherapy that attempt to influence more enduring personality structures and the presumed vulnerability to react to stress with affective symptomatology.

References

Azima, H. (1961). Psychodynamic and psychotherapeutic problems in connection with imipramine (Tofranil) intake. *Journal of Mental Science* 107:74–82.

Bellak, L., and Rosenberg, S. (1966). Effects of antidepressant drugs on psychodynamics. *Psychosomatics* 7:106–114.

Breuer, J., and Freud, S. (1950). *Studies in Hysteria.* Boston: Beacon.

Covi, L., Lipman, R. S., DeRogatis, L. R., et al. (1974). Drugs and group psychotherapy in neurotic depression. *American Journal of Psychiatry* 131:191–198.

Festinger, L. (1957). *A Theory of Cognitive Dissonance.* Evanston, IL: Row Peterson.

Frank, J. D. (1965). *Persuasion and Healing: A Comparative Study of Psychotherapy.* Baltimore, MD: Johns Hopkins University Press.

Friedman, A. S., et al. (1972). Drugs and family therapy in the treatment of depression. American College of Neuropsychopharmacology, December.

Gottschalk, L. A., Gleser, G. C., Wylie, H. W., et al. (1965). Effects of imipramine on anxiety and hostility levels. *Psychopharmacologia* 7:303.

Klerman, G. L., DiMascio, A., Weissman, M. M., et al. (1974). Treatment of depression by drugs and psychotherapy. *American Journal of Psychiatry* 131:186–191.

Klerman, G. L., and Gershon, S. (1970). Imipramine effects upon hostility in depression. *Journal of Nervous and Mental Disease* 150:127–132.

Kramer, M., Whitman, R., Baldridge, B., et al. (1968). Drugs and dreams: III. The effects of imipramine on the dreams of depressed patients. *American Journal of Psychiatry* 124:1385–1392.

Luborsky, L., Chandler, M., Averbach, A. H., et al. (1971). Factors influencing the outcome of psychotherapy: a review of quantitative literature. *Psychological Bulletin* 75:145–185.

Meerloo, J. A. (1955). Medication into submission: the danger of therapeutic conversion. *Journal of Nervous and Mental Disease* 122:353.

Ostow, M. (1962). *Drugs in Psychoanalysis and Psychotherapy.* New York: Basic Books.

Paykel, E., Klerman, G. L., and Prusoff, B. (1970). Treatment setting and clinical depression. *Archives of General Psychiatry* 22:11–21.

Sarwer-Foner, M. S. (1960). *The Dynamics of Psychiatric Drug Therapy.* Springfield, IL: Charles C Thomas.

Seitz, P. F. (1953). Experiments in the substitution of symptoms by hypnosis. *Psychosomatic Medicine?* 15:405.

Szasz, T. S. (1957). Some observations on the use of tranquilizing drugs. *AMA Archives of Neurology and Psychiatry* 77:86.

Weiss, E. (1944). Clinical aspects of depression. *Psychoanalytic Quarterly* 13:445.

Weissman, M. M., Klerman, G. L., Paykel, E. S., et al. (1974). Treatment effects on the social adjustment of depressed patients. *Archives of General Psychiatry* 30:771–778.

Wikler, A. (1957). *The Relation of Psychiatry to Pharmacology.* Baltimore, MD: Williams & Wilkins.

12

Countertransference Aspects in the Treatment of Schizophrenia

STEVEN T. LEVY, M.D.

Emphasis is placed on largely unconscious aspects of the therapeutic relationship that determine the inappropriate or untimely use of psychotropic drugs, particularly on the therapist's response to the regressive modes of relating and sharing emotional experience that characterize therapeutic work with schizophrenic patients. Case examples illustrate the use of drugs to establish interpersonal boundaries, to disavow frightening feelings within the self, and to renounce forbidden regressive pleasures—thus defending against the regressive pull of the developing symbiotic relationship. The effect of postpsychotic depression on the therapeutic relationship is explored with regard to the dynamics of psychotropic drug usage in treatment.

It is not the purpose of this chapter to question the value of psychotropic agents in the treatment of schizophrenia. There are many studies that demonstrate the effectiveness of phenothiazines and related drugs in the management of psychotic patients. The relative merits of pharmacotherapy versus both supportive and insight-oriented psychotherapies, both alone and in combination with drugs, have been extensively investigated (see especially Davis 1975, Feinsilver and Gunderson 1972, Grinspoon et al. 1972, Karon and Vanden Bos 1972, May 1968, 1971). That no consensus among investigators has been reached is in part due to difficulties in controlling for variables both within and across studies. I believe that for certain patients, a psychoanalytically oriented, investigative psychotherapy, with the goal of increased self-understanding and personal growth, can be successful even in the face of vulnerability to psychotic disorganization (Levy et al. 1975). It is the treatment of such cases which is the subject under discussion here, particularly as it relates to the concomitant use of psychotropic drugs.

During the course of therapeutic work with schizophrenic individuals, therapists are often confronted with feelings within themselves that lead them, for reasons largely outside their awareness, to consider using pharmacologic agents. This is in contrast to the consciously planned use of medication as an adjunct to insight psychotherapy. Whenever medications are used during psychotherapy, their meaning and usefulness to patient and therapist must be continuously scrutinized to prevent medications becoming a vehicle for the unconscious avoidance of the therapeutic task (Langs 1973, Linn 1964, Ostow 1962). In my own work, as well as in supervising the work of others, I have found that at certain junctures during therapy with schizophrenic patients, a consideration of adding or changing drugs becomes an almost predictable event that signals a disruptive but not necessarily detrimental alteration in the therapeutic relationship. Inexperienced therapists, in particular, are prone to use the complex controversies around what constitutes the best treatment for schizophrenia to justify using or changing drugs at this point, and suddenly question whether initial therapeutic hopes and goals were realistic given such severely impaired patients.

The following clinical vignette illustrates how the issue of medications may enter the treatment situation and result in the therapist not responding appropriately to the patient.

Case 1

Miss A., a 23-year-old single woman, was evaluated and referred for time-limited psychoanalytic psychotherapy with an advanced psychiatric resident. The following information is abstracted from the intake worker's case summary. Miss A. complained of feelings of "deadness" and "vagueness," insomnia, and trouble organizing her thoughts. She had recently worked as a waitress, having dropped out of college owing to feelings of anxiety, confusion, and inability to concentrate. Within a year of dropping out of school and returning home to live with her mother, Miss A. had a psychotic episode for which she was hospitalized for 7 months. After discharge, she moved to another city because living with her family was thought by the hospital staff to be too stressful.

Miss A. was one of six children, whom she described as "scattered all over the country." Her parents, both educators, were divorced when she was 11 years old. After that time, the patient lived with her mother and rarely saw her father. The evaluation report ended with the following statement: "The patient feels badly about her inability to function at a higher level. She is frustrated at her difficulty in communicating but, in fact, expresses her feelings quite well. She has been on a variety of drug regimens, none of which were helpful."

The therapist, Dr. T., reported that, even prior to beginning the treatment, he felt anxious about working in psychoanalytic psychotherapy with a severely impaired patient who had recently been psychotic. Miss A. arrived at her first session dressed boyishly, without make-up, looking somewhat unkempt. She began by relating that she had "cracked up" while away at college. She had dropped out of school and was admitted to a hospital in her home town. Miss A. then added that she didn't "focus on one thing a lot." She described her current living arrangement with a girlfriend. She next detailed some of her family history and mentioned her parents' divorce. This was followed by a long pause. The therapist had not said anything yet, and reported that the patient seemed very anxious about his listening quietly. In fact, Dr. T. attributed the long pause to his inability to think of what to say after her "giving a history."

Miss A. now became somewhat agitated and said that she knew treatment would go badly, that she couldn't think properly, that she had really been in need of treatment for a long time, but that now it was too late. She said rather dispairingly that she used to function well prior to her crack-up. Dr. T. asked what she meant by "crack-up" and she responded by saying that she felt foolish and was thinking about her friend sitting in the waiting area. She next said, "You're not going to get anywhere this way." Dr. T. replied that he heard Miss A. saying she would waste his time.

He reported in supervision that he said this under the impact of the patient's anxiety, which he described as unbearable. When asked how this made him feel, he said he felt somewhat paralyzed, dissatisfied with his comments as well as with his silence. In fact, he hadn't meant to say that the patient might waste his time. He had actually wanted to make an empathic remark about her concerns that treatment might not help her. He admitted that his comment related to his wondering at this time whether this way of treating her was appropriate. He thought that he should stop groping around and put her on medicine.

He asked the patient whether she had been on drugs in the past. Miss A. replied that she hadn't been honest in talking about herself. She didn't live away from home while at college. She commuted every day from home to school, a 100-mile trip. She couldn't leave home; couldn't leave mother. She next added that she had been seeing a psychologist while at school and had asked for medicine. She next recounted several of her experiences with medication. She told Dr. T. that medicines made her numb and she wished Dr. T. would talk more. She paused and then said she thought Dr. T. had his own problems.

During this session, the therapist experienced the patient as frightening and unbearably anxious. He felt much the way she did, not being able to collect his thoughts or respond appropriately. He wondered whether it was too late and thought about medication. The patient recognized his difficulties, told him that medicines didn't help, and said that what she needed was talk. The next several sessions were occupied with both the patient and the therapist trying to be more comfortable with each other. The patient repeatedly both asked for drugs that would make her feel better and said that the people she knew who had been on medication for long periods looked hollow. She seemed to have taken in the therapist's ambivalence about drugs and was working this over internally.

Dr. T., after exploring his reactions in supervision, told the patient that medications had not helped her in the past and that he thought working on her problems by talking together would be more helpful. Miss A. looked relieved and described her current life as "being on the outside looking in. But I do it, I don't let things register." Dr. T. asked her to elaborate on not letting things register. She responded, "Yes, because it doesn't matter. There has to be like a frame of reference—something to refer back to. Something that you're going to stay with. Ask me another question. See, the thing I have in my head, I have like a dialogue. Your inner voice; but it's not there to refer back to. It's just not there. It's just a whiny, irritating, little—"

We see in this vignette how the therapist used the issue of medication to deal with his own anxieties. The patient's immediate response to the therapist's introducing medication into the therapeutic field is to confess her dishonesty; next she provides information that drugs do not help, and finally points out that she wants the therapist to help her by talking. In subsequent sessions, the patient is preoccupied with medicines. She has incorporated the therapist's ambivalence and works to create a more helpful treatment relationship. In psychotherapy with schizophrenics and to a lesser degree with neurotic individuals, the patient is prone to take in relatively sick aspects of the therapist (Langs 1976, Searles 1958) and to make curative efforts on his behalf (Langs 1975a, 1975b, 1976, Little 1951, Searles 1975).

When the therapist resolved his ambivalence about being able to treat the patient and made a clear statement to her, the patient was obviously relieved and commenced to describe with greater detail and clarify aspects of her inner experience. Her comment about the need for "a frame of reference—something to refer back to" describes what she needs the therapist to provide if she is to stay with the work. I believe she correctly perceived the therapist's ill-timed and anxiety-ridden introduction of the medication issue as a threat to the therapeutic frame which required immediate restorative efforts (Langs 1975b).

Symbiotic Relatedness and the Therapeutic Relationship

The nature of the relationship between schizophrenic patient and therapist regularly takes on a particular cast that recapitulates a pathologically extended, unsuccessfully mastered, phase of early development commonly referred to as the symbiotic phase. The role and importance of symbiosis in normal and pathological development has been extensively explored by Mahler (1968). In this chapter, I use symbiotic relatedness to refer to the patient–therapist relationship when it is characterized by a severe degree of loss of self-object differentiation reflecting a significant diffusion of ego boundaries between patient and therapist. This boundary diffusion greatly facilitates projective and incorporative modes of identification which come to dominate the treatment relationship (see especially Heimann 1955, Klein 1946, Langs 1976, Malin and Grotstein 1966).

It is most important to remember that, in therapeutic work with adult schizophrenics, symbiotic relatedness exists simultaneously with less regressive modes of relating. Symbiosis is a childhood phenomenon that cannot be totally replicated in adulthood. The nonpsychotic part of the adult schizophrenic patient (Bion 1957, Katan 1954) is available to perceive and respond to both the patient's and the therapist's participation in the regressive exchange and merging of feelings and ideas. Symbiotic relatedness is at times experienced by both patient and therapist as terrifying, and at other times as comforting and gratifying (Searles 1961). The patient needs a therapist who can shift back and forth between symbiotic relatedness and a more mature, better differentiated patient–therapist relationship, even if the patient himself is not as readily able to make these shifts. Incapacity to accept the patient's symbiotic mode of related-ness deprives the patient of the opportunity to resolve important early fixations (Little 1957, Searles 1961). However, the therapist must ultimately be able to use the nonsymbiotic aspects of the relationship to understand the patient and correctly formulate and interpret the unconscious meanings of the patient's experiences and fantasies.

The therapist's need to shift back and forth between symbiotic modes of relatedness and a more detached, analytic position, relates to the meaning of countertransference in the treatment of schizophrenic patients. Kleinian ana-lysts, particularly Winnicott (1949), Little (1951, 1957), and Heimann (1950), point out the special importance of countertransference problems in work with schizophrenics. Countertransference is seen by these authors as a legitimate, and at times exclusive means of understanding the patient. I disagree that what these authors describe should be called countertransference in the same sense as the more traditional view of countertransference—that is, the interference of the therapist's unconscious needs and conflicts with his ability to understand and treat the patient.

Reich (1960, 1966) has clarified the relationship between empathy and countertransference in a manner that seems useful in this connection. She conceptualizes empathy as a series of transient identifications with the patient which the therapist employs in understanding the patient's experience. These consciously intended trial identifications must be distinguished from the thera-pist's unconsciously determined identifications and projections. The latter rep-resent countertransference problems in the therapist, in that they interfere with, rather than promote, emphatic understanding. This is not to say that more classically defined countertransference problems cannot be used, if carefully analyzed, to aid in the therapeutic work. However, the focus is then on clarifi-cation and understanding of unconscious fantasies and attitudes rather than on the mere experience of mutual incorporations and projections. The shifts back and forth between symbiotic relatedness and a more objective analytic position in work with schizophrenic patients is related to Reich's concept of trial identification. When the therapist is not in conscious control of these shifts, or fears losing his control over them, the search for countertransference problems is warranted.

Proper understanding of aspects of symbiotic relatedness within the therapeutic relationship helps to clarify the complex interaction between psychotherapy and drug therapy in question here. The manner in which the therapist is drawn into a symbiotic relatedness, at times against his will and outside of his awareness, will be described below. Schizophrenic patients and their therapists, in the course of their work together, come to share many ideas and feelings that seem to obscure, and at times obliterate, their interpersonal boundaries. Both parties, in effect, become caught up in the confusion and tragedy of psychosis. Elements of symbiotic relatedness can be observed even in the earliest meetings between patient and therapist. It is during this early phase of treatment that the therapist most often begins to wonder about medications. The patient, long accustomed to the intrusion of primitive ideas into his thinking and interpersonal relationships, especially with equally, if less obviously, disturbed family members, begins to stir up feelings in the therapist for which the latter feels totally unprepared.

Searles (1959a) has discussed aspects of this process as "the effort to drive the other person crazy," and has clarified much about its motivation and mechanisms. The therapist may begin to experience many of the patient's psychotic ideas and disturbing affects as his own. Schizophrenic patients readily project their own distortions, feelings, and conflicts into the therapist. In addition, such patients are very quick to respond, usually in an exaggerated way, to correctly perceived areas of conflict in their therapists. This can be a particularly unnerving experience for therapists unaccustomed to working with schizophrenic patients. In my experience, the therapist's use of pharmacologic intervention at this time represents an unconscious attempt to firmly localize in the patient both that which has been projected into the therapist by the patient (Grinberg 1962), as well as those conflicts within the therapist accurately perceived and accentuated by the patient. The prescribing of medicines is then used as tangible evidence of the interpersonal boundaries between patient and therapist, repudiating any shared ideas and feelings that reveal a growing symbiotic relatedness with its regressive pull on both participants.

The fact of their own readiness to be drawn into symbiotic modes of relating comes as a great surprise to most therapists as they begin work with schizophrenic patients. It is usually thought that for nonpsychotic individuals, the ideas, affects, and modes of relating characterizing both preverbal developmental periods and psychotic states are deeply repressed and unavailable to consciousness without considerable effort. On the contrary, the ease with which new parents, for instance, enter into nonverbal, intense, and mutually gratifying relationships with their infants serves as evidence that relatively well-adjusted individuals, given the right circumstances, have easy access to regressive modes of relating.

In therapeutic work with schizophrenic patients, however, the appearance of symbiotic trends is often an unexpected development, particularly early in the course of treatment. Therapists may find themselves harboring murderous and sadistic thoughts toward patients and important people in their patient's lives, without recognizing that this represents an incorporation of their patients' own hostility and sadism. Therapists may spend sessions daydreaming, only half-listening or half-heartedly trying to engage withdrawn or mute patients. This usually reflects the therapist's defensive flight from the patient's frighteningly aggressive or even more frightening needful and loving impulses. Therapists of schizophrenic patients often entertain the idea that they are able to read their patients' minds. Patients wishing to be magically understood may suggest this by leaving out pertinent parts of a train of thought and then accepting whatever the therapist fills in regardless of its accuracy. Such patients may adopt the therapist's manner of speech and thought, leading the therapist to feel he completely understands and can even anticipate the patient's train of thought; Deutsch (1942) describes related phenomena in her discussion of the "as-if" personality.

Case 2

Miss R., a 28-year-old single woman, was referred by her former therapist because he felt that therapy had come to a standstill, that the patient tended to act out in a bizarre manner, and that the patient needed a therapist with more experience in working with schizophrenic patients. The patient had been very attached to her former therapist and resented being transferred to a new doctor. She began treatment by describing her withdrawal from the world. She no longer had friends, hated her parents, spent hours staring at the walls of her room, and spoke of her life as empty. During the first 6 months of twice-weekly psychoanalytic psychotherapy, she became progressively more withdrawn during sessions, rarely showing much enthusiasm about any ideas she grudgingly admitted to having during the hours. One exception arose when she spoke of her horse, of which she was passionately fond. She described her horse as the only thing to which she felt close, and believed that she completely understood what her horse was thinking and feeling. She treated the therapist as an unwelcome intruder but unfailingly attended sessions. "Only my horse means anything to me." She rarely responded to what the therapist said and spoke little of herself, taking the view that the therapist already understood her completely. She elaborated occasionally on a point he brought up, in a way that seemed to complete his thoughts, but then would fall silent or report that she was daydreaming about riding her horse. Mostly she said nothing at all, and after a while the therapist found himself falling in with the patient's silence.

During these silences the therapist would often daydream about the patient and her family. The patient described her mother as depressed, overtly intrusive, and controlling. She portrayed her father as perpetually angry and uninterested in her mother. She was disgusted with her father because he was, in her eyes, "too seductive" toward her. She felt uncomfortable around him because he was always embracing her, his hands straying toward her breasts and genitals. During one particular session, the patient and therapist had been sitting quietly for 30 minutes. The therapist remembered feeling extremely angry about the patient's father during this silence. He recalled his fantasy of exposing this father, a prominent and respected community leader, as a "disgusting, incestuous fraud." The patient commented at this point, suddenly breaking the silence and startling the therapist with her rare verbalization, that she wished the hour would end so she could get to the stables. The therapist remarked angrily that someday she would have to give up this horse of hers, that people also had something to offer. The patient again fell silent. The therapist thought it ridiculous to feel jealous "toward the patient's horse." He thought the therapy was going nowhere, that "nothing was happening." He decided the patient needed medication to "help get things moving."

This brief clinical illustration illustrates the means by which the therapist takes in the patient's problems. The therapist felt disgusted, murderous, jealous, and ridiculous, while the patient, having emptied these feelings into the therapist, sat quietly wishing to be riding in the country. In supervision, the therapist was able to understand that his wish to medicate arose not from a desire to get things going in the patient, but to stop things from going in himself. The therapist had incorporated the patient's conflicts, experiencing them as his own. He felt out of control, unable to step back from the therapeutic interaction and objectively evaluate what was happening in order to interpret to the patient the feelings she felt unable to contain. His wish to medicate reflected his countertransference inability to use the projective-incorporative process as a means of understanding because he was unable to shift back to a more objective analytic position.

Regressive Gratification

An important issue to consider in understanding countertransference problems and the use of drugs during psychotherapy with schizophrenic patients is the gratification, often not immediately obvious, which is a part of psychosis and symbiotic relatedness. There can be no question that psychosis and the modes of interpersonal interaction characterizing the relationships of schizophrenic individuals must be viewed, at least from the angle of adaptation to society at large, as maladaptive and tragic. However, elements of symbiosis as a severely regressive process are also deeply satisfying and thus tenaciously maintained (Searles 1959b, 1961). This is true for schizophrenics and pertinent to our discussion, for their therapists as well. To return to an earlier analogy, parents of infants regularly greet the milestones of development (communicative use of language, etc.) with nostalgic sadness, recognizing each developmental achievement as a harbinger of the end of very special rewards and gratifications that are only reluctantly relinquished as separation-individuation proceeds. The prolonged use of baby-talk by parents after the child is available for more meaningful communication supports this notion. As treatment begins with schizophrenic patients, and particularly as therapists struggle to make emotional contact with difficult-to-reach patients, they discover to their surprise formerly repudiated regressive yearnings in themselves, which their patients are all too ready to gratify.

Case 3

A supervisee reported, somewhat hesitatingly, that he secretly looked forward to his therapy hours with a particularly regressed schizophrenic patient. He had agreed to include this patient in a caseload of primarily neurotic and borderline individuals with considerable trepidation, recognizing that work with this patient would be difficult and demanding. He reported, however, that after the restrained and often tedious hours with his better integrated patients, he found himself enjoying the no-holds-barred encounters that his schizophrenic patient demanded of him. Although the therapist often ended these therapeutic hours feeling drained and confused, he nevertheless enjoyed and valued these experiences, much to his own surprise. He recognized these crazy hours as a rare opportunity for him to experience ideas and feelings within himself from which he felt cut off in other settings.

He reported that he often thought about medicating his patient, several times made a decision to do so, but never seemed to find an opening. It gradually became clear during supervision that his wish to medicate the patient arose from guilty feelings about enjoying his patient's engaging him in primitive modes of relatedness. Using drugs was a means of disturbing the symbiosis, communicating to the patient that this craziness has got to stop. By doing so the therapist was hoping to renounce in himself gratifying aspects of symbiotic relatedness about which he felt guilty. His reluctance to in fact medicate the patient is evidence of just how powerful are the gratifications inherent in the regressive relationships formed with schizophrenic patients. It further became clear that, in wishing to treat the patient with drugs, the therapist was treating what he viewed as his own craziness manifest in his enjoyment of his patient's bizarre and uninhibited mode of relationship.

The therapist's fear and guilt concerning gratifying aspects of symbiotic relatedness are common motives for introducing phenothiazines during psychotherapy. Drugs may also be used for the opposite reason, to perpetuate symbiosis. Searles (1959b) has noted that in long-term psychoanalytic psychotherapy with chronically psychotic patients, therapists must be wary of blocking their patients' movement away from undifferentiatedness and toward increased personality integration, owing to the therapist's unconscious wish to maintain the rewards of symbiosis. Here drugs are used to block the patient's growth in a variety of ways. Medication may represent an abandonment of hope about increased self-understanding through insight, a communication to the patient that his impulses are too dangerous to express without being dampened by drugs, or a warning to the patient that changes he is making are intolerable to the therapist. A third possibility needs mention here, namely, that drugs may be withheld when their use would be appropriate. This often happens to keep the patient disorganized and thus maintain regressive gratifications. At other times, the therapist may inappropriately withhold drugs in order to join the patient in splitting off the patient's bad self and denying its existence, particularly its aggressive components. In summary, drugs may be inappropriately used or inappropriately withheld to maintain or repudiate regressive gratifications, depending on the therapist's countertransference response to his involvement in regressive forms of relatedness.

Postpsychotic Depression

An important clinical phenomenon pertinent to the dynamics of psychotropic drug usage with recovering psychotic patients is the syndrome referred to as postpsychotic depression (PPD). The PPD syndrome was found to occur in as many as 50 percent of recovering schizophrenic patients in a recent study (McGlashan and Carpenter 1976a; for a review of the literature about PPD, see McGlashan and Carpenter 1976b). In this syndrome, the patient, who while psychotic seems particularly alive, fascinating, and accessible to influence, perhaps excessively so, gradually becomes withdrawn, stubbornly uncommunicative, monotonous, and painful to be with during therapeutic sessions. The therapist who begins work with an acutely psychotic patient is often surprised and dismayed by the appearance of severe depressive symptomatology and is frequently moved to consider using psychotropic drugs at this juncture in therapy.

The dynamics active in therapists confronted with the appearance of severe depressive symptoms following an acute psychotic episode are illustrated in the following vignette:

Case 4

The therapist reported to the author his work with a 22-year-old man who had recently experienced his first psychotic episode, which lasted approximately 6 months. Therapy began while the patient was still psychotic and actively involved with feelings of extraordinary intellectual and physical endowment. He saw himself as a champion scientist, athlete, and lover, and he regaled his therapist with the details of his grandiose ideas.

The therapist, while anxious about his inexperience in doing psychoanalytic psychotherapy with schizophrenic individuals, spoke of his work with enthusiasm and guarded optimism. He expressed both surprise and pleasure at his growing rapport with a patient whom he would heretofore have viewed as incomprehensible and too impaired to enter into a therapeutic alliance. As treatment proceeded, the patient began to express wonder and astonishment at the therapist's own unique qualities, his great perceptiveness, patience, and wisdom. The therapist, while made uncomfortable by the transference idealization and feeling somewhat apprehensive about the patient's reactions should he fail to live up to the patient's expectations, reported on his work with interest and affective involvement.

After about 3 months, the therapist began a supervisory hour by reporting that he was having particular difficulty with another patient with whom he had been working for some time. He noted that therapy with his schizophrenic patient had settled down and was proceeding in an orderly and comfortable manner. After hearing something of the current problems with his troublesome patient, I requested that we return to the therapist's work with the case we had previously been discussing, suspecting that the introduction of troublesome material from work with a new patient represented a commentary on even more troublesome developments in work with the previous patient. In fact, what was hidden behind "proceeding in an orderly and comfortable manner" was painfully tedious and often discouraging work with a depressed, withdrawn, almost mute patient who seemed to be mourning the loss of his omnipotent psychotic feelings. The therapist, who had come to share in a real way the patient's former psychotic ideas and feelings, was himself discouraged, resentful, and feeling hopeless about recapturing the excitement that had been part of the treatment process while the patient was closer to psychosis. In fact, he had changed the patient's phenothiazine to an "activating" phenothiazine, and had added an antidepressant to the drug regimen.

Without commenting on the psychopharmacological soundness of such a decision, some discussion of the psychological forces effecting this decision is warranted. In reviewing with the therapist his reactions to the patient's postpsychotic depression and his thoughts about why he chose to avoid further exploration of therapeutic problems with this patient in supervision, the following themes emerged.

First, the therapist's conviction that he could help the patient was built on shaky ground. He was much influenced by the attitudes of many that schizophrenic individuals are irretrievably impaired and doomed to chronic emotional desolation. For the therapist, the appearance of the patient's feelings of emptiness with the gradual abandonment of protective narcissistic fantasies confirmed his worst fears of an irreversible progression toward burnt-out, chronic schizophrenia. In fact, the therapist admitted that he had, at times, covertly supported and encouraged the patient to maintain his omnipotent ideas in hopes of forestalling what seemed like the inevitable appearance of painful depressed feelings in both himself and his patient.

A second theme that emerged concerns the character of the depression which often follows psychosis. In exploring why the therapist felt disinclined to use supervision to help him deal with the depression which had come to characterize the treatment, the therapist noted that some of his reluctance was related to ambivalent feelings about using drugs in this case. He had the distinct feeling of "treating myself rather than the patient." He noted that his patient failed to take the familiar demanding posture of other depressed patients he had treated, and in fact tended not to complain so much as wish to be left alone. The therapist felt he was intruding on the patient, that he was more upset at the end of each session than the patient, and that his patient had somehow tricked him into believing he could be of help. (No doubt he had similar feelings toward his supervisor for encouraging him to treat this schizophrenic patient.)

The therapist had prescribed the drugs to define who was in distress and to allow himself to feel he was doing something useful for the patient. The therapist was fearful he might otherwise attack the patient for not establishing the kind of relationship he had hoped would follow after the mutual excitement of psychosis. The patient's need to keep the therapist at a distance was experienced by the latter not as an outgrowth of the patient's previous overly close, confusing, anxiety-ridden relationships with deeply disturbed and intrusive parents, but rather as a rejecting, depriving act on the patient's part. The therapist, in retrospect, viewed his own prescribing of medicines at this point as a disguised, hostile, rejecting counter-attack, which he felt his patient and his supervisor would interpret as an abandonment of a psychotherapeutic, investigative stance.

The patient accepted the prescriptions from the therapist without comment. He missed the next session, his first absence since beginning therapy. Upon his return, he began describing his troubles at home. His mother had put him out of the house and he spent the night with his father, whom mother had divorced 10 years earlier. He said he didn't feel at home in either mother's or father's house. He couldn't look people in the eye and tell them how he felt without getting scared. He felt it was hard to talk to his mother because she never believed him and was always preoccupied with her own feelings. He said he didn't know whether "talk therapy" was for him. His mother couldn't understand him and nagged him about getting a job. She felt that the patient's coming to see the therapist was "no indication of illness." He reported missing the session because he was job hunting. He asked his mother to come in his place. "She's a talker." Next he mentioned how different he was from his brother. The patient's mother was always comparing him to his more outgoing brother. She accused the patient of being lazy like his father. After a pause, the patient asked the therapist how the medicines worked. He hadn't filled the prescriptions but was meaning to.

The patient responded to the untimely offer of drugs by talking about being misunderstood by his mother. People kept wanting him to be something he wasn't, more talkative, more outgoing. Mother couldn't understand because her feelings got in the way. He felt put out. We see that the patient correctly perceived the therapist's distress and many of his reasons for prescribing drugs. Although not expressed directly, his perceptions were communicated as displaced observations about people in his family.

Eventually the therapist came to understand the patient's depressive withdrawal as a needed retreat that gave him time to bear the pain of having had a severe psychotic break, to slowly relinquish very important grandiose views of himself, and to partially disengage himself from very destructive family interactions. The patient felt his wishes for personal growth dangerous and, by his withdrawal, was preserving a much needed therapeutic relationship, albeit at a distance greater than seemed comfortable for the therapist. Young therapists generally underestimate their importance to their schizophrenic patients, particularly when the latter are withdrawn and depressed. In this case, the therapist felt that one reason he had put the patient on medication was to justify meetings which the patient was more than willing to attend anyway. This clinical example, while it by no means exhausts the list of dynamic factors which determine the nature and timing of pharmacologic interventions during postpsychotic depression, does illustrate many salient issues which complicate psychoanalytic psychotherapy with recovering schizophrenic individuals.

Conclusions

The introduction of drugs of proven value in the management of psychotic decompensations requires an integration of pharmacologic and psychotherapeutic treatment modalities which is far from complete. Factors other than sound clinical and pharmacological judgment contribute to decision making about prescribing psychotropic drugs in the setting of psychoanalytic psychotherapy with schizophrenic patients. Of particular importance in this regard are the nature and intensity of shared emotional experiences characteristic of work with these patients. The therapist, partly due to the patient's own mode of relating and partly due to the therapist's genuine wish to make contact with and understand his difficult-to-reach patient, reaches deep into his own regressive and largely repudiated store of feelings, memories, and modes of relating, for a common ground upon which to establish a relationship based upon shared experience. Kernberg (1975) refers to an analogous process in work with borderline patients as empathic regression.

As discussed earlier, trial identifications play an important role in this empathic process. The therapist's difficulty in negotiating the shifts back and forth between these trial identifications and a more objective, analytic position results in many of the disturbing feelings leading to the unnecessary or untimely use of drugs. The schizophrenic patient's ability to rapidly establish a mode of relatedness characterized by intense and ubiquitous projective and incorporative identifications often leaves the therapist unable to determine the origin of his own thoughts and feelings. The therapist's unconscious attempts to deal with this problem by prescribing drugs is a form of countertransference frequently observed in work with schizophrenic patients. The widely accepted appropriateness of using antipsychotic agents in this patient group makes this form of countertransference problem particularly likely to occur. As illustrated in the clinical material, the therapist may use the prescribing of drugs as a concrete enactment of establishing interpersonal boundaries, a disavowal of frightening feelings, a guilty renunciation or secret fostering of forbidden regressive pleasures, or a means of establishing control over a seemingly uncontrollable situation. The frequency with which psychotropic agents are used during the course of psychoanalytic psychotherapy with schizophrenic patients, when contrasted with the paucity of information in the scientific literature about the interaction of these different modes of treatment, points out the need for continued analytic investigation of the psychological determinants which play a decisive role in the nature, timing, and outcome of this interaction. This discussion will hopefully lead to further investigation and debate about this important and little-studied clinical problem.

References

Bion, W. R. (1957). Differentiation of the psychotic from the non-psychotic personalities. *International Journal of Psycho-Analysis* 38:266–275.

Davis, J. M. (1975). Overview: maintenance therapy in psychiatry. I. Schizophrenia. *American Journal of Psychiatry* 132:1237–1245.

Deutsch, H. (1942). Some forms of emotional disturbances and their relationship to schizophrenia. *Psychoanalytic Quarterly* 11:301–321.

Feinsilver, D. B., and Gunderson, J. G. (1972). Psychotherapy for schizophrenics—is it indicated? A review of the relevant literature. *Schizophrenia Bulletin* 6:11–23.

Grinberg, L. (1962). On a specific aspect of countertransference due to the patient's projective identification. *International Journal of Psycho-Analysis* 43:436–440.

Grinspoon, L., Ewalt, J. R., and Shader, R. I. (1972). *Schizophrenia, Pharmacotherapy and Psychotherapy*. Baltimore: Williams & Wilkins.

Heimann, P. (1950). On countertransference. *International Journal of Psycho-Analysis* 31:81–84.

———— (1955). A combination of defense mechanisms in paranoid states. In *New Directions in Psycho-Analysis*, ed. M. Klein, P. Heimann, and R. E. Money-Kyrle, pp. 240–265. London: Tavistock.

Karon, B. P., and Vanden Bos, G. R. (1972). The consequences of psychotherapy for schizophrenic patients. *Psychotherapy: Theory, Research and Practice* 9:111–119.

Katan, M. (1954). The importance of the nonpsychotic part of the personality in schizophrenia. *International Journal of Psycho-Analysis* 35:119–128.

Kernberg, O. F. (1975). *Borderline Conditions and Pathological Narcissism.* New York: Jason Aronson.

Klein, M. (1946). Notes on some schizoid mechanisms. *International Journal of Psycho-Analysis* 27:99–110.

Langs, R. (1973). *The Technique of Psychoanalytic Psychotherapy.* Vol. 1. New York: Jason Aronson.

_____ (1975a). The patient's unconscious perception of the therapist's errors. In *Tactics and Techniques in Psychoanalytic Therapy,* vol. 2, ed. P. Giovacchini, pp. 239–250. New York: Jason Aronson.

_____ (1975b). The therapeutic relationship and deviations in technique. *International Journal of Psychoanalytic Psychotherapy* 4:106–141.

_____ (1976). *The Bipersonal Field.* New York: Jason Aronson.

Levy, S. T., McGlashan, T. H., and Carpenter, W. T., Jr. (1975). Integration and sealing over as recovery styles from acute psychosis: metapsychological and dynamic concepts. *Journal of Nervous and Mental Diseases* 161:307–312.

Linn, L. (1964). Use of drugs in psychotherapy. *Psychiatric Quarterly* 38:138–148.

Little, M. (1951). Counter-transference and the patient's response to it. *International Journal of Psycho-Analysis* 32:32–40.

_____ (1957). "R"—the analyst's total response to his patient's needs. *International Journal of Psycho-Analysis* 38:240–254.

McGlashan, T. H., and Carpenter, W. T., Jr. (1976a). An investigation of the postpsychotic depressive syndrome. *American Journal of Psychiatry* 133:14–19.

_____ (1976b). Postpsychotic depression in schizophrenia. *Archives of General Psychiatry* 33:231–239.

Mahler, M. (1968). *On Human Symbiosis and the Vicissitudes of Individuation.* Vol. 1: *Infantile Psychosis.* New York: International Universities Press.

Malin, A., and Grotstein, J. (1966). Projective identification in the therapeutic process. *International Journal of Psycho-Analysis* 47:26–31.

May, P. R. (1968). *Treatment of Schizophrenia.* New York: Science House.

_____ (1971). Psychotherapy and ataraxic drugs. In *Handbook of Psychotherapy and Behavior Change: An Empirical Analysis,* ed. A. E. Bergin and S. L. Garfield. New York: Wiley.

Ostow, M. (1962). *Drugs in Psychoanalysis and Psychotherapy.* New York: Basic Books.

Reich, A. (1960). Further remarks on countertransference. *International Journal of Psycho-Analysis* 41:389–395.

_____ (1966). Empathy and countertransference. In *Annie Reich: Psychoanalytic Contributions,* pp. 344–360. New York: International Universities Press, 1973.

Searles, H. F. (1958). The schizophrenic's vulnerability to the therapist's unconscious processes. In *Collected Papers on Schizophrenia and Related Subjects,* pp. 192–215. New York: International Universities Press.

_____ (1959a). The effort to drive the other person crazy—an element in the aetiology and psychotherapy of schizophrenia. In *Collected Papers,* pp. 254–283. New York: International Universities Press.

_____ (1959b). Integration and differentiation in schizophrenia: an over-all view. In *Collected Papers,* pp. 317–348. New York: International Universities Press.

_____ (1961). Phases of patient–therapist interaction in the psychotherapy of chronic schizophrenics. In *Collected Papers,* pp. 521–559. New York: International Universities Press.

_____ (1975). The patient as therapist to his analyst. In *Tactics and Techniques in Psychoanalytic Therapy,* vol. 2, ed. P. Giovacchini, pp. 95–151. New York: Jason Aronson.

Winnicott, D. W. (1949). Hate in the countertransference. *International Journal of Psycho-Analysis* 30:69–75.

13

The Challenge of Integration

PAUL M. GOLDHAMER, M.D.

The use of psychotherapy and pharmacotherapy in combination remains a neglected area of study. In spite of evidence validating the
combined treatment psychiatrists often avoid this approach. When
combined treatment is employed, insufficient attention may be devoted to the important interactive effects.

Patients may react to the prescription of medication with a variety
of transference feelings such as acceptance, rejection, manipulation
and narcissistic injury. Discussion of interpersonal issues precipitated
by the use of medication can improve not only the doctor–patient
alliance but also the patient's symptomatic experience.

The initiation or discontinuation of medications must be carried
out with sufficient attention to the patient's realistic concerns and
transference distortions. The neglect of a negative transference reaction aroused by the prescription of a medication can result in a
resistance to treatment. Case examples and discussion in the article
illustrate such phenomena.

Psychiatrists need to be aware that their decision to prescribe
medication may be influenced by their own unconscious conflicts
surrounding the use of medication. They may prescribe or fail to
prescribe motivated by their latent fantasies.

Attention to the interactive effects of combined therapy is viewed
as essential in order to aid patients in the dual goals of symptom
alleviation and enrichment of interpersonal experience.

The use of psychotherapy and pharmacotherapy in combination remains a
neglected area of study (Shader and Greenblatt 1982). A frequent misconception
exists that psychiatric drugs can be prescribed with or without psychotherapy.
In fact, a psychotherapeutic relationship is created whenever a patient presents

to a physician in emotional distress and the physician prescribes a drug. Systematic study of this relationship, particularly the aspects of transference and countertransference, can contribute to our understanding of mental processes and to our therapeutic efficacy. Are the effects of the medications we prescribe enhanced or diminished by this doctor–patient relationship?

Psychotherapy and Pharmacotherapy Integration

Klerman (1966, 1975) has written extensively on the combined treatment of depression with drugs and psychotherapy. He has speculated about eleven models whereby psychotherapy and pharmacotherapy interact. Rounsaville, Klerman, and Weissman tested these models in a clinical trial of psychotherapy and tricyclic antidepressants alone and in combination, as treatment for ambulatory depression (Rounsaville et al. 1981). The combination was more effective than either treatment alone, confirming previous reports (Weissman 1979), and the data provided no evidence to support the various hypotheses of negative interactions. This study refutes the hypothesis of a general negative interaction but does not illustrate how interactional effects can influence individual cases. Specifically, it does not reveal how transference issues, precipitated by the use of pharmacotherapy, are handled in psychotherapy.

Subsequent discussion and examples of transference and countertransference reactions in this chapter will show that interactive effects, including negative and positive placebo effects, can be detected in individual cases. Their detection can lead to effective psychotherapeutic interventions that enhance the value of treatment.

Marmor (1981) reviewed the adjunctive use of drugs in psychotherapy. He points out that very little mention of the use of drugs is made in psychoanalytic writings. He reviews the major indications for the use of drugs in psychotherapy, as summarized by the Group for the Advancement of Psychiatry (1975). He concludes that medications are most useful in dynamic psychotherapy to alleviate symptoms on a short-term basis, and to enable a patient to be more accessible to psychotherapeutic exploration. He emphasizes that drugs should be used adjunctively, not as an alternative to dealing with the sources of a patient's problems.

Ostow (1960, 1966) has also written on the use of drugs in psychoanalysis. He believes that medications can improve ego control in certain patients and allow the use of psychoanalytic treatment in instances where it would otherwise be contraindicated.

Sarwer-Foner describes transference and countertransference implications of the use of medications (Sarwer-Foner and Koranyi 1960). He has studied the meaning to patients of the experience of receiving medications, particularly neuroleptic medications. He has found that certain patients are psychologically disturbed by the effects of medications, and implies that they be contraindicated in many such cases.

Resistance to Combined Treatment

In spite of evidence validating the efficacy of combined treatment, psychiatrists often avoid this approach. Docherty and colleagues (1977) have written about the conceptual difficulties of combining the two modalities. Each requires a specific mental set. The danger exists of ignoring one method to maintain cognitive congruence.

Some specialists in pharmacotherapy contend that psychotherapy is unnecessary or even dangerous, in that it leads patients to remain preoccupied with "unhealthy conflict-laden" subjects. These psychiatrists believe that an emphasis on psychotherapy can discourage patients from appreciating the necessary role of medications (Klerman 1966, 1975). On the other hand, psychotherapists may withhold drugs viewing the prescription of medications as promoting an undesirable magical attitude among patients.

Psychiatrists in their training are seldom exposed to teachers who advocate a combined approach, or to models and articles elaborating on such approaches. Consequently when combined therapy is employed, psychiatrists may experience a sense of unease at deviating from orthodox procedure. This may lead to insufficient attention being devoted to the important interactive effects.

Transference Issues

Transference is defined as an unconscious phenomenon in which the feelings, attitudes, and wishes originally linked with important figures in one's early life are projected onto others who have come to represent them in current life (Hinsie and Campbell 1970). Freud first viewed transference as a threat to psychoanalytic treatment. One of his greatest discoveries was that in every case transference, rather than a threat, can become a tool to understand and effect the most secret compartments of mental life (Freud 1916–1917).

Case 1

Mr. A., a 25-year-old married man, was referred to a psychiatrist because of incapacitating agoraphobic symptoms. His symptoms began two years prior to the commencement of treatment and increased after his marriage six months before treatment. He had a controlled and manipulative mother who discouraged expression of affect and blamed the children for her periodic heart attacks. The patient was unaware of anger at his mother, but disclosed his strong feelings against teachers and employers who were authoritarian and manipulative. Diagnosis was obsessive-compulsive personality and phobic neurosis.

Treatment included systematic desensitization and pharmacotherapy with imipramine. The patient reacted adversely to both modes of treatment. He developed marked intolerable side effects to the medications which required their discontinuation. He perceived the dispensing of medication as a manipulative attack on his state of equilibrium. He frequently expressed his fear of "rocking the boat" and of being forced to undergo change against his will. In psychotherapy he became aware of his anger at his manipulative mother and his guilt at expressing this anger. His transference impression of the therapist as a manipulative mother figure was gradually modified by the therapist's interpretations and by the corrective emotional experience of dealing with a nonintrusive therapist. Now he was more receptive to new ideas but still severely agoraphobic. At this time medication was reinstituted. He experienced no side effects and rapid progress ensued.

This case illustrates the virtuous circle created by the optimal combination of psychotherapy and pharmacotherapy. Psychotherapy worked through intense transference feelings precipitated by the use of medications. This allowed the appropriate medication to be employed, which resulted in symptom relief and made the patient even more accessible to psychotherapy. Without discussing in therapy the patient's reaction to the medications, the negative transference reaction could have doomed the treatment to failure.

In chronic schizophrenia, the use of maintenance neuroleptics to prevent relapses has been repeatedly demonstrated Davis (1975). As well, the importance of patients' compliance with a medication regime (in this and all other psychiatric and medical illnesses) has been amply documented. In fact significant failure to take prescribed medications occurs in between 25 percent and 50 percent of outpatients (Blackwell 1973).

Long-acting intramuscular neuroleptics were hailed as a major advance in the treatment of chronic schizophrenia. It was thought that intramuscular delivery of medications would ensure compliance and lower the relapse rate. Yet studies comparing oral and intramuscular fluphenazine have not consistently shown a difference in the relapse rate (Rifkin et al. 1977, Schooler et al. 1980).

One explanation is that forced compliance with a medication regime can result in a negative transference reaction, which reduces the positive pharmacologic impact of the medication (Goldhamer 1981). Chronic schizophrenic patients are particularly sensitive to intrusion and overprotection, and often respond to the compulsory medication as an unwelcome intrusion. Hogarty has reported that relapsers taking fluphenazine decanoate relapse with symptoms of anxiety and depression rather than exhibiting typical schizophrenic symptoms (Hogarty et al. 1979). The anxiety and depression may occur because the more florid psychotic manifestations are controlled by the medication, but may also be present as an expression of the patients' negative transference.

With such patients it is proposed that the relapse rate can be reduced by (1) educating them about their illness and its consequences; (2) encouraging them to participate in decision making concerning type and dose of medication; (3)

working with families to lessen the hostility directed towards the patient; and (4) discussing with the patient his feelings about intrusion (Goldhamer 1981).

When a physician prescribes a medication, powerful unconscious fantasies are aroused in doctor and patient. The patient may fear the omnipotent parent-doctor. He may have fantasies of being poisoned, manipulated, coerced, seduced.

The other side of the issue is the patient's hope for a magical cure delivered by the good doctor. The patient may wish to become dependent on the doctor in a passive childlike fashion. This transference pattern recreates an old situation; the suffering child turns to his parent to have his suffering relieved, to be comforted, to be instructed (Sarwer-Foner and Koranyi 1960).

A universal wish on the part of the patient is to be loved and understood by the doctor. The medication can be experienced as a gift signaling the doctor's concern and indicating he understands the degree to which the patient has been suffering.

Again this gift can arouse ambivalent feelings. The patient may feel rejected and dismissed. He may feel the doctor is prescribing a medication believing him to be too sick to control his own behavior, or he may think the doctor is giving him pills instead of listening to him. The prescription may thus represent a narcissistic injury for one patient, while in another instance the successful alleviation of painful symptoms by a drug may instill hope and confidence in a despairing individual.

Therapist Issues

Psychiatrists need to be aware that their decision to prescribe medication may be influenced by their own unconscious needs and conflicts. Countertransference issues require careful scrutiny. A decision to give medications may indicate an inability on the part of the therapist to accept the necessarily slow pace of psychotherapy. The therapist may need to prove to himself and the patient that he is omnipotent. This places a heavy burden on the patient. As well, the therapist may not be able to tolerate painful affects of sadness and anger, and medicates to treat his own anxiety. The therapist may find the passive role of the psychotherapist frustrating, and prescribe because of his own need to be active. This is illustrated in the well-known phenomenon of the physician who listens to his patient's somatic complaints, cannot make a diagnosis of a physical illness, but feels he must do something for the patient, and so prescribes a tranquilizer.

By prescribing powerful drugs, the doctor may be asserting his authority over the patient. More frequently, he may be expressing his wish to please the patient, and to be loved and admired. At times medications are given as an alternative to time and attention, and represent a distancing maneuver or rejection.

Case Examples and Discussions

Several case vignettes will illustrate some of the above features.

Case 2

Mrs. B., is a 31-year-old married woman who has sought therapy, complaining of anxiety and depressive symptoms. She wished relief from her symptoms, and also expressed a desire to understand herself—why is she prone to depression, why can she not choose a career for herself, why does she dread not only failure but also success?

After 2 months of twice-weekly psychotherapy, depressive symptomatology was prominent preventing the patient from progressing in her life or in therapy. The therapist introduced the possibility of antidepressant medications, explaining their purpose. Mrs. B. expressed apprehensive feelings. "Pills may lead me to present an image of myself that is superficial and overly optimistic." Medications were prescribed and one month later the patient stated, "I am better, but is it me or the pills that deserve the credit?"

This patient verbalized commonly experienced feelings. She was afraid that in prescribing medications, the therapist did not want to listen to her pessimistic feelings, and she would have to present cheerful feelings to please him. These fears were discussed and related to her fears of displeasing her parents. When she made rapid symptomatic improvement, she continued to worry that the improvement was for the therapist's sake. She did not have a feeling of mastery and success. Her difficulty in feeling successful required further psychotherapeutic work.

Case 3

Ms. C. saw her first psychiatrist, complaining of depressive feelings. She recalls the doctor telling her that she was talking as if it were about someone else. He injected her with medication that allowed her to talk more freely. She cried profusely and felt relieved. After two such sessions antidepressant medications were prescribed and therapy sessions became shorter and less frequent. She improved rapidly. Therapy was terminated. She moved to another city and relapsed.

She came to see another psychiatrist and discussed the painful losses she had suffered in the past few years. In discussing her previous therapy, she felt the first doctor had given her the injections because he was impatient and critical of her. As well, she felt the sessions were shortened because he did not want to listen to her.

The new doctor prescribed antidepressant medications and arranged to meet the patient for weekly psychotherapy sessions. For one month the patient was unable to cry. Finally she burst into tears and revealed her fears that this therapist was also demanding immediate progress and would reject her. Her rejection fears were worked through with particular attention to the significance of termination for this woman.

Issues dealing with transference and termination were not adequately resolved in the first therapy. Consequently, she responded to that treatment with temporary improvement followed by relapse on termination. In the second therapy she held back her tears and her progress, feeling angry at what she experienced as a demand to perform, and feeling fearful that when she did perform, she would be quickly dismissed.

Case 4

Mr. D. consulted a psychiatrist because of the sudden onset of jealous feelings, concerning his wife, which he realized to be irrational. He was offered psychoanalysis but refused it, as he insisted on a more rapid form of treatment. He was referred to a second psychiatrist, who examined him and found significant depressive features. This doctor suggested that Mr. D. accept a trial of antidepressant medications. The patient expressed various reservations but agreed. In ensuing visits he revealed that he felt humiliated at having to see a psychiatrist and accept medications. He disclosed his fear of "giving in to feelings." He was ashamed of his jealousy, anger, and sadness. Further, he believed that his subordinate, dependent role in therapy indicated unacceptable weakness in a man. Gradually, he came to accept the need to take medications, and concurrently, became more accepting of "weaknesses" in himself. Depressive symptoms cleared and further psychotherapy led to a less perfectionistic personality.

Mr. D. regarded psychiatric treatment as a narcissistic injury. He refused psychoanalytic exploration but cautiously accepted a pharmacotherapy approach, undoubtedly motivated by his considerable distress. Discussion of his fears concerning medications and psychotherapy allowed him to pursue treatment, and also led to uncovering of his fears of dependency and inadequacy. Symptomatic improvement and careful transference interpretations encouraged him to look more deeply into his psychic make up and to accept himself more fully.

Case 5

Mr. E. is a 30-year-old man who had been seen for over one year when antidepressant medications were proposed. He was explained their purpose and mode of action. In response to questioning he was told that they were not stimulant drugs that would induce a temporary high, but rather were antidepressant medications that would correct a pathologic state. He agreed to take the pills, and he improved in a few weeks. The following exchange occurred at that point between patient and doctor:

Mr. E.: Depression was part of me. You are taking it away. I am losing my freedom.

Doctor: The depression was inhibiting you from being yourself. The medications allow you to be yourself.

Mr. E.: The medications then are removing my inhibitions, and these inhibitions were me as well.

In this dialogue Mr. E. expresses his fear of loss of freedom. Having experienced extremely manipulative parents such a fear was not surprising. The therapist had already discussed the mode of action of the medications. Now a more empathic response acknowledging Mr. E.'s fear of manipulation would have been preferable. Instead he argued with the patient, revealing his own discomfort at being perceived as a manipulator.

Whenever medications are introduced, the therapist must explain his thinking, allow the patient time to consider the issues, and respond to his realistic concerns. The patient's associations including dreams, questions, feelings and memories in the subsequent sessions will reveal transference as well as reality concerns. Transference distortions should be noted by the therapist and interpreted, particularly when a negative transference might result in a resistance to treatment.

The therapist must also be tuned in to countertransference reactions, so that these are not acted out to the patient's detriment. Unconscious conflicts in the therapist can result in inappropriate prescription of medications, lack of sensitivity to the patient's reaction to medications, or alternatively in the inappropriate withholding of medications. A therapist may be reluctant to prescribe a necessary treatment because he feels this would imply that his psychotherapeutic efforts have failed.

The discontinuation of medications is also an activity that must be thoroughly discussed with a patient. The patient needs ample opportunity to ask questions and to express his fears and hopes. Reassurance can be given to the patient that discontinuation of medications will not necessarily coincide with termination of the therapy. Indeed, it is generally inadvisable for the two modalities of treatment to end simultaneously.

Conclusion

Medications can be seen as alleviating symptoms and psychotherapy as improving interpersonal relationships and enhancing self-knowledge. Symptom alleviation will influence the therapist–patient relationship, and discussion of the therapist–patient relationship will influence the patient's symptomatic experience. It must not be forgotten that the act of prescribing medications is part of the interpersonal relationship that needs to be scrutinized. A psychotherapist would not fail to recognize the significance of such changes in therapy as vacations, missed sessions, or termination, and would evaluate their effects. Similarly, he must evaluate the consequences of his prescribing medication and not regard it as a time to assume a new role, that of the authoritarian doctor.

Malan (1979) has systematically researched the methods and outcome of short-term dynamic psychotherapy. He has found that positive outcome correlates with attention to transference and termination issues. It is my contention that medication prescription in no way lessens the need for such attention.

Ostow (1966) has written that even with the most competent prescription of medications, there remains ample opportunity for human suffering. The same may often be said of psychotherapeutic efforts. Only an optimal combination of the methods, and an awareness of their mutual interaction, can best serve our patients' interests.

References

Blackwell, B. (1973). Drug therapy patient compliance. *New England Journal of Medicine* 289:249–254.

Davis, J. M. (1975). Overview, maintenance therapy in psychiatry: schizophrenia. *American Journal of Psychiatry* 132:1245–1247.

Docherty, J. P., Marder, S. R., Van Kammen, D., and Siris, S. (1977). Psychotherapy and pharmacotherapy: conceptual issues. *American Journal of Psychiatry* 134:529–533.

Freud, S. (1916–1917). Introductory lectures on psychoanalysis. *Standard Edition* 16:431–447, 1963.

Goldhamer, P. (1981). Relapse in schizophrenia. *Archives of General Psychiatry* 38:842–843.

Group for the Advancement of Psychiatry (1975). *Pharmacotherapy and psychotherapy; paradoxes, problems, and progress.* Vol. 9, Rep. No. 93. New York: Group for the Advancement of Psychiatry.

Hinsie, L. E., and Campbell, R. J. (1970). *Psychiatric Dictionary.* 4th ed. New York: Oxford University Press.

Hogarty, G. E., Schooler, N., Ulrich, R., et al. (1979). Fluphenazine and social therapy in the aftercare of schizophrenic patients. *Archives of General Psychiatry* 36:1283–1294.

Klerman, G. L. (1966). Psychoneurosis: integrating pharmacotherapy and psychotherapy. In *Successful Psychotherapy,* ed. J. L. Claghorn, pp. 69–91. New York: Brunner/Mazel.

——— (1975). Combining drugs and psychotherapy in the treatment of depression. In *Drugs in Combination with Other Therapies,* ed. M. Greenblatt, pp. 67–83. New York: Grune & Stratton.

Malan, D. H. (1979). *Individual Psychotherapy and the Science of Psychodynamics.* Boston: Butterworth.

Marmor, J. (1981). The adjunctive use of drugs in psychotherapy. *Journal of Clinical Psychopharmacology* 1:312–315.

Ostow, M. (1960). The use of drugs to overcome technical difficulties in psychoanalysis. In *The Dynamics of Psychiatric Drug Therapy,* ed. G. J. Sarwer-Foner, pp. 443–463. Springfield, IL: Charles C Thomas.

——— (1966). The complementary roles of psychoanalysis and drug therapy. In *Psychiatric Drugs,* ed. P. Soloman, pp. 91–111. New York: Grune & Stratton.

Rifkin, A., Quitkin, F., Rabiner, C. J., and Klein, D. F. (1977). Fluphenazine decanoate, fluphenazine hydrochloride given orally, and placebo in remitted schizophrenics. *Archives of General Psychiatry* 34:43–47.

Rounsaville, B. J., Klerman, G. L., and Weissman, M. M. (1981). Do psychotherapy and pharmacotherapy for depression conflict? *Archives of General Psychiatry* 38:24–29.

Sarwer-Foner, G. J., and Koranyi, E. K. (1960). Transference effects, the attitude of the treating physician, and countertransference in the use of neuroleptic drugs in psychiatry. In *The Dynamics of Psychiatric Drug Therapy,* pp. 392–491. Springfield, IL: Charles C Thomas.

Schooler, N. R., Levine, J., Severe, J. B., et al. (1980). Prevention of relapse in schizophrenia, an evaluation of fluphenazine decanoate. *Archives of General Psychiatry* 37:16–24.

Shader, R. I., and Greenblatt, D. J. (1982). Editorial: pharmacotherapy and psychotherapy. *Journal of Clinical Psychopharmacology* 2:1.

Weissman, M. M. (1979). The psychological treatment of depression: evidence for the efficacy of psychotherapy alone, in comparison with and in combination with pharmacotherapy. *Archives of General Psychiatry* 36:1261–1269.

14

Medication Consultation and Split Treatment During Psychotherapy

DAVID A. KAHN, M.D.

In split treatment a patient simultaneously sees both a psychotherapist and a pharmacotherapist. Research indicates that medication and psychotherapy have additive value when used together in the treatment of depression and probably in other disorders as well. However, little is known about the presumably common technique of separate therapists administering these treatments. Complex interpersonal issues arise, reflecting both ideological and transferential attitudes toward medication as well as the intricacies of triangular relationships. Establishing a three-way therapeutic alliance, awareness of competitive countertransference feelings, and recognition of covert issues other than medication in the request for consultation are examples of areas where special attention can help the treatment succeed.

The use of medication during psychotherapy raises interesting issues. I will discuss one way in which medication may be introduced, by consultation and subsequent split treatment. In split treatment a patient essentially has two ongoing therapists: a psychotherapist and a pharmacotherapist. (The latter term is more descriptive than psychopharmacologist). This differs from combined treatment, where one psychiatrist administers both psychotherapy and medication. Psychotherapists seem increasingly willing to recommend concurrent medication for certain patients. One might guess that their decision to employ split or combined treatment depends mainly on their training. This is obvious with nonphysicians; Beitman and colleagues (1984) have estimated that up to 210,000 patients per month are seen in split treatment between psychiatrists and nonmedical therapists in private practice. It is also common and understandable for medical psychoanalysts to ask more pharmacologically experienced colleagues to medicate their patients. At times, even an analyst knowledgeable about medication may prefer split treatment over introducing new parameters.

(For brevity, throughout this article the use of the term psychotherapy will include psychoanalysis.)

I have served as the pharmacotherapist in many rewarding split treatments and have been interested in the dynamic interplays within the triangle of a patient and two therapists. My focus in this article will be the treatment of patients with depressive, anxiety, or character disorders, representative of a typical office practice. Although split treatment also occurs in many hospital and community clinic settings where multidisciplinary teams treat primarily psychotic patients, that most important area is beyond my scope here.

Review of the Literature on Combined Treatment

In the three decades since the advent of neuroleptics and antidepressants, many authors have explored the effects of combining these with psychotherapy. Fewer explicitly address the interpersonal complexities of split treatment or medication consulting (Beitman, Chiles, and Carlin 1984, Chiles, Carlin, and Beitman 1984, Roose 1988). However, the work on combined treatment is relevant, particularly concerning the philosophical tension between the approaches of medication and psychotherapy.

Sarwer-Foner published the proceedings of the first conference to examine this area (1960). Analytic or social milieu treatments were held the only effective treatments for severe illness, although their curative mechanisms were admittedly unclear. Medication was thought not to cure underlying disease in a physiologically specific way but only to stabilize florid symptoms and clarify transference phenomena so that patients would be more amenable to psychological treatment.

Ostow (1962) elaborated on the concept that drugs worked primarily to help patients tolerate the curative stresses of psychoanalysis, cautioning that pharmacologic relief could lead to premature termination. Two examples illustrate his hierarchical view: First, "drugs should not be used in psychoanalysis or psychotherapy unless they are essential to protect the patient or to protect the treatment. If treatment can be successfully conducted without drugs, none should be given" (p. 147). Second, "Ordinarily in analysis we try to avoid taking such steps to make the patient comfortable lest we cut off the flow of analytic material. A comfortable patient has little motivation . . ." (p. 181). Despite his reservations, Ostow pioneered the use of combined therapy. Foreshadowing neurobiologic theories, he postulated that drugs regulate libidinal energy upward or downward and described antidepressants and neuroleptics respectively as energizers or tranquilizers.

Controlled studies of combined treatment emerged in the 1970s, encouraged by thoughtful critiques of research methodology by the American Psychopathological Association (Spitzer and Klein 1976) and the Group for the Advancement of Psychiatry (1975). Initial studies were performed in many illnesses (reviewed by Greenblatt 1975) with landmark work in schizophrenia (Goldstein et al. 1978, Hogarty et al. 1986, Leff and Vaughn 1981) and outpatient unipolar depression (DiMascio et al. 1979, Weissman et al. 1979, The Boston–New Haven Collaborative Study). Promising research areas today include addictions, eating disorders, and anxiety disorders.

Combined treatment of borderline personality is a matter of great interest and controversy. Medication, but not psychotherapy, has been the subject of controlled studies (Cowdry and Gardner 1988, Goldberg et al. 1986, Soloff et al. 1986) though psychotherapy remains the standard treatment. Combined treatment is advised by some authorities when there is comorbidity with a major affective or psychotic disorder (Cole et al. 1984, Gunderson 1984, Marcus and Bradley 1987). There has even been a provocative debate as to which treatment should be regarded as primary and which adjunctive (Goldberg and Schulz 1988, Gunderson 1988).

Most research in combined treatment suggests that psychotherapy and drugs work additively on different aspects of illness; psychotherapy appears most helpful in social functioning, while medication treats abnormalities of mood and thought content. Numerous authors have sought to reconcile the historical competition between treatments (e.g., Beitman and Klerman 1984, Docherty et al. 1977, Goldhamer 1983, Greenhill and Gralnick 1983, Klerman 1983, Marmor 1981, Ward 1984). Among the more interesting, Karasu (1982) suggested that psychotherapy helps chronic "traits," whereas medication treats acute "state" symptoms. Myerson (1982) differentiated between neurophysiologic deficits that a patient "can't change" without medication and resistance that "won't change" but can be treated with analysis.

The Boston–New Haven Collaborative Study of depression provided the best scientific exploration of how medication and psychotherapy interrelate (Rounsaville et al. 1981). The researchers tested the hierarchical view that therapy is superior to drugs and that drugs interfere with therapy. They distilled four traditional hypotheses of negative interactions: (1) drugs could be a negative placebo, increasing dependency and prolonging some kinds of psychopathology; (2) drug relief of symptoms could reduce motivation for further therapy; (3) drugs could eliminate one symptom but create others by symptom substitution if underlying conflicts remained intact; (4) drugs could decrease self-esteem by leading the patient to believe he or she was not interesting enough for insight-oriented work. They also examined the reverse position, that psychotherapy could be harmful in patients sick enough to need medication, either by promoting regression or by encouraging the patient inappropriately not to use drugs. Careful statistical evaluation of outcomes in large samples receiving different treatment combinations revealed no negative interactions. On the contrary, their work supported the theory that the two treatments are additive, not conflicting.

Despite these advances, some writers on combined treatment still show a moralistic preference for psychotherapy, reserving drugs only for psycho-therapy failures. For example, Sarwer-Foner wrote in a 1983 essay approving of the limited use of combined treatment (Sarwer-Foner 1983):

> It is clear that one will not give pharmacotherapy to a patient unless one believes that the symptoms the patient presents and the disease process producing the symptoms cannot be mastered or dealt with by the patient in psychotherapy at that moment in time or space. If this assumption is not correct—if the patient can, in fact, with the help of the physician, correct and master the intrapsychic problems causing the symptoms and the suffering then the psychotropic medication . . . is not really needed. . . . [T]he patient may perceive the act of taking the medicine as proof that he cannot handle his symptoms without it. [pp. 167–168]

Psychotherapy is clearly portrayed as a virtuous treatment, medication as a necessary evil. The main objection is not side effects or toxicity; the objection is that the act of taking medication may be psychologically destructive to a patient's autonomy and self-esteem and to the therapist–patient relationship.

The history of ideological warfare between partisans of talking therapies and drug therapies is too lengthy to review here. Current psychiatric research emphasizes the integration of mental life and neurophysiology, and the interactions between constitution and environmental influence. Within certain constraints, each part molds the expression of the other in shifting causal patterns. The tension between medication and psychotherapy seems archaic; perhaps the deep cultural legacy of mind–body dualism, rooted in traditional religion and later Cartesianism, best accounts for its persistence.

In split treatment an ideological antipathy toward medication (or psycho-therapy) on the part of either the patient or doctors creates obvious conflict. Such a view, however, is not necessarily transferential except in a reductionist sense. Certainly, patients and doctors have strong feelings and fantasies about medication (as with psychotherapy) that may be profitably explored on a symbolic level as transference and countertransference. Often, however, individuals experience their biases about treatment as intellectually or morally based convictions. Within the limited framework of consultation it is rarely possible to change such beliefs. Attempts by the consultant either to interpret them as resistance or to pseudoeducate about "chemical imbalances" are usually doomed to alienate the patient and referring psychotherapist.

The Triadic Therapeutic Alliance

The aim of consultation is to determine whether a particular patient in psychotherapy might benefit from the addition of medication. If the individual patient meets diagnostic criteria similar to those of research populations where medication has proven useful, an attempt is made to engage the patient in a complete trial of pharmacotherapy and continue the indicated psychotherapy without premature termination of either.

I believe that success in split treatment depends on the patient and the pair of doctors forming a three-way therapeutic alliance in which all share a common "reality" view of the illness and treatment plan. Studies suggest that outcome in psychotherapy is strongly related to the presence of a therapeutic alliance (Hartley 1985). It is reasonable to extend this concept to the pharmacotherapist who has become a factor in the psychotherapy. While the term is meant for a dyad, I propose applying it to the triad. A triadic therapeutic alliance requires, along with the right personal "match" (Luborsky and Auerbach 1985), respect between therapists for each other's technique, and sharing of this feeling by the patient. Therapeutic alliance differs from positive transference, which contains unconscious distortions. However, it is vulnerable to negative transference and countertransference storms.

Practical Techniques in Split Treatment

From the time the patient first calls the consultant, care must be taken to foster a three-way alliance. If the patient initiates contact, the pharmacotherapist should find out on the telephone who wanted the consultation. If the idea was the patient's, it is crucial to learn whether the call was made with the knowledge and approval of the therapist. It is unwise and often unethical to see the patient otherwise, except in the rare case where it can be clearly ascertained that the patient is legitimately dissatisfied and not just acting out. I use the patient's referral source as my guide, that is, whether the patient has received my name from a trusted friend or a colleague of mine. A psychotherapist may also call inappropriately, for example, with the unspoken aim of ending treatment and shifting responsibility. Again, my own guide is personal knowledge of the therapist or a referral from a trusted source.

Prior to the consultation the two therapists should discuss several items besides history. First, how is psychotherapy or analysis going? One may learn of hidden transference or countertransference problems that bear on the meaning of the consultation. The point in treatment at which consultation occurs, the beginning or middle (or unconsciously intended end) is also significant; I will return to this later. Second, who should give the patient the conclusions of the consultation? Should this wait in any case until the patient has discussed the consultation in therapy? This may be important if the patient has strong feelings about medication. Finally, who will prescribe and monitor the medication? Supervision of the psychotherapist by the pharmacotherapist is sometimes preferable to split treatment.

At the consultation itself there are two tasks. The first is making a diagnosis using phenomenological criteria such as those in *DSM-III-R* that will lead to a decision about medication. The second is to elucidate psychodynamic factors that may influence compliance and placebo reactions. The consultant's interview technique reflects these goals. It is useful to educate the patient as to the kind of information needed and to explain that the interview style differs from the flow in a therapy session. While the patient's associations are of interest, the consultant should explain that the interview will impose a greater structure of questions and interruptions to elicit certain symptoms. Following Roose (1988), I have found it very helpful to clarify that I will need to learn mainly what the patient feels rather than why he feels it and that medications may treat specific symptoms regardless of their etiology. This approach avoids the unwinnable debate over whether symptoms are "biological" or "psychological" in origin. Roose (1988) eloquently cautions against confusing the psychic meaning of symptoms with their etiology. Beyond symptoms, I also take a psychosocial history and explore dynamic issues; if this surprises the patient, I explain that the information helps us both know what we can and cannot expect from medication and what taking medication will mean. Patients may open-mindedly wonder about the compatibility of medication and psychotherapy. It may reassure patients to describe the effects as additive and emphasize that more can be accomplished in therapy (and in life) when disabling symptoms are under control.

If treatment ensues, I review certain ground rules that differ from those the patient has become accustomed to in psychotherapy. I set a flexible schedule of office visits (anywhere from weekly to monthly until stable) and encourage the patient to make phone calls at both regular and as-needed intervals. Other differences in the framework of treatment include answering most questions directly, obtaining informed consent, and having physical contact for limited examinations.

Regarding confidentiality, the patient must give permission for the therapists to talk to each other. Material is exchanged in both the acute phase and during later decisions about continuing medication. To certain patients it must be made explicit that the therapists cannot keep secrets from each other (such as noncompliance, delusions, or suicidal plans) that would endanger treatment. A final aspect of confidentiality is that if I wish to interview the patient's family at any point, I ask permission first from the psychotherapist in case it would undermine the framework of therapy.

Problems

Objections to Medication

Roose (1988) points out that consultation often goes most smoothly during the initial evaluation phase of psychotherapy. The therapist who considers early on the potential role of medication for appropriate indications has erased the mind–body dichotomy and avoided a competition between treatments.

Requests for consultation in the middle of treatment, often after a few years, are much more problematic (except in the rare instance where a new disorder has developed). In one type of situation there have been good indications for medication all along but either the patient or therapist has opposed the idea. The objector later relents if progress has been unsatisfactory. The opposition on either side may be based both on character problems that predispose toward transference fears of medication, as well on the kinds of ideological problems I discussed earlier. The two causes of opposition need to be handled differently. The consultant's approach must also take into account whether it was the patient or the therapist who initially objected to medication. Two case examples illustrate these problems.

Case Example 1

A 42-year-old housewife in psychotherapy for 4 years with a psychologist referred herself for antidepressant medication. She had first complained of depression to her internist, who started her on amitriptyline 50 mg per day with benefit and referred her to the psychologist. The internist had continued prescribing the same dose although melancholic symptoms recurred after several months. The patient felt that the psychologist helped her significantly with self-esteem and various family problems and remained in therapy with him. By the third year of therapy, however, she began to ask him about having her internist increase the amitriptyline. The psychologist objected, telling her it would be a crutch that would keep her away from deeper issues. At her continued insistence he obtained my name from an analytic supervisor of his who happened to be a psychiatrist; she called me a year later. I called the psychologist before the first appointment; he clearly thought medication would harm therapy. When I saw the patient, she was peeved at her therapist but had no desire to stop what had otherwise been a valuable treatment. I felt she needed more vigorous medication. To avoid catching her in the crossfire between her therapist and me, I decided to avoid a dramatic change and advised her to stay on amitriptyline (a drug I usually do not prescribe) but to raise the dosage gradually over a month. I told her that her internist had made a good initial plan and that we should stick with it, thus allying myself with the source of her referral to the psychologist. I explained that I disagreed slightly with her therapist because I had often seen depressed patients get more out of therapy when they took medication. I offered to call him to discuss my opinion; she agreed to this. A higher dose of medication helped her symptoms, which her therapist soon acknowledged with approval. After several months I was able to switch her over to nortriptyline to reduce her side effects; a year later she remained improved and in therapy.

Case Example 2

A 38-year-old businessman was in analysis for 4 years for depression and obsessional personality. Lack of intimacy with his wife, insomnia, anxiety, and marked anhedonia were his chief symptoms. Early on his analyst advised a medication consultation. The patient refused; self-reliance and abstention from medication had always been admired in his family, and he felt now that he should solve his problems without a crutch. He equated medication with failure of analysis. However, after the 1987 stock market crash he became so anxious that he finally agreed to the consultation. He made his reluctance immediately known to me. His objections were a blend of characterologic conflicts over castration and dependency mixed with an intellectualized view that analysis and medication were incompatible. I realized there was no point trying to persuade him and simply said that while I agreed with his analyst's assessment, medication was not mandatory and that he should make his own decision. He decided to try medication and had a gratifying response to imipramine, not only in reducing his depression and anxiety but also in softening his rigid, aloof character style.

In dealing with the patient's resistance to medication, I left interpretation of unconscious material to the analyst and avoided a power struggle over intellectual questions. These steps may have helped form a three-way alliance, enabling the patient to follow his analyst's advice. Also of interest, the change in chronic personality traits highlights the difficulty separating so-called biological and psychological symptoms.

Therapeutic Stalemate

Therapeutic stalemate may prompt consultation in the middle of treatment, with a hidden desire of therapist or patient to quit. Medication may represent a devaluing threat and a defense against examining transference. The consultant who overlooks these possibilities risks becoming part of the problem. As in the following example, psychotherapy consultation is often more appropriate.

Case Example 3

A 43-year-old woman was referred by her female therapist of 3 years. The therapist of the woman's husband first suggested the consultation to see if a drug-treatable depression was at the root of severe marital problems. The husband told his wife who told her therapist, who called me. I found no cause for medication. However, the patient complained angrily to me that her therapist was too competitive in career issues and directive concerning the marriage. Prior therapy with an older male for 20 years had been supportive and nurturing, ending at the therapist's death. I advised against medication and urged the patient to discuss her anger directly with her therapist. The two shortly agreed on changing to a new therapist. An added complication in this case was that the therapists of both patient and husband were distinguished senior analysts. The husband's therapist had recommended a well-known psychopharmacologist who was also a respected analyst and therefore likely to focus on the problems in the treatment itself.

The patient's therapist chose me, a relative unknown. Flattered at first, I realized that I was part of a plan to avoid subtler issues. I was mildly anxious and felt out of turn offering an unsolicited opinion. Fortunately the patient herself came to grips with the stalemate in the course of airing her feelings. On follow-up a year later she had made progress with a new therapist without medication.

Transference and Countertransference Triangles

Triangular transference problems may arise during split treatment. In one scenario, the patient uses the defense mechanism of splitting object images of the two therapists, idealizing one and devaluing the other, and/or telling different things to each (Sarwer-Foner 1983). Roose (1988) notes that a strong reaction to the consultant often betrays a side of the transference not being expressed in therapy.

Though split treatment might be expected to impair therapy in patients who use the defense of splitting, Gunderson (1984) believes it may aid in treating borderline personality if the patient must split in order to preserve any positive feelings about themselves and others. In the inpatient setting, he advocates a therapist–administrator split to protect the therapist from the anger generated by limit setting on the part of the ward administrator. He extends this principle to medication, where he feels that medication side effects and failures could explode into negative transference and make psychotherapy impossible; both for inpatients and outpatients he recommends having a separate doctor prescribe medication. Dr. Lewis Opler (personal communication) described to me the treatment of a very ill borderline patient that seemed to succeed by a daisy chain of shifting positive and negative transferences to a series of three capable psychiatrists.

Case Example 4

This female, now 28, received combined psychotherapy and medication from her first psychiatrist at age 15. She gradually became disenchanted and began to idealize a medication consultant she had seen intermittently on referral from her therapist. She eventually switched to the consultant for psychotherapy, and then after 3 years repeated the process with a new consultant. The patient has gradually improved, remaining in treatment by always preserving one therapist as a good object. The series of referring doctors were friendly colleagues, which allowed continuity and perspective. All agreed that treatment would not change the patient's defensive structure; instead they made the best of the situation and allowed her to progress at her own pace in other areas of her life.

Defensive splitting is more often a hazard than a help, however. Treatment especially founders when a patient with a severe personality disorder has overtly magical expectations of drugs or a history of addiction. Gratification by the consultant's prescription can turn the psychotherapist into a bad, withholding object and prevent examination of the negative transference. The following case illustrates a classic disaster.

Case Example 5

A 49-year-old divorced woman with severe dependent, histrionic, and narcissistic features was referred by her female psychiatrist for possible hypomania. She had had an episode of major depression 25 years earlier and episodic benzodiazepine abuse since then. Though I agreed she might have hypomania, standard antimanic drugs were of no help except for clonazepam (a benzodiazepine), which, with strict limits on use, aided sleep. For a year the patient continued twice-weekly psychotherapy and saw me every other week. The unusual frequency of our sessions was dictated by continual distressed phone calls to me cataloging ongoing anxiety, dysphoria, and insomnia. She spent most of her therapy session angry at her therapist and most of our medication session trying to tell me about her romantic disappointments. When I pointed out this pattern she said she could not talk to her therapist and found me much more helpful. She deteriorated over the course of the year, finally threatening to stop psychotherapy and see me alone. Of course I told her that this was unacceptable. I also began to think that her hypomanic-appearing symptoms might be manifestations of her personality defenses and not a true bipolar disorder. Her therapist and I then jointly recommended hospitalization for a better evaluation and a potentially hazardous trial of an antidepressant. During a brief hospital stay, by consent of all involved I referred her for combined therapy and medication to a new, male psychiatrist. Over the next year he weaned her from most medication and worked more successfully with her splitting defenses to the point where she returned to work for the first time in years. In retrospect, the frequency of our appointments and my problems limiting our discussions to medication were signs of a destructive split transference and lack of a three-way alliance. Blind spots in my countertransference led me to collude with this seductive patient's acting out of oedipal and preoedipal conflicts.

Countertransference may arise not only toward the patient but also toward the other therapist in the split treatment triangle. Psychotherapists and pharmacotherapists who are ideologically biased may feel defeated if their modality does not "win." Ideology aside, competitive feelings on any ground may catch the patient in the middle. In the worst scenario, countertransference struggles between the two therapists may reduce the patient to a narcissistic object by which to prove a point. Although such florid situations are rare, both therapists should be aware of subtle forms.

Another variation, intergenerational countertransference, arises when a young, recently trained psychiatrist consults for a senior colleague, such as a supervisor, who remains an unresolved oedipal figure (Roose 1988). Although the consultant has expertise to offer about medication, as a student in other respects he or she has a unique opportunity to learn by viewing up close the work of this teacher. Yet this intimacy can also lead to competitive fantasies undone by an anxious, overly deferential posture that hinders giving the best advice.

Problems of Responsibility

Severely ill patients may require an active intervention such as family meetings or hospitalization. Ethical and legal factors dictate that the pharmacotherapist and psychotherapist clarify their roles as early as possible if such events appear likely. When the psychotherapist is not hospital based or a physician, the responsibility to manage the crisis may fall on the pharmacotherapist by default. The change in roles, apart from the inherent nature of the crisis, may be very disruptive to treatment. The pharmacotherapist who has had far less contact with the patient during more normal times suddenly becomes the central figure. The patient may feel abandoned by the psychotherapist; maintaining contact through hospital visits or phone calls is crucial, as is continued communication between therapists. Hidden dynamics may burst forth, particularly if family becomes involved. For example, a family skeptical of the role of psychotherapy in the long-term treatment of a manic-depressive may try to undermine the indicated split treatment plan and shift the goal entirely toward medication management.

Another ethical and legal dilemma arises when the consultant has realistic doubts about the psychotherapy after considering distortions in the patient's report, competitive feelings, and so forth. As a member of a professional community, it would be natural for the consultant to weigh the nature of the relationship with the referring therapist against the risks facing the patient. Careful screening of referral sources can help avoid uneasy collaborations. Optimally, the medication consultant with a broad perspective will know when to recommend that the course of psychotherapy be reviewed by another consultant.

Too rarely addressed is the related question of when the patient sent for split treatment should be transferred to one doctor for combined treatment instead. Split treatment usually occurs by accident, typically when a nonpsychotic, nonsuicidal patient is referred for psychotherapy without assessment for potential medication needs. Thereafter, most psychotherapists who themselves do not prescribe medication will not give up a patient just because medication becomes needed. The split treatment that ensues is expedient; the patient and therapist may have formed a comfortable relationship, at least temporarily benefiting the patient, and a financial arrangement has been entered into, benefiting the therapist. Split treatment ideally should be seen as a coherent plan with specific advantages and disadvantages rather than as a serendipitous "turf" process. In reality, its existence reflects both economic factors and the academic divisions of the mental health field. Properly executed, though, it can succeed admirably in bringing relief to certain patients and the pleasures of collaboration and learning to practitioners.

References

Beitman, B. D., Chiles, J., and Carlin, A. (1984). The pharmacotherapy–psychotherapy triangle: psychiatrist, nonmedical psychotherapist, and patient. *Journal of Clinical Psychiatry* 45:458–459.

Beitman, B. D., and Klerman, G. L., eds. (1984). *Combining Psychotherapy and Drug Therapy in Clinical Practice.* New York: Spectrum.

Chiles, S. A., Carlin, A. S., and Beitman, B. D. (1984). A physician, a nonmedical therapist, and a patient: the pharmacotherapy–psychotherapy triangle. In *Combining Psychotherapy and Drug Therapy in Clinical Practice,* ed. B. D. Beitman and G. L. Klerman, pp. 89–101. New York: Spectrum.

Cole, J., Salomon, M., Gunderson, J., et al. (1984). Drug therapy in borderline patients. *Comprehensive Psychiatry* 25:249–262.

Cowdry, R. W., and Gardner, D. L. (1988). Pharmacotherapy of borderline personality disorder. *Archives of General Psychiatry* 45:111–119.

DiMascio, A., Weissman, M. M., Prusoff, B. A., et al. (1979). Differential symptom reduction by drugs and psychotherapy in acute depression. *Archives of General Psychiatry* 36:1450–1456.

Docherty, J., Marder, S., Van Kammen, D., and Siris, S. G. (1977). Psychotherapy and pharmacotherapy: conceptual issues *American Journal of Psychiatry* 134:529–533.

Goldberg, S. C., and Schulz, S. C. (1988). Pharmacotherapy for patients with borderline personality disorder. (Letter). *Archives of General Psychiatry* 45:195–196.

Goldberg, S. C., Schulz, S. C., Schulz, P. M., et al. (1986). Borderline and schizotypal personality disorders treated with low-dose thiothixene vs placebo *Archives of General Psychiatry* 43:680–690.

Goldhamer, P. (1983). Psychotherapy and pharmacotherapy: the challenge of integration, *Canadian Journal of Psychiatry* 28:173–177.

Goldstein, M. J., Rodnick, E. H., Evans, J. R., et al. (1978). Drug and family therapy in the aftercare of acute schizophrenics *Archives of General Psychiatry* 35:1169–1177.

Greenblatt, M., ed. (1975). *Drugs in Combination with Other Therapies.* New York: Grune & Stratton.

Greenhill, M. H., and Gralnick, A., eds. (1983). *Psychopharmacology and Psychotherapy.* New York: Macmillan.

Group for the Advancement of Psychiatry (1975). *Pharmacotherapy and Psychotherapy: Paradoxes, Problems and Progress.* Vol. 9. Report No. 93. New York: Group for the Advancement of Psychiatry.

Gunderson, J. (1984). *Borderline Personality Disorder.* Washington, DC: American Psychiatric Association Press.

———— (1988). In reply (a letter). *Archives of General Psychiatry* 45:196.

Hartley, D. E. (1985). Research on the therapeutic alliance in psychotherapy. In *Annual Review,* vol. 4, ed. R. E. Hales and A. J. Francis, pp. 532–549. Washington, DC: American Psychiatric Press.

Hogarty, G. E., Anderson, C. M., Reiss, D. J., et al. (1986). Family psychoeducation, social skills training, and maintenance chemotherapy in the aftercare treatment of schizophrenia *Archives of General Psychiatry* 43:633–642.

Karasu, T. B. (1982). Psychotherapy and pharmacotherapy: toward an integrative model. *American Journal of Psychiatry* 139:1102–1113.

Klerman, G. L. (1983). Conceptual issues in combined treatment. In *Psychopharmacology and Psychotherapy.* ed. M. H. Greenhill and A. Gralnick, pp. 13–20. New York: Macmillan.

Leff, J., and Vaughn, C. (1981). The role of maintenance therapy and relatives' expressed emotion in relapse of schizophrenia: a two-year follow-up. *British Journal of Psychiatry* 139:102–104.

Luborsky, L., and Auerbach, A. H. (1985). The therapeutic relationship in psychodynamic psychotherapy: the research evidence and its meaning for practice. In *Annual Review*, vol. 4, ed. R. E. Hales and A. J. Francis, pp. 550–561. Washington, DC: American Psychiatric Press.

Marcus, E., and Bradley, S. (1987). Concurrence of axis I and axis II illness in treatment-resistant hospitalized patients. *Psychiatric Clinics of North America* 10:177–184.

Marmor, J. (1981). The adjunctive use of drugs in psychotherapy. *Journal of Clinical Psychopharmacology* 1:312–315.

Myerson, P. (1982). Won't or can't change? *Journal of Clinical Psychopharmacology* 2:58–62.

Ostow, M. (1962). *Drugs in Psychoanalysis and Psychotherapy.* New York: Basic Books.

Roose, S. P. (1988). Psychoanalysis and Medication. *Bulletin of the Association for Psychoanalytic Medicine* 28:89–92.

Rounsaville, B. J., Klerman, G. L., and Weissman, M. M. (1981). Do psychotherapy and pharmacotherapy of depression conflict? *Archives of General Psychiatry* 38:24–29.

Sarwer-Foner, G. J., ed. (1960). *The Dynamics of Psychiatric Drug Therapy.* Springfield, IL: Charles C Thomas.

_____ (1983). An overview of combined psychopharmacology and psychotherapy. In *Psychopharmacology and Psychotherapy*, ed. M. H. Greenhill and A. Gralnick, pp. 165–180. New York: Macmillan.

Sarwer-Foner, G. J., and Koranyi, E. K. (1960). Transference effects, the attitude of the treating physician, and the countertransference in the use of the neuroleptic drugs in psychiatry. In *The Dynamics of Drug Therapy*, ed. G. J. Sarwer-Foner pp. 392–420. Springfield, IL: Charles C Thomas.

Soloff, P. H., George, A., Nathan, R. S., et al. (1986). Progress in pharmacotherapy of borderline disorders. *Archives of General Psychiatry* 43:691–697.

Spitzer, R. L., and Klein, D. F., eds. (1976). *Evaluation of Psychological Therapies.* Baltimore: Johns Hopkins University Press.

Ward, N. G. (1984). Psychological aspects of medication management. In *Combining Psychotherapy and Drug Therapy in Clinical Practice*, ed. B. D. Beitman and G. L. Kerman, pp. 37–65. Spectrum: New York.

Weissman, M. M., Prusoff, B. A., DiMascio, A., et al. (1979). The efficacy of drugs and psychotherapy in the treatment of acute depressive episodes. *American Journal of Psychiatry* 136:555–558.

15

Psychoanalytic Perspectives on the Use of Medication for Mental Illness

DONALD B. NEVINS, M.D.

The author examines the use of psychoactive medication from the psychoanalytic perspective. He notes that medication has psychological meaning and acquires additional mental representation, and that pharmacotherapy interventions may obscure the differentiation between direct effects of medication on patients and neurotic conflicts in patients. He discusses specific factors involved in the decision to prescribe medication, including the patient's and the clinician's own readiness to use medication, medical countertransference, and common pharmacotherapy interventions (suggestion, manipulation, and inexact interpretation). A case report illustrates issues involved in combined psychoanalytic and neurobiologic treatment.

Prescribing psychotropic medication has become widespread during the past 30 years by a generation of psychiatrists trained to apply neurobiologically active agents to treat symptoms of major mental illness. Recently there has been movement to integrate biologic treatment with psychoanalytic understanding and psychotherapeutic strategies (Elkin et al. 1988a,b). The purpose of this report is to examine, from the psychoanalytic perspective, considerations involved in the use of psychoactive medication for the treatment of mental illness. Following a brief review of the literature, I will discuss some general psychological issues, specific factors involved in the decision to prescribe medication, medical countertransference, and common pharmacotherapy interventions and their implications. A case report will illustrate issues that may arise in the course of combined psychoanalytic and neurobiologic treatment.

Literature Review

A review of the literature should consider the methodologies and levels of abstraction used to infer relationships between the clinical setting (objective behavior, subjective affect, cognition, states of awareness, and doctor–patient interactions) and the domains of neuroscience (psychopharmacology, medication effects, and physiochemical changes). The levels at which medications affect the neurobiologic system may not be related directly to: (1) the transduction of physiologic brain events into psychological meanings (Reiser 1984); (2) changes in the subjective experience of patients (Docherty et al. 1977) or shifts in their psychological functioning; or (3) methods of observation or clinical interpretation, clinical generalization, clinical theory, and metapsychology within the psychological system (Waelder 1962).

Sarwer-Foner (1957, 1960, 1961, 1963, 1983) postulated that chemical changes affect activity–passivity conflicts and may cause the sudden removal of behavioral defenses, with the result that "secondary psychodynamically determined reactions [become] grafted onto . . . neurologically determined responses" (1961, p. 628). Other early investigators (Azima 1961, Ostow 1962) reported changes in libidinal and aggressive drives in conjunction with drug administration. According to Azima (1961), the economic position best explains the alteration of psychic energy by chemical substances. More recent studies of the mood-stabilizing agent lithium carbonate presented evidence for its effect on mania (Loeb and Loeb 1987). These studies hypothesize that the medication reduces the intensity of unconscious and conscious phallic sexual drives, thereby reducing the preemption of ego and superego functioning.

Klerman (1975, 1976, 1978) has questioned the assumption that the combined treatment of depression is not effective; his data indicated that drug therapy facilitates psychotherapeutic accessibility. No evidence was found to support the previously held concepts of a negative placebo effect on the psychotherapeutic relationship, drug-induced reduction of symptoms as a motive for discontinuing psychotherapy, deleterious effects of pharmacotherapy on psychotherapy outcome, premature undermining of defenses, or symptom substitution. However, psychoanalytic measures or inferences obtained from the psychoanalytic situation were not used to arrive at these descriptive conclusions.

In the treatment of schizophrenic psychosis, the transference may be concretized and focused onto the drug as distinct from displacements onto the prescribing physician. May (1976) drew attention to the "significance that drug prescribing and taking has for a . . . patient" (p. 33), including motives ascribed to the person giving the drug. May concluded, "There is, in effect, negative and positive transference to a drug, which is just as irrational as transference to the psychotherapist" (p. 33).

Clinical observers have commented on how the prescription of medication may elicit transference phenomena (Goldhamer 1983), even to the medication itself (Gutheil 1982). The medication may also serve as a transitional object (Hausner 1985–1986), and using medication may have a symbolic meaning (Docherty 1980, Gutheil 1978). The withholding of medication has also been studied (Gutheil 1978). Other authors have described effects of medication on the psychotherapeutic relationship: the problems encountered by the clinician in simultaneously relating to the patient as "both a person and as a disordered biological system" (Docherty 1980, p. 2); the obscuring of countertransference responses, including the arousal of unconscious fantasies and conflicts in the clinician (Goldhamer 1983); and the use of medication to establish interpersonal boundaries and to defend "against the regressive pull of the developing symbiotic relationship" (Levy 1977, p. 15).

General Psychological Issues

Psychological meanings are conveyed and mental representations are acquired by the recommendation to use medication, as well as in the act of taking medication and in the psychopharmacologic effects of medication. To the depressed patient, these factors may imply the sanctioning of punishment for misdeeds, a self-accusatory confirmation of deficiency and inferiority, the assumption of another burden, a self-reproachful sign of personal powerlessness and helplessness, a reinforcement of passive frustrating masochistic tendencies, a pardon, a concrete embodiment of hope and support, a "flight into the pharmacotoxic states" (Radó 1928, p. 429), or a further disappointing resignation to painful loneliness and isolation now that medication may replace human relationships. To the manic patient, these factors may imply an unnecessary and unwelcome interruption in the search for gratification, a debilitating constraint on grandiose creative power and inspiration, a threat to the elated feeling of well-being and to the denial of depression (i.e., a premature and intolerable confrontation with reality), or a muting of sensitivity, alertness, sociability, and sexual drive. To the schizophrenic patient, these factors may imply the loss of magical omniscient control, a penetrating and confusing merger, body-image distortion, a further push toward regressive self-engulfment and narcissistic preoccupation, or a restitutive incorporation into auditory hallucinations with voices signaling their displeasure by prohibiting the medication.

Because significant psychotherapeutic issues arise within the matrix of the doctor–medication–patient relationship, this matrix can be viewed as a target function (Irwin 1974) and, as such, can have broader explanatory and clinical power than a more restrictive target symptom or target diagnosis. Issues arising in medication usage may provide opportunities for psychotherapeutic understanding. According to Gutheil (1978), the prescribing of medication is "as rich in potentially useful affects, fantasies, and associations as any other aspect of the therapeutic process" (p. 225). Thus psychopharmacology can be viewed "as part of the fabric of therapy" (p. 225). Furthermore, the transference can prove instrumental for dealing with the mental representation of medications, the dynamic and economic shifts accompanying their use, their psychological functions, the seemingly adverse medication effects, and patient compliance (Nevins 1977).

In contemporary practice, psychiatrists often prescribe needed medication for the patients of nonmedical psychotherapists. This situation raises questions about the splitting of the transference. Freud's (1958) observation may be pertinent: "For when all is said and done, it is impossible to destroy anyone *in absentia* or *in effigie*" (p. 108). This division of responsibility may interfere with understanding of the subsequent effect of treatment on symptoms, and it may circumvent exploration and integration of combined psychoanalytic and neurobiologic treatment. There is a need for systematic treatment outcome studies of patients with different prescribing and treating clinicians.

The Decision to Medicate

The decision to use psychotropic medication—itself a dramatic, substantive, and powerful therapeutic modality—requires careful consideration. At least five specific factors are involved in this decision: (1) the context of the initial contact between clinician and patient, (2) the evocative influence of the patient on the clinician, (3) the paradigm that guides the clinician, (4) the natural science model, and (5) clinicians' views of their own and their patients' roles in treatment.

The Context

The clinician's initial contact with a patient frequently occurs when the patient is struggling with regressive symptoms and levels of functioning. In addition to the patient's need for symptom relief, the clinician's decision to medicate may be influenced by social and legal pressures. Clinicians are increasingly confronted with community expectations and standards. Stone (1984) has noted that failure to administer biologic treatment for certain mental disorders, such as depression, may be viewed as negligent and thus may subject the practitioner to the threat of legal malpractice.[1] Furthermore, an appeals court, in deciding a case involving insurance payment, upheld a ruling in which bipolar affective disorder was judged a physical illness, with its treatment costs to be reimbursed at a higher rate than treatment for mental illness (*Arkansas Blue Cross and Blue Shield v. Doe* 1987).

The appeal and constraints of medical orthodoxy may also influence the decision. Clinicians may align themselves with scientific recognition and respectability by using quantifiable biologically active substances within the biomedical model. Gutheil (1982), however, has denoted as "the delusion of precision" the view of "medication as having the virtues of concreteness, specificity, precision, and straightforwardness" (p. 322). Exclusive reliance on serum lithium levels or on "therapeutic windows" (e.g., serum nortriptyline levels) as inclusive measures may be such instances of misleading belief systems.

---

[1] A recent debate has highlighted the issues of the putative right to biologic treatment and lack of establishment of psychoanalytic treatment efficacy (Klerman 1990) and the potential adverse consequences of standardized clinical procedures (Stone 1990).

Factors that may contribute to a readiness to use a biologic solution are not inherently problematic, provided the choice rests with the clinician without preemption of alternatives or the illusion that the medication will provide, for the clinician, a complete understanding of the patient's biopsychosocial functioning.

The Evocative Pull

The clinician's use of medication may be influenced by a protective response to the patient's evocative unconscious wishes and motivations. Consider the excited, omniscient, elated, seductive, merging, gratification-seeking wishes of the manic patient; the empty, lonely, fragmented disorganization covered by the bizarre restitutive efforts of the schizophrenic patient; or the reproachful, clinging, insatiably and relentlessly punishing, immobilized, ambivalently devouring strident appeals, failings, and exigent yearnings of the depressed patient. The mode of expression of the patient's complaints, and their meaning to the clinician, must be consciously factored into the decision to medicate.

The Conceptual Paradigm

Every clinician is guided by a paradigm (Kuhn 1970), or organizing explanatory system, which is acknowledged as the foundation for clinical practice. The present-day psychiatrist organizes data most parsimoniously to explain descriptive phenomena (DSM-III-R 1987), thereby defining what should be studied and treated and emphasizing control of target symptoms. However, the units of observation corroborating the neurobiologic descriptive model, if viewed as all-inclusive measures, run the danger of "enumerative inductivism," that is, "the view that any observation entailed by a hypothesis 'supports' it, and that the greater the number of such positive instances of a hypothesis [that are collected] the greater the degree of empirical 'support' " (Edelson 1984, p. 1).

Exclusive reliance on medication can obscure other factors that contribute to treatment outcome. Furthermore, if the clinical puzzle does not fit the paradigm, the aberrant factors may be unrecognized, disregarded, or even disavowed (Kuhn 1970). These attitudes, which are appropriate for narrowing the parameters of research criteria, can jeopardize a specific treatment regimen; that is, if a patient's experience is not responsive to pharmacologic manipulation, the clinician may regard that lack of response as a misdiagnosis, irrelevant to treatment outcome, or dismiss it as simply a problem of everyday living.

The Natural Science Model

In psychopharmacologic treatment as it is frequently practiced, the patient is the sole object of study. The clinician is left out of the equation. Yet it is the clinician who organizes behavioral data into a diagnostic syndrome and implements pharmacologic therapy. It is the clinician who assesses the indications for medication and monitors patient compliance, serum levels, pharmacologic side effects, duration of drug usage, and symptom response.

This approach is modeled on experimental science. However, despite the fact that in ordinary patient care, clinicians "constantly perform experiments" that are "designed, executed, and appraised" (Feinstein 1967, pp. 21–22), such as in laboratory work, clinical medicine is essentially a *natural* science. Accordingly, everything that pertains to the patient's condition and treatment is data (G. L. Engel, personal communication, December 10, 1981), including the behavior and attitude of the clinician/experimenter. Excluding the clinician fails to fully consider the natural situation. Such exclusion removes the clinician's own scientific instrument and capacities, the "human equipment" (Feinstein 1967, p. 29), as a valuable object of study and source of data. To view the patient as a physiologic apparatus, the clinician as psychologically inert, and the interaction as unaffected by this mutual refraction threatens to artificially modify the data.

Roles of Clinician and Patient

Viewing the clinical situation as a process involving an engaged, rather than a nonparticipating, observer-clinician emphasizes the relevance of clinicians' beliefs in both their own and their patients' roles. Balint (1972) described the "apostolic function" whereby each clinician possesses "a vague, but almost unshakably firm, idea of how a patient ought to behave when ill. . . . *It was almost as if every doctor had revealed knowledge of what was right and what was wrong for patients to expect and to endure, and further, as if he had a sacred duty to convert to his faith all the ignorant and unbelieving*" (p. 216). Psychiatric clinicians who are committed to a clinical attitude based exclusively on biologic mechanisms can ignore psychological factors in either doctor or patient; they can regard countertransference as an irrelevant distraction; and they can replace ambiguity with conviction.

Medical Countertransference

The role of medical countertransference is central to a full understanding of medication usage. As explicated by Lewin (1946), medical training introduces physicians to their first patient, the cadaver. As the accommodating prototypal model for future clinicians, the cadaver is entirely passive, compliant, and "unresistant to the dissector's intentions" (p. 195). To avoid identifying with the patient as a human being, medical students can pretend that they are emotionally detached from the cadaver. More than 40 years ago, Lewin cautioned that "the heat which rises from so many useless clashes between the proponents of 'organic' and 'psychological' medicine might not appear, if it were realized that the main issue was a matter of preference, an emotional preference for the dead or the live patient" (p. 197). His prophetic insight is equally applicable to our modern psychiatry, and the passionate insistence that major mental illness is entirely biologic in origin, to be treated pharmacologically to the exclusion of meaningful psychotherapy, may represent such a preference.

A clinician's readiness to medicate may be influenced by unconscious or conscious identification with the patient. At some level, clinicians recognize patients' needs and may therefore modify treatment to transiently (and safely) feel like the patient. By the use of medication, clinicians may seek to maintain a link to their patients by substantively and symbolically placating, satisfying, or indulging them, thereby sustaining therapist–patient ties. Medication may thereby provide a plausible compromise, serving as a "reflexive acceptance of the role which the patient is forcing on [the clinician]" (Sandler 1976, p. 46). Clinicians may thus offer a solution to their patients' distress while distancing themselves from unpleasant aspects of transient identification with patients.

There is also a universal primitive unconscious sense of danger experienced by individuals in the presence of sick people (Lewin 1946). There may be plausible exigencies that obscure this component of the clinician's motivation for self-protection. For example, clinicians can justify their insistence that the agitated, depressed patient take medication because the illness renders the patient ruminative, self-doubting, indecisive, and immobilized to pursue goal-directed behavior. The clinician steps in, decides, and both are relieved.

Furthermore, clinicians may derive comfort from theoretical models that explain the beneficial effects of medication. For example, in the treatment of schizophrenia, neuroleptics have been hypothesized to diminish disproportionate perceptual input and central nervous system activation, thereby reducing jamming of the central nervous system and the resulting psychotic disintegration (Lehmann 1974). When medication is considered a prerequisite to psychotherapy to reduce the schizophrenic patient's inner disorganization, such theory may serve to rationalize the therapist's own withdrawal from the patient.

Pharmacotherapy Interventions

Pharmacotherapy can be instituted with unstated attitudes about the mind, which, in turn, may have consequences for psychotherapy. Three types of interventions (Bibring 1954) are commonly employed: (1) suggestion, (2) manipulation, and (3) inexact interpretation.

Suggestion

With suggestion, the clinician attempts to induce in the patient, without the patient's conscious participation, a set of attitudes and beliefs and an emotive stance toward the medication. It may be labeled an "antidepressant" (rather than the more descriptive term, "psychic energizer"), an "antipsychotic" (rather than the more neutral term "neuroleptic"), or an "antimanic" (rather than the more phenomenologic term "mood stabilizer"). Thus the medication appears to oppose depression, psychosis, and mania. The emphasis shifts from an auto-plastic orientation toward an alloplastic, or other-than-self, solution. In so doing, there is an implicit recognition of a "friendly paranoi[d]" (Glover 1931, p. 410) view of the illness process. The patient's depression/psychosis/mania is an alien force that must be eliminated. The clinician's view of the symptom as an enemy to be expunged in battle by the antisymptom drug weapon has its psychological correlate. By magically designating the symptom as an invading enemy (Reider 1955), the clinician imparts the expectation that the patient will, in time, renounce the exorcised disturbers (e.g., "it takes approximately 3 weeks to achieve an effective serum level").

When clinicians incorporate hypotheses into their explanations of medica-tion, patients may experience the message concretely as unquestioned truth. How is a depressed patient to process the statement, "This antidepressant medication is given to correct a disturbance in brain chemistry"? Statements involving scientific terminology invite additional concretizations. These hypoth-eses are replete with phrases such as "chemicals going across spaces," "finding their way to receptors where keys fit," "blocking of reuptake," or with analogies to disturbances in metabolism such as a diabetic individual's need for insulin. These explanations may stimulate a patient's unconscious fantasies or confirm pathogenic beliefs of personal defectiveness, deficit, or vulnerability. Major mental illness does not confer immunity from neurotic conflicts, compromises, and distortions. Accordingly, neurotic disturbances may be intensified and neurotic components obscured by medications, particularly when the symptom-reducing effects are substantial. There may even be an additional element of trauma. The patient's fantasy (e.g., I am defective) and the experienced or suggested reality (e.g., I require lithium carbonate indefinitely to function) may be interpreted as confirming, thereby reinforcing the patient's original fantasy and contributing to a readiness to be medicated.[2] This fantasy may be expressed alternatively as an obligatory refusal to take medication, in part serving defen-sive functions (e.g., I do not want a crutch; what I need is a proper diet).

Closely aligned to suggestion is the *placebo effect,* that "therapeutic proce-dure . . . [that] has an effect on a patient, symptom, syndrome, or disease, but which is objectively without *specific* activity for the condition being treated" (Shapiro 1961, p. 75). The clinician's unambiguously positive attitude toward medication, "an ingredient compounded into every prescription" (p. 77), may be internalized and, as an introject (Schafer 1968), have a felt presence within the patient. The clinician's faith, beliefs, and needs interact with transference-based

---

[2]This theory is consistent with Greenacre's view (1971) wherein "the basic fantasy will . . . be a fusion of the genetically determined instinct representation with whatever responding stimulations the environment has to offer. These may reinforce the endogenous elements in the nuclear fantasy" (p. 278). She added, "Fantasies that are brought one way or another into activity in outer reality and meet there an . . . intensified form of apparent confirmation and assume, thereby, the cloak of the trauma are particularly likely to be repeated . . . in activity" (p. 283) and to be confusing.

responses in the patient, such as magical expectations and trust, as well as with the patient's desire to please the clinician. By accommodating the clinician, patients are providing their own counterpart to the placebo effect.[3]

Manipulation

Manipulation occurs when the clinician employs "emotional systems *existing in the patient*" to produce "favorable attitudes toward the treatment situation or to remove obstructive trends" (Bibring 1954, pp. 750–751, italics added). The clinician's understanding of and attitude toward symptoms may be central. Are symptoms regarded as the product of intrapsychic conflict or of physiologic deficiency (Wexler 1971)? In depression, self-punitive trends may combine with pathogenic beliefs of injury to yield a conviction that something wrong has already happened and that reparation is necessary (Brenner 1976). Self-criticism by the depressed patient may combine with neurotic factors to modify, for example, what is, in the clinician's view, a biochemical disturbance, so that it is experienced by the patient as a psychological defect. A positive symptomatic change at the descriptive level may be transformed into a silent negative therapeutic reaction that confirms defectiveness, unworthiness, and a need to make reparation.

Inexact Interpretation

A third type of intervention in pharmacotherapy is a form of inexact interpretation (Glover 1931). By prescribing psychoactive medication, clinicians may convey to patients the view that biologic mechanisms provide the exclusive explanation of symptoms and treatment courses. Clinicians may intend—or patients may experience—such explanations as unacknowledged interpretations that enhance denial and repression. In psychotherapy, patients may internalize their clinician's attitudes or "interpretations." As Glover (1931) noted, "The physician encourages the patient by demonstrating his own capacity for repression"—and denial; "he says in effect, 'You see, I am blind [here the entire explanation is genetic or biological]; I don't know what is the matter with you: go and be likewise' " (p. 405).

There are also considerations of the transitional object and transitional phenomena (Winnicott 1953). Medication may allay anxiety in the patient's "state of intimate separation" (Stone 1961, p. 86) from the clinician. The clinician-medication unit may function as an introject that the patient experiences as an inner presence existing within "the confines of his body or mind or both" (Schafer 1968, p. 72). This emotional relationship with the clinician-medication unit, which the patient subjectively experiences either continuously or intermit-

---

[3]The concept of placebo (a term derived from *placere, to please*) is frequently viewed as stemming primarily from the clinician's own desire to please.

tently, may be enhanced by long-term drug administration (e.g., lithium treatment for bipolar illness). Periodic laboratory examinations that yield data such as serum lithium levels may sustain this tie.

Case Report

Ms. A., a 34-year-old artist with a history of occasional substance use (marijuana, wine), sought treatment for symptoms of depression. During a period of 2 years, she had become increasingly dysphoric and irritable, with progressive vegetative depressive symptoms of sleep disturbance, early morning awakenings, diurnal mood variation, periods of crying, weight loss, and diminished energy, sexual drive, and appetite. Ms. A. brooded over her capacity to care for her toddler son and to love her husband. She found it increasingly difficult to concentrate. This condition was superimposed on chronic low self-esteem wherein she felt defective, inadequate, unworthy, unwanted, unlovable, and flawed. She was unable to complete a professional degree. She feared exposure and avoided displaying her artistic abilities, preferring to remain unobserved in the background.

Ms. A.'s diagnosis was major depression with melancholia superimposed on a dysthymic disorder (depressive neurosis). In addition to exploratory psychoanalytic therapy (three times a week), she received psychoactive medication (desipramine, stabilized at 200 mg per day; serum level: 209 ng/ml; reference therapeutic range: 40–280 ng/ml). When I prescribed the medication, I indicated to her that the medicine, in conjunction with the psychoanalytic therapy, might alleviate her vegetative depressive symptoms. Psychoanalytic therapy allowed us to explore Ms. A.'s experience of and response to the medication. The process helped her to recognize that her understanding, although plausible, was not unequivocal and that her "experience of the situation is based to a greater or lesser degree on determinants within [herself]" (Gill 1984, p. 165). The patient's verbalizations about the medication were treated like other associations. By prescribing the medication and then inquiring into its effects, however, I was, in a real and concrete manner, entering into her psychophysiological life. Furthermore, my use of psychoactive medication introduced de facto suggestive and manipulative elements (Bibring 1954) into the treatment process.

Initially, Ms. A. viewed the effects of combined treatment with uncertainty and confusion. Although she had previously been convinced that something was wrong with her, she had believed that her discomfort had both organic *and* psychological origins. Once medication was prescribed, however, her conscious focus changed, and she attributed her ailment solely to a physical cause. Compounding this interpretation was her belief that she had previously deceived herself by thinking that there was a psychological element when the problem was *only* organic. Her previously disquieting uncertainty was thus relieved by shifting and concretizing her ambivalence onto a physical condition. In addition to negating the psychological conflict, she could no longer blame alcohol and marijuana (i.e., externalize her problem) because she had quit using these substances. Rather, she viewed her depression as caused by her "chemistry . . . an allergy to something that is irritating me . . . a physical reason like diet or hypoglycemia" (a medical condition). Medication, she said, would do away with the "physical reason . . . clear up the part that is not me . . . eliminate all that is wrong with me." The medication thus served initially to disavow, purge, and suppress recognition of psychological "dis-ease," conflict, and causality, and to commemorate a belief in bodily deficit.

As Ms. A.'s depression showed early signs of improvement, her responses indicated additional transference-based meanings. She reported feeling better but wondered whether she should be using medication. Equating chemical substances (marijuana, wine) with prescribed psychiatric medication, she noted her previously unsuccessful efforts at self-cure. She recognized the amelioration of symptoms and enhanced functioning, yet feared an increasing dependency. Although at first she was attracted to the prospect of psychoactive medication ("an easy answer"), she now found herself relying on it. This reliance "reinforced . . . [that] there is something wrong with me." Although Ms. A. initially viewed her medication as a crutch, she began to worry about whether she could have managed or felt the same without the medication. This doubt intensified her feelings of deficiency, her conflicts over autonomy and closeness, and her fears of loss of control and of the unconscious. However, the treatment process was reassuring and protective, and she perceived it as preventing her from doing something drastic or irrational. Increasingly, Ms. A. experienced the medication as an extension of the analyst. Furthermore, she externalized the presumed deficit in herself, as represented by the medication, and adopted a passive attitude. It was "no longer me" nor her "responsibility." Rather, she would be taken care of by a fusion of the analyst and the drug. She believed it was simply up to her to let the analyst know how she felt and, by this arrangement, she would become intact. Medication would resolve her physical problem so that she could address the mental problems, a situation in which she was now assured of the analyst's presence.

Ms. A. became troubled, however, by the idea of "taking something I don't know anything about." Her complaint that she also knew little about the analyst led to an elucidation of an additional transference theme. Characterologically, she made efforts to observe others while remaining "invisible" in the background, and she saw the analyst as a possible threat to her privacy. She began to have phobic concerns about therapy, which were initially expressed in relation to the medication. She questioned whether the desipramine caused her to hallucinate, because she experienced a strange feeling of dreaming soon after sleep onset.[4] She feared that someone was in her room and that she would fall off her bed. In her dream, Ms. A. was trying to get away from someone but was unable to move. She alluded to the transference by disclosing that she had started sleeping in a separate bedroom. Mutual tension had ensued: Her husband felt that she had "closed the door" on him sexually; she felt that he had "closed the door" on her emotionally.

Within 14 weeks of attaining the stable medication dosage, Ms. A. noted that she had become more articulate and "less hobbling." She disclosed that she had become more active, assertive, penetrating, and excited toward her husband, but she felt that her efforts were producing no lasting effect. She also wanted a response from me. However, she then became apprehensive about her recent revelations to me and wanted to take them back—"smooth it over." She reported a second dream in which she was with her son at a petting zoo in an amusement park. Everyone seemed unconcerned, although a crocodile with *soft* skin was snapping at people! In her dream, she had incorporated the "smooth" day residue into its manifest content, serving to hide and reverse what she believed to be wrong with her. Nonchalant on the surface, she was hard and menacing underneath. She feared that if she exposed her toughness, I would regard her as a repugnant and devouring person (the way she perceived herself) and take flight.

As the transference unfolded, Ms. A. began to doubt her ability to remember significant events, including previous states of mind. She wondered whether her mind was playing tricks on her or if she was deceiving herself. She reported a third dream, in which she was trapped and falling off the bed. This time, however, she could not move because she was drugged. The scene shifted to a party where she was with people she distrusted, and she herself was in a partially drugged state. The other people there seemed concerned that she was sick, but she could not arouse their interest to elicit help. She tried to discover what they were up to. They walked by, brushing against her, scraping her arm, and giving her an injection like a smallpox vaccination. My inquiry about whether she experienced the medication (i.e., desipramine) as harmful or protective led to our more direct exploration of transference resistance, neurotic conflict, cognitive processing, and recall of traumatic memories, revealing that she experienced the medication as having subdued her and muted her feelings. She held things in check and resisted spontaneity because she was unsure of what would "come out" or how I would react to her exposures. Like the crocodile in the second dream, she could appear nonchalant yet be menacing underneath: "Can't

---

[4]Depression has been noted to be accompanied by shortened REM latency (Kupfer et al. 1978), although medication effects cause suppression of REM. The hypnopompic experience bore psychological resemblance to the Isakower phenomenon (Isakower 1938).

let me see my strong side . . . it's safer to smooth it over . . . and be missing something." This insight led her to suspect something perverse in herself. Just as the neurosis may represent a negation of the perversion (Freud 1953), Ms. A. defended against her belief in a bodily defect with a fear of exposure and with the putative effects of the medication, which in turn necessitated submission, punishment, the muting of her exhibitionism, and the numbing of her desires.

Further explication of the function of Ms. A.'s self-deception followed. The medication had previously served as an inexact focus for uncertainty and self-deception, as was the case when, early in the treatment process, she concluded that she had erroneously construed her illness as both physical and psychological. Now, apprehensively, she wondered whether she characteristically and actively attempted to re-create events and to "reorder" her memory. She recalled, as a young adult, placing herself in a situation in which she could have been raped, only to subsequently rear-range the events in her mind and then to wonder what had really happened and how she had "made it safe." Similarly, there was recall, reconstruction, and initial working through of earlier childhood experiences, including her father's abandonment of the family when he learned that she was a girl, her intense desire to disavow her gender identity and become a boy, her sexual exploitation by a pedophilic uncle, and her repeated fondling by a grade-school teacher during preadolescence.

Discussion

Psychoactive medication produces neuropharmacologic changes that suddenly affect the patient's mental apparatus. Waelder's (1976) principle of multiple function could be extended to a consideration of the ego's function "actively to assimilate" the effects of medication "into its own organization" (p. 71). The introduction of psychotropic medication confronted my patient with psychological tasks. Initially, she responded passively to this imposition by concluding that her problem was caused by an innate physical deficit, which served an economic function accompanied by an awareness of unresolved characterologic residues of self-deception. Ms. A. believed that people could not trust her because she was untrustworthy, an attitude consistent with a narcissistic withdrawal through which she attempted to secure the pardon of her superego (Radó 1928). Furthermore, although psychotropic medication initially alleviated Ms. A.'s symptoms, it also laid the groundwork for a masochistic attitude by eliciting passivity toward an innate defect, a depressive dynamic originally described by Abraham (1968).

Ms. A.'s neurovegetative symptomatic improvement led to conflict between relief from depression and a shift in mental representation, which, in turn, was expressed in the transference. She responded defensively to her "need" for medication and the attendant impairment of self-esteem by introjecting the analyst/drug. The clinician-medication unit, which served as both a need-satisfying object and a "needed functional capacity" (Dorpat 1977, p. 21), would counter the state of helplessness associated with Ms. A.'s basic depressive response, thereby providing "a vehicle for . . . [attaining a] state of well-being" (Joffe and Sandler 1965, p. 398), with accompanying feelings of safety and security.

Ms. A.'s response to the pharmacologic effects of medication and the symbolic meaning of being medicated were assimilated into her character structure, where they aroused neurotic conflicts and were then organized and expressed as transference resistances. The clinician-medication unit trapped her so that she was unable to move. She expressed further passive–active conflicts in relation to her defended exhibitionistic-scopophilic instincts. She "smoothed" over her ambivalent and orally tinged, devouring, hidden genital defectiveness, a component of her depressive symptomatology. Likewise, to the extent that the medication served as a plausible inexact explanation for the muting and sub-duing of her desires rather than of her characterologic hiding, the components of self-deception, negative oedipal conflicts, and reordering of events were initially obscured. Similarly, the psychological issues central to Ms. A.'s psychosexual development and her traumatic history of early paternal rejection and sexual molestation were expressed in relation to the medication and were reenacted as a transference resistance.

For Ms. A., being medicated during psychoanalytic therapy acquired psy-chological representation and was accompanied by dynamic and economic shifts. Issues related to character structure, to the dynamics of the transference, and to the psychodynamics of depression were expressed in relation to medication.

References

Abraham, K. (1968). Notes on the psycho-analytical investigation and treatment of manic-depressive insanity and allied conditions. In *Selected Papers of Karl Abraham,* trans. D. Bryan and A. Strachey. pp. 137–156. New York: Basic Books.

Arkansas Blue Cross and Blue Shield v. *Doe,* 733 F.2d 429 (S.W. Cir. 1987).

Azima, H. (1961). Psychodynamic and psychotherapeutic problems in connection with imipramine (Tofranil) intake. *Journal of Mental Science* 107:74–82.

Balint, M. (1972). *The Doctor, His Patient and the Illness.* 2nd ed. New York: International Universities Press.

Bibring, E. (1954). Psychoanalysis and the dynamic psychotherapies. *Journal of the American Psychoanalytic Association* 2:745–770.

Brenner, C. (1976). *Psychoanalytic technique and psychic conflict.* New York: International Universities Press.

Diagnostic and Statistical Manual of Mental Disorders (1987). 3rd ed., rev. Washington, DC: American Psychiatric Association.

Docherty, J. P. (1980). Psychotherapy and pharmacotherapy: clinical problems. *Yale Psychological Quarterly* 3:2–11.

Docherty, J. P., Marder, S. R., Van Kammen, D. P., and Siris, S. G. (1977). Psychotherapy and pharmacotherapy: conceptual issues. *American Journal of Psychiatry* 134:529–533.

Dorpat, T. L. (1977). Depressive affect. *Psychoanalytic Study of the Child* 32:3–25. New Haven, CT: Yale University Press.

Edelson, M. (1984). *Hypothesis and evidence in psychoanalysis.* Chicago: University of Chicago Press.

Elkin, I., Pilkonis, P. A., Docherty, J. P., and Sotsky, S. M. (1988a). Conceptual and methodological issues in comparative studies of psychotherapy and pharmacotherapy. Vol. 1: Active ingredients and mechanisms of change. *American Journal of Psychiatry* 145:909–917.

—— (1988b). Conceptual and methodological issues in comparative studies of psychotherapy and pharmacotherapy. Vol. 2: Nature and timing of treatment effects. *American Journal of Psychiatry* 145:1070–1076.

Feinstein, A. R. (1967). *Clinical judgment.* Baltimore: Williams & Wilkins.

Freud, S. (1953). Three essays on the theory of sexuality. *Standard Edition* 7:123–245.

—— (1958). The dynamics of transference. *Standard Edition* 12:97–108.

Gill, M. M. (1984). Psychoanalysis and psychotherapy: a revision. *International Review of Psycho-Analysis* 11:161–179.

Glover, E. (1931). The therapeutic effect of inexact interpretation: a contribution to the theory of suggestion. *International Journal of Psycho-Analysis* 12:397–411.

Goldhamer, P. M. (1983). Psychotherapy and pharmacotherapy: the challenge of integration. *Canadian Journal of Psychiatry* 28:173–177.

Greenacre, P. (1971). The influence of infantile trauma on genetic patterns. In *Emotional growth: psychoanalytic studies of the gifted and a great variety of other individuals,* vol. 1, pp. 260–299. New York: International Universities Press.

Gutheil, T. G. (1978). Drug therapy: alliance and compliance. *Psychosomatics* 19:219–225.

—— (1982). The psychology of psychopharmacology. *Bulletin of the Menninger Clinic* 46:321–330.

Hausner, R. (1985–1986). Medication and transitional phenomena. *International Journal of Psychoanalytic Psychotherapy* 11:375–398.

Irwin, S. (1974). How to prescribe psychoactive drugs. *Bulletin of the Menninger Clinic* 38:1–13.

Isakower, O. (1938). A contribution to the patho-psychology of phenomena associated with falling asleep. *International Journal of Psycho-Analysis* 19:331–345.

Joffe, W. G., and Sandler, J. (1965). Notes on pain, depression, and individuation. *Psychoanalytic Study of the Child* 20:394–424. New York: International Universities Press.

Klerman, G. L. (1975). Combining drugs and psychotherapy in the treatment of depression. In *Drugs in Combination with Other Therapies,* ed. M. Greenblatt, pp. 67–81. New York: Grune & Stratton.

—— (1976). Psychoneurosis: integrating pharmacotherapy and psychotherapy. In *Successful Psychotherapy,* ed. J. L. Claghorn, pp. 69–91. New York: Brunner/Mazel.

—— (1978). Combining drugs and psychotherapy in the treatment of depression. In *Depression: Biology, Psychodynamics and Treatment,* ed. J. O. Cole, A. F. Schatzberg, and S. H. Frazier pp. 213–227. New York: Plenum.

—— (1990). The psychiatric patient's right to effective treatment: implications of *Osheroff* v. *Chestnut Lodge. American Journal of Psychiatry* 147:409–418.

Kuhn, T. S. (1970). *The Structure of Scientific Revolutions.* 2nd ed. Chicago: University of Chicago Press.

Kupfer, D. J., Foster, F. G., Coble, P., et al. (1978). The application of EEG sleep for the differential diagnosis of affective disorders. *American Journal of Psychiatry* 135:69–74.

Lehmann, H. E. (1974). Physical therapies of schizophrenia. In *American Handbook of Psychiatry,* vol. 3, ed. S. Arieti (2nd ed., pp. 652–675). New York: Basic Books.

Levy, S. T. (1977). Countertransference aspects of pharmacotherapy in the treatment of schizophrenia. *International Journal of Psychoanalytic Psychotherapy* 6:15–30.

Lewin, B. D. (1946). Counter-transference in the technique of medical practice. *Psychosomatic Medicine* 8:195–199.

Loeb, F. F., and Loeb, L. R. (1987). Psychoanalytic observations on the effect of lithium on manic attacks. *Journal of the American Psychoanalytic Association* 35:877–902.

May, P. R. A. (1976). Psychotherapy and pharmacotherapy of schizophrenia. In *Successful Psychotherapy*, ed. J. L. Claghorn, pp. 24–42. New York: Brunner/Mazel.

Nevins, D. B. (1977). Adverse response to neuroleptics in schizophrenia. *International Journal of Psychoanalytic Psychotherapy* 6:227–241.

Ostow, M. (1962). *Drugs in Psychoanalysis and Psychotherapy.* New York: Basic Books.

Radó, S. (1928). The problem of melancholia. *International Journal of Psycho-Analysis* 9:420–438.

Reider, N. (1955). The demonology of modern psychiatry. *American Journal of Psychiatry* 111:851–856.

Reiser, M. F. (1984). *Mind, Brain, Body: Toward a Convergence of Psychoanalysis and Neurobiology.* New York: Basic Books.

Sandler, J. (1976). Countertransference and role-responsiveness. *International Review of Psycho-Analysis* 3:43–47.

Sarwer-Foner, G. J. (1957). Psychoanalytic theories of activity-passivity conflicts and of the continuum of ego defenses: experimental verification, using reserpine and chlorpromazine. *Archives of Neurology and Psychiatry* 78:413–418.

———— (1960). Recognition and management of drug-induced extrapyramidal reactions and "paradoxical" behavioral reactions in psychiatry. *Canadian Medical Association Journal* 83:312–318.

———— (1961). Some comments on the psychodynamic aspects of the extrapyramidal reactions. *Revue Canadienne de Biologie* 20:623–629.

———— (1963). On the mechanisms of action of neuroleptic drugs: a theoretical psychodynamic explanation. In *Recent Advances in Biological Psychiatry*, vol. 6, ed. J. Wortis, pp. 217–232. New York: Plenum.

———— (1983). An overview of combined psychopharmacology and psychotherapy: summing up and critical comments. In *Psychopharmacology and Psychotherapy*, ed. M. H. Greenhill and A. Gralnick, pp. 165–180. New York: The Free Press.

Schafer, R. (1968). *Aspects of Internalization.* New York: International Universities Press.

Shapiro, A. K. (1961). Factors contributing to the placebo effect: their implications for psychotherapy. *American Journal of Psychotherapy* 18(Suppl.):73–88.

Stone, A. A. (1984). The new paradox of psychiatric malpractice. *New England Journal of Medicine* 311:1384–1387.

———— (1990). Law, science, and psychiatric malpractice: a response to Klerman's indictment of psychoanalytic psychiatry. *American Journal of Psychiatry* 147:419–427.

Stone, L. (1961). *The Psychoanalytic Situation: An Examination of its Development and Essential Nature.* New York: International Universities Press.

Waelder, R. (1962). Psychoanalysis, scientific method, and philosophy. *Journal of the American Psychoanalytic Association* 10:617–637.

———— (1976). The principle of multiple function: observations on overdetermination. In *Psychoanalysis: Observation, Theory, Application: Selected Papers of Robert Waelder*, ed. S. A. Guttman, pp. 68–83. New York: International Universities Press.

Wexler, M. (1971). Schizophrenia: conflict and deficiency. *Psychoanalytic Quarterly* 40:83–99.

Winnicott, D. W. (1953). Transitional objects and transitional phenomena: a study of the first not-me possession. *International Journal of Psycho-Analysis* 34:89–97.

16

Depression: When Is Psychotherapy Not Enough?

SHEPARD J. KANTOR, M.D.

Any patient in analytic psychotherapy may simultaneously have two illnesses, one psychologic and one biologic, and these two illnesses may have independent origins and may require separate and concurrent treatments. This concept, which is embodied in the multiaxial diagnostic categories of *DSM-III,* has represented a major advance in psychotherapeutic thinking.

The introduction of medication has profound effects on ongoing treatment, which must be analyzed. Technically, it should be regarded as would the introduction of any parameter; that is, it is dealt with by interpretation. In fact, the introduction of medication can facilitate the psychotherapeutic process.

Traditionally, analysts have focused on the metapsychology of depression; the author instead views the mental productions of patients in a major depression as a consequence of altered central nervous system chemistry. These biologic instabilities can in turn compromise development in children and adolescents.

Traditionally, there have been two contexts in which to consider depression when it occurs in the course of an ongoing psychoanalysis or psychoanalytically orientated psychotherapy. It has been viewed as a transference manifestation (that is, a reflection of something occurring between the analyst and the patient), or it has been viewed purely intrapsychically, instances of which might be aggression turned against the self, or ego reactions to failures to live up to one's ideals or moral standards. Although either of these dynamics are possible, and other formulations might be brought forth depending on the details of any particular patient's treatment, therapists must now consider the possibility that the depression has arisen as an independent illness that must be understood in a biologic and not an analytic context, and it must be treated medically and not analytically.

Unfortunately, it is at this juncture that biologically and analytically oriented therapists often part company with biologists and those with a psychoanalytic orientation; the former focuses on the depressive illness as a medical condition requiring antidepressants, and the latter focuses on a range of dynamic formulations that would require interpretation.

In recent years, certain affective states have been viewed in a medical/biologic context and not in terms of psychology. There is now general agreement as to the clinical characteristics of major depressive disorder: weight loss, loss of appetite, sleep disturbance, decreased sexual interest, diurnal variation in mood, impaired concentration, diminished interest in surroundings, and depressed or dysphoric mood. In some patients, suicidal thinking is prominent, whereas others who are equally depressed may not be at all suicidal. This condition may occur as a single episode or as a recurrent illness.

The Effect of Medication on Ongoing Treatment

Given that the patients I discuss are in analytically oriented treatment, the occurrence of a biologic illness, its course, how medication is prescribed, who prescribes it, and what the relationship is between the primary therapist and the psychopharmacologist, all become issues in psychotherapy. Greenfeld (1985), in his book about the treatment of psychotic patients, discusses some of these factors in great detail. What he says about the therapy of psychotic patients is also applicable to work with patients suffering from affective disorders.

He assumes that the primary responsibility for psychotherapy or analysis is in the hands of the therapist and the medication is in the hands of the psychopharmacologist. However, this can only work optimally if the two know what the other is doing. This means that the psychopharmacologist must know something about therapy and the therapist something about medication. Are medications being changed too frequently? Are plasma levels of medication of benefit and have they been obtained? Are side effects being attended to? Is the patient becoming preoccupied with "side effects" that are unlikely to be medication related? Should medication be continued after the patient is well and for how long? Is the patient complying with medication? If not, are there psychological factors that must be analyzed before the patient is willing to accept medicine? In addition to questions like these, the therapist must be prepared for managing transference splitting and fantasies about the relationship between his or her two therapists. I will try and illustrate some of these concerns with clinical material.

What issues does the patient confront in having to take medication? I recently saw a young actress in consultation for mood instability. My recommendation that she have a therapeutic trial of lithium carbonate upset her greatly. She was unable to begin medication until she worked intensively with her therapist on issues related to the severe manic-depressive illness of her mother. The patient had lived in dread of carrying the same diagnosis and prognosis as her mother, and it was not until the irrational components of this were analyzed that she could attempt medication.

For some patients, compliance is interfered with because they do not like the idea that they are taking medicine. For them, being on medication means that they have some type of insanity and avoiding medication serves to deny this. Others state that taking medication makes them feel powerless. A type of powerlessness is well described by Bursten (1985), who discussed two patients who, rather than being relieved that they had a treatable biologic condition, were alarmed that they had an illness beyond the control of their will. For them, avoiding medication avoided the notion that they were out of control.

Major differences of opinion between the treating therapist and the psychopharmacologist can be detrimental to the patient.

A recovered alcoholic man, actively participating in Alcoholics Anonymous, (AA) became severely depressed. When referred he had become nonfunctional at work and in his marriage. History revealed two previous untreated depressive episodes. It seemed clear that he would benefit from medicine. However, the AA sponsor who accompanied him, taking a rather extreme and rigid stand on the general AA policy concerning avoidance of medications, in effect forbade the patient to take any. After the consultation in which I met with both the patient and this sponsor, the patient went home and tore up his prescriptions. Fortunately, this was a substitute sponsor and on return from vacation his usual sponsor voiced the opinion that although he felt medications were to be avoided, taking antidepressants was the patient's decision. The patient, continuing his participation in AA and telling no one, took medication and was fully recovered in 2 weeks.

For another patient, differences of opinion between her therapist and the consultant ended treatment.

A 21-year-old woman was referred at the urging of her family after 6 weeks of four-times-a-week psychotherapy had not benefited her condition. Six weeks before that had begun, she had interrupted a summer abroad because she had become unable to function—she could not eat, do her schoolwork, or cope, and felt that she had "lost her feelings." She said that for the first time in her life, "Nothing meant anything to me." During 6 weeks of psychotherapy, her therapist found her to be vague and nebulous. She could not talk and seemed to show thought blocking. He felt she was repressing a great deal. When asked about this after her recovery, she described herself during that period as having lacked imagination and added, "Thoughts just wouldn't come to my mind."

At the time of the consultation, she appeared severely withdrawn and depressed, was sleeping and eating poorly and said about herself, "I feel

neutral; I don't feel things; Things don't effect me the way they used to."
Although she was not suicidal, she thought, "Death wouldn't be that
different from the way I am now." Unable to decide between my recommendation for medication and her therapist's contrary recommendation,
she returned to college in another city and resumed treatment with a
previous therapist. Independently he started her on medication and she
promptly improved. Two months later she returned, wishing to continue
medication under my supervision while she resumed therapy with her
former therapist. He, however, refused to treat her if she remained on
medication. At that point she began psychotherapy with me. This initially
focused on her illness and how it had affected and might continue to affect
her life. Concerns about where she ended and her illness began were
prominent as were her feelings about her family's reaction to the illness.
Her mother blamed her: "It's anger turned against yourself. Get treatment,
find out why you have such anger and get yourself better!" Her father's
initial attitude was that she should pull herself together, complete her
schoolwork, and not be so self-indulgent.

     As with other patients suffering from affective disorders, issues related
to her personality disorder, such as her masochistic attachment to a boyfriend, her failure to live up to her intellectual potential, and sexual fantasies
and dreams of which she had recently become aware, were all noted, but
their exploration was deferred in view of the patient's struggle with the
recognition of her affective disorder and its impact on her life.

Medication as a Parameter

     Those who discuss the subject of parameters usually cite Freud's having
commanded a phobic patient to enter a feared situation as an example of a major
departure from interpretive technique. As defined by the American Psychoanalytic Association, the term *parameter* applies to an aspect of technique that
departs from interpretation as the exclusive tool (More and Fine 1968). Its use is
circumscribed by four caveats: (1) its introduction should only be undertaken to
prevent the psychoanalytic process from coming to a standstill; (2) it should not
make a return to standard technique impossible; (3) it should become dispens-
able after fulfilling its usefulness; and (4) the patient should be able to gain insight
into its function.

     In my view, the occurrence of an episode of major depression during the
course of therapy represents something not accessible to analytic intervention
that has intruded on the psychotherapeutic treatment. It needs to be treated as
a medical condition, either by the physician-therapist or by a consultant working
in concert with the nonphysician-therapist. Technically, the introduction of
medication should be regarded as would the introduction of any parameter and
would have to be handled accordingly.

     Kurt Eissler (1980) has extensively discussed the use of parameters. He states, "A parameter is irreconcilable with psychoanalytic technique if it would convert the transference into a relationship per se inaccessible to psychoanalytic interpretation" (p. 385). Therefore, when a parameter is introduced, "the meaning which this parameter has had for the patient and the reasons which necessitated the choice of the parameter must retrospectively be discussed, that is to say, interpretation must become again the exclusive tool to straighten out the ruffle which was caused by its use" (p. 400).

Providing that the therapist thoroughly explores and interprets issues related to the facts and implications of the patient's biologic illness, the psychological consequences of having to take medication, and fantasies about the therapist's or consultants actual prescription of medication, the psychotherapeutic or psychoanalytic process should not be interfered with. In fact, the introduction of medication can facilitate the psychotherapeutic process, often by bringing to light areas of previously unexamined psychological life.

This can be exemplified by another case.

A 33-year-old woman had been in psychotherapy for 3 years. Medication had been discussed over the years as the psychotherapy had not benefited her moods, but the patient had been reluctant to obtain a consultation. This time the therapist insisted, and the consultation was reluctantly pursued. At the time of the consultation, her concentration was poor and she was functioning less well than usual. Her sleep, appetite, and sexual interest were all impaired, and she was spontaneously tearful at work where she was a highly functioning professional.

When placed on antidepressant medication her mood improved considerably. Her chronic obsessional worrying, very much exacerbated by her depression, had diminished. Her appetite improved, she was no longer crying at work, and her concentration was better. As to the impact of all this on her treatment, she said, "Now I talk about what the worrying means, I used to just voice the worries. Now I see their connection to my mother. She worried all the time. Worrying has been a memorial to her."

This patient was also able to gain insight into her initial reluctance to take medication. "My mother demanded that I be perfect. Perfect people don't take medication."

Another patient illustrates ways in which medication can eliminate behavioral manifestations of a biologic illness, which, because of their origin, had been previously uninfluenced by psychotherapeutic work.

This 47-year-old woman had been in twice-weekly psychotherapy for 2 years. She had entered treatment because of marital difficulties and a depressed mood. According to her therapist, she initially appeared to have an anxiety neurosis with oedipal dynamics. During the course of psychotherapy her depression waxed and waned. Treatment focused on issues of separation, marital discord, difficulties at work, especially arguments with coworkers. Neither her mood nor her difficulties with co-workers and supervisors seemed to be influenced by psychotherapy. After 18 months of therapy, she had a severe depression. Imipramine helped her substantially, but the question of a subtle bipolar illness prompted the psychiatrist to urge a consultation. At that time she gave a history of severe 2-week depressions each fall, less severe depressive episodes several times each year, and a 10-day period 7 years previously of "cockiness" that she had never had before. In addition, her difficulties at work seemed a result of periods of irritability that came and went without apparent reason.

A lithium trial was begun. She continued to work in psychotherapy on marital, separation, and job-related issues. However, once lithium was instituted, there were no further episodes of fighting at work. She reported herself as no longer being so easily provoked, and consequently there were no more cycles of provocations and lashing out followed by the subsequent need to rationalize her behavior. Both she and her therapist felt that when she was depressed or upset, she was less overwhelmed by affect and could work more effectively in psychotherapy. She also experienced herself as having become more stable in her moods.

The issue of whether positive feelings engendered by the use of medication adversely effect the transference is raised by another case.

A 26-year-old medical student with overwhelming depression and anxiety was referred for a consultation when, because of her symptoms, she was considering dropping out of medical school. The patient had had four previous episodes of illness characterized by poor sleep, poor appetite, weight loss, loss of interest in her surroundings, and failure to be concerned about her personal hygiene. Five years of psychotherapy had not helped either her anxiety or her incapacitating bouts of depression, and she decided to switch therapists. The psychiatrist with whom she began a new course of treatment felt her moods should be treated with medication but did not wish to manage the medications herself. With antidepressant medication, her symptoms markedly improved and she no longer doubted her capacity to pursue her medical studies. The patient's fantasy about her therapist and the medicating physician was that of idealized parental surrogates working together for her benefit. How wonderful she thought her new therapist to be for making the correct diagnosis!

What are the consequences of such an intervention for transference? Or, to directly address one of Eissler's concerns: does such an intervention make a return to psychoanalytic technique impossible? Of course the patient will have positive feelings engendered by the therapist's prescribing or recognizing a disorder for which medications need to be given and for feeling better, often in a dramatic way. But this should no more interfere with the treatment than the patient's recognizing real life benefits from psychotherapeutic work.

For instance, a woman who overcomes her impulse to terminate a basically satisfactory relationship because the work of treatment has enabled her to better understand the neurotic components to this impulse, will of course be very appreciative of her therapist's work. No one would suggest that such positive feelings would represent an interference with treatment.

Similarly, the beneficial effects of the accurate diagnosis and treatment of a patient's affective disorder would be expected to intensify positive transferential feelings. Over valuation of the therapist's referral for drug treatment could be worked with analytically, as would any other grandiose inflation of the therapist's abilities. Alternatively, in patients who must resist the expression of positive feelings toward the therapist, this would provide further material that could be worked with in treatment.

Mortimer Ostow (1957, 1961, 1966, 1987) is an analyst who over the past 25 years has consistently written about the concurrent use of drugs and psychoanalytic treatment. He makes a number of clinical observations that are as relevant now as when they were written. These include the ideas that little analytic work is possible when a patient is in a state of severe depression and that in some states of depression, most, if not all, clinical improvement is attributable to medication. He states, "I doubt that the demonstrations of the ego maneuvers and defenses, the pointing up of superficial connections among symptoms, symptomatic behavior and external events, and directing attention to problem areas are sufficient to control the pathogenic tendencies" (1957, p. 458).

Concurring with Eissler, Ostow states, "Everything which happens in the transference can be prepared for and interpreted and the additional analytic material that issues can only facilitate, not retard definitive psychotherapy," and adds, "While the patient may use the drug cure to reinforce his resistance to psychotherapy, I should not have been able to justify to myself withholding an instrument that would prevent a possible suicide, merely in order to ensure *better treatment* if the patient survives" (Ostow 1961, p. 15). Finally, Ostow stresses, "The classical theory of psychoanalytic psychodynamics is valid only within certain limits . . . [we should not] ignore its deficiencies, or struggle to patch them up or mask them, rather than make the changes that reality requires" (Ostow 1987, p. 279; see Chapter 8, this volume).

This brings us back to the main theme: that patients may have two independent illnesses with the biologic disorder arising independently of the work of an analytic treatment. The disorder's expression may be a consequence of periods of biologic vulnerabilities that have nothing to do with intrapsychic life, but rather are explainable in terms of genetic predisposition, such as fluctuating chemical states the control of which is on a biologic basis.

This, of course, raises the question of whether or not I believe intrapsychic life has anything to do with the onset of an affective episode. As I view it, people with affective disturbances demonstrate a spectrum of vulnerabilities to the onset of an episode. Any patient might have all of his or her affective episodes triggered by conflict, loss, and so on; others could have episodes unrelated to psychological issues or apparent real life stress; still others might have each type of episode.

Not long ago I saw a physician in consultation who some years previously had completed an analysis, which by her estimation and that of her analyst, had been very successful. She had had two previous depressions and now had the onset of a third, which at the time of the consultation was incapacitating. She asked whether she should resume analysis or begin another.

In view of the level of satisfaction with the rest of her life, I advised an exclusively medical approach to her current illness and suggested that she reevaluate the question of resuming analysis after this episode of depression had been successfully treated. When placed on medication, she fully recovered and chose not to resume analysis. It is now a year later and she is entirely well.

One might view this patient as having had a flight into health or a resistance to further analytic treatment. If one had more data, one might attempt to give a specific analytic explanation for the current episode of illness.

However, to do so would be to ignore Ostow's (1987) caveat, "Classical theory of psychoanalytic psychodynamics is valid only within certain limits" (p. 278). In my opinion, the episode of illness in this particular patient was beyond those limits. The unpredictable manifestation of her depressive illness occurred at a time unrelated to her psychological state and called for an other than psychological treatment.

Another patient's clinical presentation was quite the opposite.

A 50-year-old architect sought treatment for his third episode of depression, the first having occurred at age 36 and the second at age 44. Each episode had lasted several months and the symptoms each time were quite similar. He described himself as being "uptight," preoccupied with business concerns, generally negative about his work, and guilt-ridden about his behavior toward his wife and children, although they had no complaints and he did not normally have such guilty feelings toward them. Although he referred to all this as "anxiety," his wife felt that he appeared and acted depressed. He acknowledged loss of appetite and weight loss as well as early morning awakening. He felt worse in the mornings, with his tensions gradually diminishing as the day progressed. He had lost his usual interests and found himself quite tearful. His mother had received electroconvulsive therapy 30 years previously and was currently on antidepressant medication.

What was so striking about his history and current illness was that each of these three depressions had occurred in an almost identical context: prior to each episode his career had dramatically advanced. There was little doubt in my mind that these depression were psychologically triggered and from what little background information I had, seemed related to conflicts over his own father's death 13 years previously. Unfortunately, he absolutely refused psychotherapy, stating that he saw no value in it. He was placed on antidepressant medication. Though his plasma levels were low, the time course of his recovery and his relapse 3 weeks after discontinuing medication indicated a true drug response.

My own speculation is that insight-oriented therapy would have and still might serve to prevent him from having a similar stress trigger future endogenous episodes. It is also possible that preventing such situationally specific episodes might preclude or delay the onset of future endogenous episodes, which may well begin to appear in the absence of such specific psychologic circumstances. Psychotherapy might prevent future episodes by interfering with the development of "kindling," which I will describe later.

Metapsychology

Analytic theories have in common the notion that severe states of depression represent some extension of the normal personality. Cornell (1985), in his attempt to integrate biologic and psychoanalytic ideas about depression, speaks of the dynamic, structural, and genetic contributions to the depressed state. All of this implies some continuum between mild and severe states of depression. However, when he speaks of economic considerations, Cornell refers to states of endogenous depression where an individual is overwhelmed with (instinctual) forces of other than psychological dimension with which he or she is unable to cope. Ostow (1966) also talks about affective syndromes that "can be defined solely in terms of energy equilibrium, with little regard for childhood or current experience, or current psychodynamic interaction" (p. 272). In such states, characteristic defenses are evident but overstressed and ineffective.

Cornell refers to two states of qualitatively identical structural and dynamic relationships but with *quantitative* differences in the strength of affective (instinctual) forces to be mastered and regulated. "Six weeks after treatment with medication, the previously incapacitated person still has a recognizable obsessional, guilt ridden personality with underlying oral issues. Psychoanalytic therapy still provides themes of addressing the dynamic and structural problems which plague the person in everyday life" (p. 31).

He states, "Psychoanalytic theory has from the outset regarded biological factors as compatible with a psychological model of psychopathology." Echoing Ostow, he adds, "It is crucial that psychoanalytic theory not abandon quantitative concepts and not foreclose the opportunity to incorporate advances in the biological domain" (p. 32).

Freud himself viewed depression from both psychological and biologic vantage points. "While the melancholic's self criticism is a correct description of his psychological situation, what is probably a somatic factor, and one which cannot be explained psychogenically, makes itself visible in the regular amelioration in the condition that takes place towards evening" (1917, p. 253).

Although Freud specifically singled out the diurnal variation as somatically and not psychogenically determined, we would now include disturbances of appetite, sleep, and sexual interest as reflective of chemical alterations within the central nervous system. To what extent the depressed state itself is caused by psychological factors, the origins of which can be traced through the mental productions of the patient or caused by somatic factors that arise independent of psychology, is an area of current controversy.

Synthesis

Depending on one's orientation, depression may be perceived as a product of the mind and hence described in terms of such constructs as drives, defenses, compromise formation, regression, self-esteem, object loss, and identification. Depression can only be viewed as a product of the brain, characterized by such biologic variables as psychoendocrine function and neurotransmitter concentrations.

Traditionally, analysts have focused on the metapsychology of depression and emphasized such concepts as object loss, ego ideal, and aggression in explaining the phenomonology of the depressed state. I would view the mental productions of patients suffering through a major depressive episode as a consequence of altered central nervous system chemistry rather than as a primary psychological phenomena.

Brenner (1982), in his recent reformulation of the psychoanalytic theory of affect, states that the mental productions seen in depression are due to associative links between certain sensations and memory traces of conscious and unconscious experiences of depression including object loss, loss of love, and castration anxieties, the so called "calamities of childhood." He feels that the ideational content of pathologic depressive affect in any given case is but a derivative of the depressive affect of childhood origins. I would suggest that the universal calamities of childhood referred to by Brenner must cause some type of localized chemical alterations. These may be reflected in qualitative or quantitative alterations in neurotransmitter levels or may be characterized by changes in membrane receptor sites. Any of the narcissistic mortifications of life must reproduce similar chemical disturbances. These must in turn stimulate brain centers that are linked to memory traces, both conscious and unconscious, of depressive situations from every developmental level.

For patients responding to narcissistic mortifications merely with depressive affect, the chemical alterations would be minimal, without systemic manifestations and too subtle to be observable by biologic techniques currently at our disposal. These same local chemical disturbances would be produced in patients with endogenous depression. In them, however, these would trigger or be associated with more widespread central nervous system alterations. The consequences of these would be twofold: they would produce the somatic changes and psychoendocrine disturbances that are currently under such intensive study, and they would also stimulate regions of the brain responsible for the mental productions of endogenously depressed patients.

Investigators (Mishkin and Appenzeller 1987) working with primates have recently presented models whereby emotion can influence perception, learning, and associative recall. They have done this by reporting primate studies and neuroanatomic evidence that demonstrates circuitry-linking central nervous system structures responsible for perception, memory, and emotion. One can easily envision how minor biochemical disturbances at any of these sites could evoke memories and affective states that would be derivatives of childhood experiences.

Another biologic model, "kindling" (Post et al. 1982), provides an additional link between biology and psychology. Kindling is a neurophysiologic phenomenon whereby subthreshold stimuli, given over a period of time, eventually produce a full neurologic response such as a seizure. Animals who are "kindled" will subsequently seize years afterwards if they are again given a subthreshold stimulus. This paradigm, when extrapolated to affective disorders, suggests a mechanism whereby early childhood experiences such as loss and separation could result in permanent alterations of receptor function that might not become clinically evident for years or decades. This model would also account for why affective episodes tend to come with increasing frequency as a person ages and why I feel the architect I mentioned might have fewer affective episodes as he ages if therapy can head off the situationally specific episodes he has now.

One of the cornerstones of modern neurology was laid through the pioneering work of Wilder Penfield (Penfield and Perot 1963). He showed how electrical stimulation of focal areas of the brain could not only elicit motor responses but ideational material in the form of memories, visual imagery, and auditory experiences. The chemically generated signals to which I refer may function as the internal equivalent of Penfield's externally applied stimulating electrodes. They would cause patients to report feelings, recollections, and ideas generated not by conflict, fantasy, or drive derivatives, but by chemical stimuli.

Summary

In doing intensive psychotherapy or analysis with patients who suffer both personality and affective disorders, one must simultaneously maintain psychological and biologic perspectives. Cooper (1985) (see Chapter 3, this volume), when talking of patients suffering from panic disorders, states that analysts must distinguish between psychological efforts to cope with miscarried brain function and the psychological efforts to cope with disturbances of the intrapsychic world. This is also true of patients who have affective disorders. For instance, patients who suffer from untreated affective disorder often speak of their experience of themselves as being out of control. They complain that they can never predict the stability of their emotional states. This aspect of their illness must be conceptualized not as reflecting faltering defensive operations and inadequate compromise formation but as the reaction of an otherwise healthy personality to the experience of being intermittently overwhelmed by biologically generated mood states.

Cooper also states that biologic illnesses must be regarded as having influences that are both developmental and ongoing. The psychoendocrine work of Puig-Antich (1989) demonstrates the existence of endogenous depression in latency-age children, and Carlson and Kashani's (1988) recent clinical observations in preschool children support the notion that this illness can arise during periods of development. For such patients, the normal developmental tasks of childhood and adolescence may be severely compromised. For instance, extreme mood fluctuations of inexplicable origin may serve as a major disruption in the consolidation of a healthy sense of object constancy.

Before closing, I would like to briefly mention two examples of the difficulties encountered when attempting to medicate and analyze the same patient. Ostow (1961) mentions patients who may attempt to use what he refers to as the "drug cure" to reinforce their resistance to psychotherapy. The analyst must be ever alert for this. An example occurred during my analysis of a 35-year-old novelist who had entered treatment for writer's block.

> The patient had been on medication for a number of years, had a strong family history of depression, and had relapses each time the medication had been discontinued or decreased.

> During the eighth month of analysis she reported that she had an interesting experience. She had forgotten to take her evening medication, something extremely unusual for her. She knew that antidepressants suppressed rapid-eye-movement sleep and that stopping tricyclics was often associated with vivid dreams and nightmares. Thus she thought that the nightmare she experienced that night, something to do with being beaten up, could be explained pharmacologically. As such, she dismissed its content as little more than a biochemical quirk and began to associate to the reasons she might have had for forgetting that night's dose of medicine. I told her that although her pharmacology was correct, and that we did need to understand why she missed a dose of medicine, the actual content of her dream could not be dismissed and needed to be analyzed.

> Her associations to this led to the recurring nature of dreams in which she was chased and attacked or beaten. Over time these dreams have become more explicit and their interpretation has led to a better understanding of a number of masochistic acts, which could be directly related to guilt over aggressive fantasies for which she felt the need to be punished. This work has diminished the extent of her writing inhibition.

Finally, it goes without saying that the analyst's awareness and understanding of his or her countertransference reactions are central to any intensive analytic treatment. This may be particularly complicated when one is simultaneously medicating and analyzing a patient in whom the recurrence of a depressive episode raises the question of whether the pharmacologic or the analytic interventions have not been adequate. This dilemma is exemplified by another case.

The patient, a 30-year-old professor, had a long history of recurrent endogenous depressions. He had shown dramatic responses to antidepressant medication and, like the novelist I mentioned earlier, had relapses whenever the medication was stopped. He had entered analysis because of general social awkwardness and a pervasive and ongoing sense of low self-esteem, which he could clearly differentiate from his bouts of endogenous depression. During the sixth month of analysis, while on tricyclic medication and finishing a major publication the completion of which would virtually guarantee him tenure, he was abruptly and unexpectedly rejected by his girlfriend. Over the next several weeks he became profoundly depressed, was unable to meet work deadlines, began feeling worthless and hopeless about his life and his future, and, though not suicidal, thought he would be better off dead.

How was this to be understood? Was his worsening mood related to conflicts over the successful culmination of his quest for tenure? Was it related to the abandonment by his girlfriend, perhaps as some regressive defense against his murderous impulses toward her? Should it be viewed as a deflated narcissistic sense of himself as a consequence of her abandonment? Was this a transference reaction the early stages of which had escaped detection? Had these or other issues been better analyzed by me, would he have become so depressed now?

Alternatively, should these psychological factors be viewed as having triggered another endogenous episode that would not be expected to respond to interpretations but needed some more adequate medical management? What would his fantasies be if I suggest a change in medication? Is my even thinking of medication at a time like this reflective of uncertainty of my own analytic ability or is it the consequences of a dispassionate evaluation of a complex clinical situation? What is the risk if I medicate when he needs more, better, or different analysis, and what is the risk if I do not medicate when that is what he really needs?

As the patient's depression deepened over the next 2 weeks and as my conviction grew that he was having another endogenous episode, I elected to increase his medication. This had a dramatic effect and he was better within 5 days. I do not mean that he was recovered from the girlfriend's rejection or that he was less conflicted about his potential career success or that his chronic sense of worthlessness had improved; rather, he was no longer so despairing that he could not function professionally, no longer felt that his life was not worth living, no longer felt that his future was hopeless, and was no longer so overwhelmed by affect that he was unable to participate fruitfully in analysis. Although the analysis resumed dealing with conflicts over his upcoming publication and the rejection by the woman, this depression prompted further exploration of his reactions to having had so many endogenous episodes throughout his life and the impact such episodes have had on his sense of self-esteem.

The recognition that patients may have major affective disorders concurrent with long-standing personality disorders is a relatively recent advance in psychiatry. More needs to be written about the complex interactions that occur in the simultaneous treatment of these patients with medications and analytic psychotherapy.

References

Brenner, C. (1982). *The Mind in Conflict.* New York: International Universities Press.

Bursten, B. (1985). Medication nonadherence due to feelings of loss of control in "biological depression." *American Journal of Psychiatry* 142:244–246.

Carlson, G. A., and Kashani, J. H. (1988). Phenomenology of major depression from childhood through adulthood: analysis of three studies. *American Journal of Psychiatry* 145:1222–1225.

Cooper, A. M. (1985). Will neurobiology influence psychoanalysis? *American Journal of Psychiatry* 142:1395–1402.

Cornell, D. G. (1985). Psychoanalytic and biological perspectives on depression: contradictory or complementary? *Psychoanalytic Psychology* 2:21–34.

Eissler, K. (1980). The effect of the structure of the ego on psychoanalytic technique. In *Psychoanalytic Explorations of Technique: Discourse on the Theory of Therapy,* ed. H. Blum, pp. 375–418. New York: International Universities Press.

Freud, S. (1917). Mourning and melancholia. *Standard Edition* 14:237–243.

Greenfeld, D. (1985). *The Psychotic Patient: Medication and Psychotherapy.* New York: The Free Press.

Mishkin, M., and Appenzeller, T. (1987). The anatomy of memory. *Scientific American* 256:80–89.

More, B. E., and Fine, B. D., eds. (1968). *Glossary of Psychoanalytic Terms and Concepts.* New York: American Psychoanalytic Association.

Ostow, M. (1957). The use of drugs to overcome technical difficulties in psychoanalysis. In *The Dynamics of Psychiatric Drug Therapy,* ed. G. J. Sarwer-Foner, pp. 443–458. Springfield, IL: Charles C Thomas.

———— (1961). The advantages and limitations of combined therapy. *Psychosomatics* 2:11–15.

———— (1966). The complementary roles of psychoanalysis and drug therapy. In *Psychiatric Drugs,* ed. I. Solomon, pp. 91–111. New York: Grune & Stratton.

———— (1987). How does psychiatric drug therapy work? *Israel Journal of Psychiatry* 24:265–279.

Penfield, W., and Perot, P. (1963). The brain's record of auditory and visual experience. *Brain* 85:595–696.

Post, R. M., Uhde, T. W., Putnam, F. W., et al. (1982). Kindling and carbamazepine in affective illness. *Journal of Nervous Mental Disease* 170:717–731.

Puig-Antich, J., Goetz, D., Davies, M., et al. (1989). A controlled family history study of prepubertal major depressive disorder. *Archives of General Psychiatry* 46:406–418.

PART IV
Case Presentations

17

An Effect of Pharmacotherapy on the Psychoanalytic Process

HAROLD W. WYLIE, JR., M.D., AND MAVIS L. WYLIE, PH.D.

A woman who had appeared suitable for psychoanalysis was persistently unable to develop an analyzable transference. Her history, as it unfolded during analysis, suggested a form of atypical depression linked to a neurochemical abnormality, which appeared to be related to her reluctance to take the emotional risk involved in examining transference phenomena. The analysis was modified by a trial of phenelzine. Changes within the analysis and in the patient's private life after the drug trial ended support the hypothesis that her affective vulnerability had inhibited her ability to engage in analysis of transference before the administration of the drug.

One of the knottier problems confronting psychoanalysis today is clarifying in an open and operational way what makes an analysis work, and for whom. (In this chapter the terms "psychoanalysis" and "analysis" are used interchangeably. Both refer to the classical Freudian psychoanalytic approach: use of the couch, a frequency of four or five sessions weekly, free association, analytic neutrality, dream work, defense and transference analysis.) Although there have been, over the past 30 years, a number of reports dealing with the characteristics of psychoanalytic patients, their analyzability, and treatment outcome, other issues related to confidentiality and the nature of the analytic process itself pose such immense problems to the construction of a good research design that, as far as we know, there have not yet been any studies which systematically examine the important question of patient selection.

Until such time as a fuller, more accurate, and reliable understanding has developed, if practicing analysts would expand their exchange of views in the literature concerning their own experiences with patient selection and the nature of the process, we could rather quickly acquire an interim body of clinical data to which we might readily refer—an important resource for comparison, criticism, and replication. If, in addition, such exchanges were to include reports of factors associated with negative as well as positive outcomes, the reservoir of data would become even more valuable. Negative outcomes are all too often inappropriately sequestered from useful inspection, like skeletons in the closet, or avoided, like black sheep. Kris (1957) observed that the assessment of a patient's analytic potential may be possible only in the course of the analysis, a fact that others (Bak 1970, Lower et al. 1972) have echoed in the intervening years. Heartened by this observation, we should not be so inhibited in our willingness to examine and report on indications that a patient in the course of analysis is not deriving maximum benefit from psychoanalytic treatment alone.

Believing that the articulation of such enigmas would serve as a pragmatic and efficient means of educating members of our profession about these dilemmas, we present the following case report in order to share such clinical observations. It is a report on an analysand who had been found initially suitable for psychoanalysis but who became, as the analysis unfolded, observably unamenable to psychoanalytic intervention alone until a pharmacological intervention was made. The treatment that followed, while conducted in a classical form, included the use of a drug and would therefore be called a modified analysis.

Case Report

Ms. A. was a 39-year-old divorced woman whose presenting symptoms included intermittent periods of depression and a persistent inability during the 7 years since her divorce to establish a satisfactory long-term relationship with a man. She regarded the latter as an especially painful reminder of her sense of aloneness. As she said, "Everyone is in pairs but me." Her lack of success in this respect appeared remarkable in view of her motivation for such a relationship, her attractive appearance, engaging manner, social credentials, excellent education, and history of many long-term friendships with both men and women. At the time she came for evaluation, Ms. A. was employed by a local university, where for several years she had worked as an administrator. She had begun to find her job "lackluster" and saw herself growing increasingly lackadaisical in it.

Ms. A.'s childhood had been spent in the suburban community of a large midwestern city. Her father's business afforded a prosperous standard of living for the family, and her mother ran their fine house in the role of full-time housewife and mother. Ms. A. was the eldest of three children; her sister and brother were 2 and 4 years her junior, respectively. She reported that she maintained frequent contact with her mother and had done so since her college days. However, aspects of this closeness appeared to be reactive, masking painfully conflicted feelings that became manifest in the contradiction between Ms. A.'s account of the respectful cordiality with which she addressed or interacted with her mother and the guiltily disdainful tone she adopted at other times when describing her mother to the analyst. Her earliest memory of this parent was of her mother's anxious preparations for the daily teatime visit of Ms. A.'s imperious paternal grandmother, who seemed to Ms. A. to dominate the household like a dowager queen.

During the evaluation, Ms. A. recalled memories of her father (who had died when she was in her late 20s), which, although ambivalent, were primarily characterized by her idealization of him. When she first spoke of him, it was affectionately and possessively, especially with regard to his early pride in her appearance and excellent school performance. However, these feelings were soon interspersed with a sense of bitter disappointment. For example, her nostalgic reminiscence of the excitement she had felt in the otherwise predominantly female household about the ritual of his evening homecoming was quickly followed by a description of the disillusionment she experienced at his later lack of interest in her during her adolescence. Upon inquiry, Ms. A. recalled that the change in her father had occurred during a period in her adolescence when he had stopped working in his business for a number of months and had remained closeted and unavailable in the house. No one in the family had discussed this then or since. Although during the evaluation Ms. A. found herself wondering whether her father had become seriously depressed (he had never been hospitalized), her speculations did nothing to attenuate her alternating feelings of anger and recrimination at his having "let me down."

During high school, Ms. A. proved herself an excellent student, popular with boys and girls and confident of her social skills. She enjoyed great success acting in school plays. However, after she completed an equally profitable first year at college, her life underwent a distinct change. Unable to recall a specific precipitant or even to describe this change in any detail, Ms. A. was only able to say that she had "just lost confidence" socially and academically. She perceived herself as increasingly less able and attractive than her collegemates—socially awkward and shy. In her words, "I seemed to miss cues and I seemed always to appear aloof." Nevertheless, through her persistent effort, she continued to be an excellent student and managed to maintain a wide range of activities. Shortly after finishing college, she married. While her marriage was considered an "excellent and enviable match" by her family's social criteria, Ms. A.'s lack of confidence remained unabated.

During the initial interviews, it became clear that Ms. A. had struggled for many years with intermittent, noncyclical episodes of depressed mood. During these episodes various of her physicians (at one time, shortly after her marriage, it was a general practitioner; later, during her second pregnancy, her obstetrician; another time, after her divorce, a psychiatrist) had each prescribed amphetamines to relieve her symptoms of fatigue and mood disturbance. In each instance the amphetamines had proved markedly effective, in contrast to a one-time trial of tricyclics, which had been notably unsuccessful, as had a brief period of psychotherapy without medication.

Information garnered in the evaluation (and amplified during her first year of analysis) seemed to indicate that Ms. A.'s unsuccessful relationships with men fell into one of two categories. There were the initially "good" relationships, which she wondered whether she had somehow played a part in inadvertently undermining, even though during the relationships she had only been aware of feeling that the men were acting in a "particularly painful and thoughtless manner" toward her. For other relationships, it became patently clear to Ms. A., once she became involved, that they were incompatible, unacceptable, and even offensive to her because of fundamental and irreconcilable differences between her own and her partners' life styles and values. In other words, her choices had been poor. During the initial interviews she expressed puzzlement about how, in the first place, she had overlooked these clues that now seemed so "clear."

In both types of relationships, despite the retrospective obviousness of warning signs, Ms. A. reported that she was "devastated" when a relationship ended and felt herself to be in a state of crisis, during which she was given to striking her fists brutally and self-injuriously against household objects or, in a passion, to scratching her skin until it bled. She described a tendency to overindulge temporarily in food (as she said, her eating habits were at the mercy, so to speak, of her love life) and occasionally to drink too much. She would subsequently feel depressed and at a loss. She had repeated the pattern so often that by the time she came to analysis, she observed that she was wary of attempting any new relationships with men.

In assessing the suitability of prescribing psychoanalysis for this patient according to the APA diagnostic criteria (1981), the analyst noted that Ms. A.'s history gave indications of persistent intrapsychic conflict together with issues of arrested development that were reflected in her symptoms. There was evidence of oedipal-level conflicts that operated through her unresolved ambivalence toward her mother (whom she both devalued and envied) and her father's memory (which she idealized and resented) and that had led her to a series of failed, masochistically tainted relationships with men. Despite the repetition of her agitated response to each rupture, there was strong evidence in the longevity and consistency of her work relationships and the long-time friendships she had maintained with both men and women to support an impression of intact ego functioning. More importantly, Ms. A.'s responsiveness to the developmental needs of her children (both of whom were excellent students and well-liked by their peers) suggested that her relationship with her own mother had involved "good enough" (Winnicott 1965) early nurturing experiences and that the mobilization of preoedipal issues was regressive rather than fixated. The fact that her children had been able to maintain a good relationship with their father, unsubverted by Ms. A. despite the divorce, added to this impression. Her history of successful motherhood combined with a capacity for self-reflection during the evaluative interviews added weight to the analyst's diagnostic sense that the characterologic container for her neurotic conflicts was essentially sound. Additionally, it was clear from Ms. A.'s history that she had an adequate capacity for sublimation and an absence of early trauma; she had also given evidence of object constancy. Further-more, it was clear from her history that she had received only temporary relief from other forms of psychiatric treatment. All in all, the analyst decided that she had the ability to establish and maintain a therapeutic relationship and could make use of analysis to complete the unfinished developmental business in her life.

Ms. A. began the analysis with enthusiasm and hope. During the first year she was forthcoming and associated freely, in this sense readily engaging in the analytic process. However, she was persistently unable to grasp the specific "as-if" characteristics of the psychoanalytic situation. Whenever the analyst brought transference phenomena to her attention, she objected, saying that "this is absurd" and that she could not "imagine such things." Although she became accomplished in observing herself outside the analytic hour, she remained intransigent about adapting the same observing capacity to feelings experienced within the hour. Like a "sector" analysis, as long as the locus of interpretations remained outside the "here and now" of the analytic hour, Ms. A. was able to make use of, accept, and talk about transference feelings in displacement. For 18 months she continued to view the analyst as a real object, stating, "I do not want to make a new relationship, any kind of relationship. . . . I don't want another rejection." In addition to being unable to approach the conflicted and erotized transference issues hidden behind her resistance (which had taken the form of this fear of rejection) and therefore being unable to establish a stable, workable transference configuration, Ms. A. was also struggling with recurrent feelings of depression.

The extended duration of Ms. A.'s reluctance to risk a therapeutic relation-ship, in combination with three other factors—depressive mood, a history of severe sensitivity to rejection, and a history of self-injurious behaviors (which became clearly illuminated in the first 18 months of the analysis)—brought to mind an article by Liebowitz and Klein (1979) on hysteroid dysphoria. Klein had written earlier on the subject:

The primary defect of hysteroid dysphorics is their affective vulnerabil-ity. . . . These patients have a pathologically heightened emotional reac-tivity to approval or disapproval, and other aspects of their behavior are expressions of this defect or attempts to compensate for it. [Liebowitz and Klein 1979, p. 558]

This could be explained by fluctuations of an endogenous amphetamine-like substance whose level is affected by interpersonal stimuli. . . . Using this model, hysteroid dysphorics may be simply suffering from an extreme of such reactivity due to an unstable control mechanism. This in turn could be explained as an inherited or an acquired defect, or as an interaction of both. [p. 561]

In their article Liebowitz and Klein presented a form of atypical depression that seemed to fit Ms. A.'s case: a chronic, nonpsychotic disturbance involving repeated episodes of abruptly depressed mood in response to feeling rejected, a history of temporary abusive reliance on food and alcohol when depressed, inappropriate love objects that are quickly overidealized, self-mutilative acts such as scratching and picking at the skin, a history of having been a performer, a high frequency of affective disorders in first-degree relatives, a history of reliance on dextroamphetamine to maintain mood and energy, and a lack of response to tricyclic antidepressants.

Because Ms. A. had, in many respects, developed a good working alliance and remained highly motivated despite her depressive feelings, and because it did not appear that the psychoanalysis alone was effective, modifying the analysis by adding a trial of the drug recommended by Liebowitz and Klein seemed appropriate. The purpose was to reduce her sense of excessive affective vulnerability, which seemed to be interfering with her ability to affectively risk approaching the interpretations of transference issues. It was hypothesized that if this interference were removed, Ms. A. would gradually be able to bring her observing self into the treatment hour to experience and analyze the transference—the feelings underlying her depressive episodes—and that she would then be able to work through in the transference neurosis the oedipal-level issues which had originally arrested her developmental processes. Eighteen months after the analysis began, following discussions with Ms. A., a trial of the antidepressant phenelzine, a monoamine oxidase inhibitor, was prescribed by the analyst. All other aspects of the analysis remained unaltered. Over a 2-week period the dose was increased from 30 mg per day to a therapeutic level of 45 mg per day. After 10 months the drug was discontinued.

The first time that Ms. A. spontaneously acknowledged the presence of transference feelings within the analytic hour occurred a month after the start of the drug trial. At that time she entered the consultation room and stumbled slightly against the door jamb as she attempted to take a direct look at the analyst. Once on the couch, she opened the hour with the account of a sexually provocative woman in the cast of an opera she had attended the previous evening. This led her to thoughts about the analyst. Without hesitation, she remarked that she found him as attractive as she did the suitable men with whom she had been afraid to seek a relationship. These thoughts were followed by her recollection of a series of memories in which she freely associated to her need to stumble through various past relationships as she had stumbled coming into the office.

From this point on, Ms. A. was able to consider the analyst's transference interpretations, first as tentative "possibilities" and then later with occasional humor, as she became actively interested in and curious about the transference phenomenon itself.

An ameliorative effect on Ms. A.'s sense of affective vulnerability was reported not long after the introduction of the drug, as she described how her general mood had improved. Coincidentally, she reported that she had begun to lose weight, reflecting a fading dependence on food. She found herself becoming more assertive in her work and enjoying what had previously begun to bore her.

During the year that followed the end of the drug trial, Ms. A. continued to analyze the aggressive as well as the libidinal components of her transference fantasies and to comprehend their interpretation. This convincingly suggests that prescription of the drug was not an "emotionally corrective experience" (Alexander and French 1946, p. 268). Her examination of rescue wishes, dreams, fantasies, and frightening thoughts previously experienced as unintelligible, alien, or unconscious to her were now brought into awareness, successfully analyzed, and perceived as meaningful aspects of herself. Outside the analysis, Ms. A. experienced a subtle but clear alteration in her relationship with her mother. This was exemplified by the development of an unambivalent appreciation of the contribution her mother's nurturance had made to her own ability to raise her two children. In a similar way, she gradually integrated her feelings about her father, arriving at a perception of the important influence of his ideals on her dogged efforts to deal with her own disabling conflicts. A year after the end of the drug trial, Ms. A. had developed a solid relationship with a "suitable" man and reported with pleasure on this as it assumed increasing importance for her.

Discussion

Although in 1985 Reiser argued for the efficacy of psychoanalytic interpretation alone in treating a patient's condition that might otherwise have been treated with a psychoactive drug, the patient in the present report did not respond to psychoanalytic interpretation. When Ms. A.'s depressive mood and sense of vulnerability were eventually conceptualized as part of a constellation of symptoms in a syndrome described by Liebowitz and Klein (1979), a specific psychoactive drug was administered. Before, during, and after the administration of the drug, the patient was seen four times a week, and except for use of the drug, the analysis was conducted strictly along classical lines. After the addition of phenelzine, Ms. A. became amenable to transference interpretations as well as to the analysis of fantasies associated with taking the drug. This lends support to the hypothesis that her "becoming amenable" was a reflection of the drug's pharmacological effect (i.e., its reduction of the affective vulnerability and alleviation of depressed mood) rather than of the psychological effect of its administration, representing a gratification of her wish to be rescued by an idealized father.

Since a major tool of psychoanalysis is the development of the transference neurosis (the vehicle by which repressed memories can be lifted from the dynamic unconscious), an abnormality in the regulation of the neurotransmitters would compound what under "normal" circumstances is a formidable task. A successful analysis depends on the ability of a patient to withstand the emotional deprivation and the adaptive regression required to permit a flowering of transference. It is an extraordinary process, the sine qua non of which is that the patient is able to undertake this new relationship under the most unusual and stressful of circumstances. Until the administration of phenelzine, Ms. A. had been unable to tolerate the sense of affective vulnerability involved in approaching crucial repressed fantasy material. This she had defensively kept out of awareness, unwilling to engage in the study of the transference, which was the only way these fantasies could be made available to her and be worked through. Both her history and her previous response to medication strongly suggested that this patient suffered a disorder of the regulation of her neurotransmitter system characterized by its instability in the face of stress. As Siever and Davis (1985) wrote, "Antidepressants, by differentially affecting distinct adrenergic receptor systems, may serve to dampen dysphoric overarousal while enhancing reinforced goal-directed behavior" (p. 1025).

There is little danger that pharmacotherapy will replace psychoanalysis, nor is it likely that chemical factors will be introduced into a classical framework as a matter of course. However, during evaluation and treatment, an adherence to psychoanalytic orthodoxy should not be cause for overlooking pertinent advances in understanding neurochemistry. As Freud (1926) predicted, there are avenues to be explored between psychoanalysis and biology.

References

Alexander, F., and French, T. M. (1946). *Psychoanalytic Therapy: Principles and Applications.* New York: Ronald Press.

American Psychiatric Association (1981). Psychoanalytic peer review. In *Manual of Psychiatric Peer Review,* 2nd ed. p. 84. Washington, DC: American Psychiatric Press.

Bak, R. C. (1970). Psychoanalysis today. *Journal of the American Psychoanalytic Association* 18:3–23.

Freud, S. (1926). The question of lay analysis. *Standard Edition* 20:231, 1959.

Kris, M. (1957). The use of prediction in a longitudinal study. *Psychoanalytic Study of the Child* 12:175–189. New York: International Universities Press.

Liebowitz, M. D. and Klein, D. F. (1979). Hysteroid dysphoria. *Psychiatric Clinics of North America* 2:555–575.

Lower, R. B., Escoll, P. J., and Huxster, H. K. (1972). Bases for judgments of analyzability. *Journal of the American Psychoanalytic Association* 20:610–621.

Reiser, M. F. (1985). Converging sectors of psychoanalysis and neurobiology: mutual challenge and opportunity. *Journal of the American Psychoanalytic Association* 33:11–34.

Siever, L. J., and Davis, K. L. (1985). Overview: toward a dysregulation hypothesis of depression. *American Journal of Psychiatry* 142:1017–1031.

Winnicott, D. W. (1965). Ego distortion in terms of true and false self. In *The Maturational Processes and the Facilitating Environment,* p. 145. New York: International Universities Press.

18

Transference and the Beta-Adrenergic Receptor

SHEPARD J. KANTOR, M.D.

This case presentation demonstrates the importance of recognizing that patients can have both character pathology and affective disorders, shows the need to assess the impact of one illness upon the other, demonstrates the importance of having both medical and psychological viewpoints in attempting to manage such patients, and shows the pitfalls that can be encountered in working with such difficult cases. The paper offers speculations about the ways in which the biologic and psychological aspects of affective disorder may be interrelated and the mechanisms of this interrelationship.

Melissa B., a 35-year-old divorced woman, began treatment with me during her hospitalization for an overdose of doxepin and digoxin. She had recently given up an extremely successful career as a music critic to move to a new city to resume her study of music. Shortly after this move, she overdosed. The intensity of her transference, the disruptiveness of her affective storms, the side effects of a variety of antidepressant medications, and the complex interplay between affective disorder and personality disorder all contributed to the extremely complicated nature of Melissa's treatment.

In presenting this case, I will focus first on the clinical material: Melissa's affective disorder, her developmental history and character disorder, and the interplay between the two during the course of a stormy 2-year analytically oriented treatment. I will then use this material as the basis from which to offer certain speculations about the interface between biology and psychology.

Affective Disorder: History and Treatment

Melissa B. described her depressions as having begun in early adolescence, if not before. Depressive episodes would begin with no apparent precipitant and last for months. When depressed, she would keep to herself, cry for hours, take to bed for days at a time, and lose all interest in her friends, family and surroundings. She was never treated for these episodes. There was also a history of bulimia and anorexia during adolescence, and she maintained a lifelong preoccupation with her weight. At age 32 she was hospitalized for 1 month for depression and treated with low doses of doxepin, which she continued until 3 months before this hospitalization. She did not think the medication helped her mood.

Melissa's maternal aunt had had severe depressions, having been hospitalized and given tricyclic antidepressants on three different occasions. One of Melissa's sisters also had episodes of depression but had refused treatment.

Melissa was maintained on digoxin for paroxysmal atrial tachycardia (PAT). Other than childhood asthma, her medical history was unremarkable. Thyroid workup, including thyroid-stimulating hormone-releasing factor (TSH-RF), was normal. There was no history of drug or alcohol abuse, central nervous system disease, or seizure disorder.

Several days after beginning nortriptyline, the patient developed resting pulses in the range of 120–130 bpm. Because she could not tolerate this, atenolol, a beta-adrenergic blocker, was added. The atenolol brought her pulse below 100 and enabled her to tolerate the antidepressant. However, she showed no improvement at nortriptyline doses of 50, 75, and 125 mg per day, each for several weeks. Her plasma levels were 50 ng/ml, 112 ng/ml and 145 ng/ml, all within the "therapeutic window." At 150 mg per day her plasma nortriptyline level was 160 ng/ml. At her urging, the drug was increased to 175 mg per day.

Despite being above the therapeutic window, she fully recovered. Her normal interests returned, her work productivity increased, and her outlook vastly improved. However, after 6 weeks, she became ataxic on 175 mg per day nortriptyline. Her plasma level at that time was 285 ng/ml. When the dose was decreased below 175 mg per day, she rapidly became suicidally depressed.

Lithium carbonate, when added to doses of nortriptyline less than 175 mg per day, was of no benefit. Both of these drugs were therefore discontinued. Melissa again became suicidal and was hospitalized. She was placed on phenelzine 60 mg per day, and after several weeks showed a full symptom remission. However, she again became ataxic and experienced orthostatic hypotension. Decreasing phenelzine caused the return of severe depressive symptomatology. The addition of lithium carbonate, when combined with less than 60 mg per day of phenelzine, was of no benefit.

The patient was then begun on trimipramine and her symptoms again resolved. She subsequently had three severe falls. It was uncertain whether these were due to trimipramine, atenolol (on which she had remained) or to the combination of the two. As she could not tolerate a tricyclic without a beta blocker because the tricyclic drugs exacerbated her PAT, both drugs were discontinued.

Her suicidal depression returned, and she was begun on alprazolam. A course of 6 months of this medication, during 2 of which she was taking 6–10 mg per day, was of no benefit. During the third month of alprazolam, phenelzine 45 mg per day was added. Alprazolam was discontinued, and she was eventually titrated to phenelzine 45 mg per day and 60 mg per day on alternate days, which resulted in a complete and sustained symptom remission for the next 6 months.

Weaning her from alprazolam took 5 months, proved extremely difficult (Kantor 1986), and contributed to the eventual disruption of treatment. This is best understood with a more full appreciation of her history and psychodynamics.

Developmental History and Psychodynamics

Melissa B., one of three siblings, grew up on a military base. Her father was a highly decorated commanding officer known for his clear-headed decisions under pressure, his force of personality, and the autocratic nature of his leadership. He liked the isolation of this remote base and had gone to some lengths to be certain that he was not reassigned to one in a more cosmopolitan area. His conviction that his family should be more self-sufficient led him to deny his wife and children permission to have more than the most superficial involvement with other military or civilian families.

Melissa's mother, a pianist who had given up her professional career to raise her family, was quiet and unintrusive to the point of being emotionally uninvolved. She acquiesced to her husband's demands for isolation with little apparent protest.

Throughout her childhood the patient felt herself to be the subject of her father's special attention. He obviously preferred her company to that of her siblings. She experienced the intensity and intimacy of their long conversations with a mixture of pleasure, excitement, and guilt. The guilt was especially intense with respect to her mother, in whom the father seemed to show little interest. Melissa felt that her mother encouraged her closeness to her father, and she thought her mother would often absent herself so that father and daughter could be together.

The patient had asthma throughout her childhood. The suffering from her illness was compounded by her parents attitude, which was that she brought the attacks on herself. At age 12 she became seriously ill with a viral pulmonary infection. This illness was of life-threatening proportions. She was debilitated and confined to bed for 3 months.

The already traumatic nature of this illness was intensified by her father's insistence, over the objections of Melissa's physicians, that she be treated at home rather than at the base hospital. Furthermore, he took primary responsibility for her nursing care, which often included examining her and bathing her "all over" when she had high fevers. She was mortified and humiliated by such behavior, felt that her life literally depended on her father's vigilance and attentiveness, and believed that she had no one to whom she could turn to change this treatment program. At the same time she was furious with her mother for not insisting she be treated at the base hospital. She had no physical sequelae and no recurrences of this illness, and her asthma went into remission in late adolescence.

The patient recalls having had affective symptoms beginning at least in her early adolescence. They soon became a major facet of her life. When depressed she would lose interest in her music and schooling, cry frequently, sleep poorly, and at times think of suicide. When these episodes passed, she was her usual outgoing, friendly, vivacious, interested self. Her father was greatly embarrassed by his daughter's moods. He would send her to her room when she got severely depressed and tearful. He was angered by her "willfulness" and seemed to feel that her symptoms were a blight on the otherwise perfect image of family happiness and tranquility he wished to project. She was often threatened with the prospect of seeing a psychiatrist but never actually referred to one. Banishment to her room for "misbehavior" was a frequent occurrence.

Melissa did well in school, left home to attend college, and married. Her marriage was characterized by her husband's physical abuse. Like her father, he would torment her about her "moodiness," telling her that she would end up in a mental hospital if it persisted. The marriage ended in divorce after 4 years.

The patient's career as a music critic began in college and flourished during the next 10 years, despite crippling bouts of depression: when she wasn't working, she was in bed feeling miserable and tearful.

During this entire period Melissa had been unsuccessful in her attempts to write her own music, a major disappointment in her life. She found 3 years of psychotherapy to be of little help with composing or with her depression. She had discussed biological depression with her therapist, who gave her modest doses of antidepressant medication but seemed to have little confidence in their usefulness. She had thought of seeking a psychiatric consultation but felt an extreme sense of loyalty to her therapist. After 3 years of treatment she was finally able to overcome this concern and move to a new city to seek help for her depression and to pursue the study of music. Several months after the move, she overdosed and was admitted to my care.

Treatment Course

After a 3-week hospitalization, twice-weekly psychotherapy was begun. However, the patient found it increasingly difficult to tolerate the days between sessions. One session after another, she would feel that she had said something that had given offense and that the therapist would abandon her. Or she would feel that what she had said was so reprehensible that the therapist would want nothing more to do with her. In an attempt to deal with her tremendous anxiety, the frequency of sessions was increased until after several months, meetings were five times a week. They were always face to face and analytically oriented.

During periods when Melissa was deeply depressed, little analytic work was possible. The content of these sessions concerned her pervasive sense of hopelessness, pessimism, and worthlessness. Suicide was constantly an issue. My role was mostly a supportive, reassuring one. The sense of the reassurances was that she had a biologic illness that had responded to medication in the past and most likely would again, and that she was not bringing on these affective states out of willfulness. When her depression was controlled by medication, analytically oriented work could proceed.

The first material to emerge after her depressive symptoms went into remission consisted of her anger toward her previous therapist for not having treated her more aggressively with medication, evidently a consequence of his not having given much weight to her biologic illness. Over the next several months, this led to an expression of anger toward her parents and of her fears that the anger was of obliterating intensity. She began to realize how guilty she felt over having such anger and wondered if perhaps she had remained in treatment with the previous therapist because she hadn't felt she deserved to get better. At this point she first spoke of the abusive treatment she had received at the hands of her husband and, for the first time, began to question why she had put up with it for as long as she had.

Melissa was then on a combination of tricyclic and beta blocker and had several serious falls. She did not report these to me until her injuries had become obvious. She feared that her falls would be perceived as psychogenic—that the therapist, like her father and her ex-husband, would think that she had brought them on willfully.

During periods of well-being, and especially as she began to see how sensitive her moods were to medication, she began to see herself as suffering from a biologic illness with which she had had to contend all her life. She also recognized that she was not merely a willfully "moody" person, as she had so often been called. This theme was repeated many times during the treatment.

It was frequently necessary to deal with Melissa's persistent concerns that the analyst wanted to get rid of her, that she was undeserving of treatment, and that the analyst was actually angry with her for being such an angry person or because she was so frequently angry at him and such a difficult case. These worries led to frequent late-night telephone calls, which were becoming an increasingly important part of the therapy.

The patient was frightened by the intensity of the anger she harbored toward her parents: toward her mother for her distance, insensitivity, and failure to protect her from her father, and toward her father for his tyrannical rule and the physical intimacy he had forced upon her during her near-fatal adolescent illness. As this was discussed, associated guilt feelings were revealed. She began to understand how the guilt fueled her chronic suicidal fantasies and how fears of losing control of her anger caused her to completely suppress her imaginative life and hence her creative artistic talents.

As the work proceeded, the patient's professional inhibitions began to diminish. She was able to spend hours with her music and wrote several pieces for which she received critical praise.

These significant gains notwithstanding, the treatment continued to be an extremely stormy one. About 18 months after treatment began, at a time when she was having severe complications from alprazolam withdrawal, I had her taken to an emergency room against her will. This came in the context of mounting suicidal threats and a late-night telephone call in which she stated that she had taken an overdose.

The patient subsequently became enraged, not for the overnight emergency room stay, which she retrospectively felt had been justified, but because I had not come to release her from the emergency room sooner than I had. For this she was furious, stating that I had totally abandoned her. She thought I was treating her just like her father, who because of her "moody" behavior had so often thrown her into her room and walked away.

Although some therapeutic work continued after this point, the therapeutic alliance was never fully restored. At times Melissa felt her anger at the therapist to be unreasonable, and she would be extremely guilt-ridden. However, for the most part her anger was uncontainable. Interpretations of the genetic and dynamic contributions to her anger were only of transient benefit. She was no longer able to maintain her sense of the transference as an "as-if" relationship, and she became increasingly convinced that the therapist had abandoned her in the emergency room because he hated her. Shortly thereafter, she fled treatment.

Discussion

Cases such as this one must be simultaneously viewed from two vantage points: the psychopharmacologic and the psychodynamic. I will turn first to the psychopharmacologic, then to the interface between psychology and biology, and then to the psychodynamics of this case.

Psychopharmacology

This patient was extremely sensitive to both the benefits and side effects of a variety of antidepressant medications. Most patients given tricyclics have negligible changes in their resting pulse rate. She, however, developed a significant and symptomatic resting tachycardia and an increased frequency of PAT. Whether her history of PAT reflects an underlying vulnerability to the beta-stimulating effects of antidepressants is uncertain, but clinically she could not be managed on a tricyclic without concurrent beta-blocking medication.

Atenolol was chosen for two reasons. Because it penetrates the central nervous system less than propranolol, it is theoretically less likely to cause depression. Equally important is this patient's history of asthma. The stimulation of respiratory beta receptors enhances dilation of the bronchioles. To block these receptors might compromise the patient's respiratory status. Unlike propranolol, atenolol at low doses is relatively selective for cardiac beta receptors and tends to spare respiratory beta receptors.

The patient's response to nortriptyline was unusual. Psychiatrists are accustomed to thinking of the therapeutic window for this drug as being sharply defined. That the patient responded at a level beyond this window is a reminder that therapeutic ranges have been established using average responses of groups of patients and that on occasion one will find a patient whose response pattern is different from the group norm.

The dramatic jump in her nortriptyline level from 160 ng/ml when taking 150 mg per day to 285 ng/ml when taking 175 mg per day explains her inability to tolerate the drug and is probably accounted for by rate-limited nortriptyline metabolism (Browne et al. 1984). In other words, the capacity of her liver microsomes to metabolize nortriptyline was completely saturated at 150 mg per day. Above that dose, she simply could not adequately metabolize the amount of nortriptyline being presented to her liver, and she became toxic.

The patient's bulimic history suggested that her depression might be responsive to monoamine oxidase (MAO) inhibitors. As with nortriptyline, she showed a narrow therapeutic index with phenelzine. However, with phenelzine, rather small adjustments in her daily dose, ultimately arriving at 45 and 60 mg per day on alternate days, provided symptomatic relief without toxicity during the last 6 months of her treatment. The characteristic ability of the MAO inhibitors to effect dramatic therapeutic responses with relatively small adjustments in oral doses is frequently observed but seldom reported in the literature.

Biology and Psychoanalytic Theory

Depending upon one's orientation, depression may be perceived either as a product of the mind and hence described in terms of such constructs as drives, defenses, compromise formation, regression, self-esteem, object loss, and identification, or as a product of the brain and characterized by such biologic variables as psychoendocrine function and neurotransmitter concentrations.

Whereas some borderline patients exhibit chronic dysphoric/depressive states, the family history of this patient (her aunt had well-documented major depressive disorder, which had been tricyclic responsive, and her sister seemed to be similarly afflicted), the episodic nature of her severe depressive states, the time course of her response to tricyclics and MAOs, one hypomanic response to MAOs, and the dramatic differences in her mood when she was on or off adequate amounts of antidepressants, would all indicate that she had a major depressive disorder.

Thus Melissa B. suffered from a borderline personality disorder with depressive and masochistic features and also from major depressive disorder. Treatment of this patient and others like her necessitates maintaining both a biological and a psychological perspective throughout the treatment.

Historically there has been a longstanding controversy regarding the relative contributions of psychology and biology to states of depression. Freud (1917) viewed depression from both vantage points: he wrote that the melancholic's self-criticism is a correct description of his psychological situation (p. 247) and at the same time stated, "What is probably a somatic factor, and one which cannot be explained psychogenically, makes itself visible in the regular amelioration in the condition that takes place towards evening" (p. 253). Whereas Freud specifically singled out the diurnal variation as somatically and not psychogenically determined, clinicians would now include disturbances of appetite, sleep, and sexual interest as manifestations of chemical alterations within the central nervous system.

To what extent the depressed state itself is caused by psychological factors, the origins of which can be traced through mental productions of the patient, or is caused by somatic factors that arise independent of psychology is an area of current controversy.

Traditionally, analysts have focused on the metapsychology of depression and emphasized such concepts as object loss, ego ideal, and aggression in explaining the phenomonology of the depressed state. I would view the mental productions of patients suffering through a major depressive episode as a consequence of altered central nervous system chemistry rather than as primary psychological phenomena.

Brenner (1982), in his recent reformulation of the psychoanalytic theory of affect, states that the mental productions seen in depression are due to associative links between certain sensations and memory traces of conscious and unconscious experiences of depression including object loss, loss of love, and castration anxieties—the so called "calamities of childhood." He believes that the ideational content of pathologic depressive affect in any given case is but a derivative of the depressive affect of childhood origins.

I would suggest that the universal calamities of childhood referred to by Brenner must cause some type of localized chemical alterations. These may be reflected in qualitative or quantitative alterations in neurotransmitter levels or may be characterized by changes in membrane receptor sites.

Any of the narcissistic mortifications of life must reproduce similar chemical disturbances. These disturbances in turn stimulate brain centers that are linked to memory traces, both conscious and unconscious, of depressive situations from every developmental level.

For patients responding to narcissistic mortifications merely with depressive affect, the chemical alterations would be minimal, without systemic manifestations, and too subtle to be observable by current biologic techniques. The same local chemical disturbances would be produced in patients with endogenous depression. In them, however, such local changes would trigger or be associated with more widespread central nervous system alterations. The consequences of these would be twofold: they would produce the somatic changes and psychoendocrine disturbances that are currently under such intensive study, and they would also stimulate regions of the brain responsible for the mental productions of endogenously depressed patients.

Investigators working with primates (Mishkin and Appenzeller 1987) have recently presented models whereby emotion can influence perception, learning, and associative recall. They have done this by providing in vivo studies and neuroanatomic evidence that demonstrate circuitry linking central nervous system structures responsible for perception, memory, and emotion. One can easily envision how minor biochemical disturbances at any of these sites could evoke memories, derivatives, and affective states whose origins lie in childhood experiences.

Another biologic model, that of "kindling" (Post et al. 1982), provides a link between biology and psychology. Kindling is a neurophysiologic phenomenon whereby subthreshold stimuli, given over a period of time, eventually produce a full neurologic response such as a seizure. Animals who are "kindled" will subsequently respond with a seizure years after they have been kindled if they are again given a subthreshold stimulus.

When extrapolated to affective disorders, this paradigm suggests a mechanism whereby early childhood experiences such as loss and separation could result in permanent alterations of receptor function that might not become clinically evident for years or decades.

One of the cornerstones of modern neurology was laid through the pioneering work of Wilder Penfield (Penfield and Perot 1963), who showed how electrical stimulation of focal areas of the brain could not only elicit motor responses but ideational material in the form of memories, visual imagery, and auditory experiences. The chemically generated signals to which I refer may function as the internal equivalent of Penfield's externally applied stimulating electrodes. They would cause patients to report feelings, recollections and ideas generated not by conflict, fantasy, or drive derivatives, but by chemical stimuli.

Psychodynamics

Intensive psychotherapy with patients having borderline personality organization is always a difficult undertaking—one in which the therapist must be prepared for intense transference reactions, affective storms, and acting out.

As with any such patient, Melissa B.'s perceptions of the treatment and the therapist were distorted by primitive defense mechanisms dominated by splitting and projection. Instinctual diffusion and her inability to discriminate between shades of affect led to distorted perceptions and extreme emotional reactions—for example, if I admitted some annoyance at yet another late-night telephone call, she imagined me to be enraged at her and thought that I would abandon her. Her inability to tolerate intense hostile and aggressive fantasies was dealt with through projective mechanisms culminating in the fantasy that I hated her. Such primitive defensive operations are characteristic of borderline patients and not seen in neurotics suffering from endogenous depressions.

Cooper (1985), in talking of patients suffering from panic disorders, states that analysts must distinguish between psychological efforts to cope with miscarried brain function and the psychological efforts to cope with disturbances of the intrapsychic world. This is particularly true when attempting to make a clinical formulation in patients who suffer from affective and personality disorders.

For instance, patients who suffer from untreated affective disorder—such as Melissa B.—often speak of their experience of themselves as being out of control. They complain that they can never predict the stability of their emotional states. This aspect of their illness must be conceptualized not as reflecting faltering defensive operations and inadequate compromise formation but as a reaction of the otherwise healthy personality to the experience of being intermittently overwhelmed by biologically generated mood states.

Cooper also states that biologic illnesses must be regarded as having influences that are both developmental and ongoing. The psychoendocrine work of Puig-Antich (Puig-Antich et al. 1984), which demonstrates the existence of endogenous depression in latency-age children, supports the notion that this illness can arise during periods of development. For patients such as Melissa B., normal developmental tasks of childhood and adolescence may be severely compromised.

For her, difficulties with object constancy could be traced to maternal deprivation and to repeated emotional abandonments by her parents. However, the affective disorder that subjected her to extreme mood fluctuations throughout her adolescence must have served as a major disruption to the consolidation of this ego function.

Transference–Countertransference

The central transference fantasy for Melissa B. was that I regarded her as her father did—that I viewed her as special, that I thought her to be willfully causing her affective states, that I was intolerant of her anger, that she was dependent on me for survival, and that I would eventually abandon her because of her anger and depression. Her limited capacity for object constancy intensified her constant fright that I would disappear. This fear was most often manifest after major affective eruptions. As treatment progressed her transference fantasies became less "as if" and subject to analytic exploration and more and more experienced as reality. Ultimately this led to the disruption of treatment.

The reality of my active interventions during the course of Melissa's treatment did in fact reinforce some of these fantasies. She had numerous uncommon, complicated, and severe side effects, which necessitated frequent consultations with internists, cardiologists, and psychopharmacologists. While their findings and recommendations were all thoroughly discussed with the patient, the final management decisions rested with me, and her dependence on me was intense. It is not surprising that she felt that if she couldn't be treated by me, she couldn't be treated by anyone.

On the other hand, the extent to which this recreated for her in fantasy the actual childhood experience of having a life-threatening illness in which her father was the primary caretaker and which was utilized by him for enacting his own incestuous fantasies must have made a major contribution to the intensity of the rage she experienced, the fears of abandonment, and the almost delusional conviction about my anger at her.

Of course the countertransference in working with borderline patients must be examined, especially when the therapist encounters relentless hostility from a patient he or she is trying to help. Professional dedication is not enough to account for the willingness to work with such patients, and each case presents a unique constellation of reactions that need to be explored.

I viewed Melissa B.'s depression as a life-threatening illness that had not been recognized or adequately treated by others. With her, at the most conscious level, I was aware of unresolved competitive fantasies connected to the previous therapist, whose treatment had failed. Certainly it would feel good to prove I was a better therapist than he. At a less accessible level was the fantasy that I could be a better father to her than her own father was, and that unlike him, I was not going to be put off by her affective storms. At a deeper level still was the notion that while her father might have been a great military commander, certainly I could prove myself the better man by showing that I was a great physician. Finally, there was a shared unconscious fantasy: she was in fact an immensely complicated patient who called upon all my professional resources—perhaps it was true, after all, that only I could treat her.

An awareness of such personal fantasies led me to consult frequently with colleagues about this case and on several occasions to urge Melissa to obtain consultations both with psychopharmacologists and psychoanalysts. Unfortunately, she refused, and in the end the treatment failed.

The recognition that patients may have major affective disorders concurrent with long-standing personality disorders is a relatively recent advance in psychiatry. More needs to be written about the difficulties encountered in undertaking intensive psychotherapy with such patients. As analytically oriented therapists work more intensively with patients they may also be medicating, the types of problems seen in the treatment of this patient may become more common. While their treatment can be extremely difficult, the utilization of one's medical and psychotherapeutic skills in the management of such patients can be beneficial to them and richly rewarding to the psychiatrist.

References

Brenner, C. (1982). *The Mind in Conflict.* New York: International Universities Press.

Browne, J. L., Perry, P. J., and Taylor, J. W. (1984). Nortriptyline capacity limited metabolism: a case report. *Journal of Clinical Psychopharmacology* 4:322–325.

Cooper, A. M. (1985). Will neurobiology influence psychoanalysis? *American Journal of Psychiatry* 142:1395–1402.

Freud, S. (1917). Mourning and melancholia. *Standard Edition* 14:239–258.

Kantor, S. J. (1986). A difficult alprazolam withdrawal. *Journal of Clinical Psychopharmacology* 6:124–125.

Mishkin, M., and Appenzeller, T. (1987). The anatomy of memory. *Scientific American* 256:80–89.

Penfield, W., and Perot, P. (1963). The brain's record of auditory and visual experience. *Brain* 86:595–696.

Post, R. M., Uhde, T. W., Putnam, F. W., et al. (1982). Kindling and carbamazapine in affective illness. *Journal of Nervous and Mental Disease* 170:717–731.

Puig-Antich, J., Novacenko, H., Davies, M., et al. (1984). Growth hormone secretion in prepubertal children with major depression. *Archives of General Psychiatry* 41:455–483.

19

Analyzing a Rapid Cycler: Can the Transference Keep Up?

SHEPARD J. KANTOR, M.D.

At one time patients with mood disturbances unresponsive to analytic interventions were viewed as having failed psychological treatments. More recently analysts have begun to view such patients as suffering from two disorders: one psychological, which has benefitted from analytic treatment and one biological, which has not. This report presents the first 12 months of the analysis of a patient whose treatment is complicated by the coexistence of Rapid Cycling Bipolar Disorder.

The chapter uses clinical material to illustrate how shifting mood states may be an episodic presence during an analysis and may be unaffected by analytic treatment. Even more important, it suggests that we must have a place in our psychoanalytic thinking for the concept that biologically generated mood states may exist that are devoid of dynamic significance, are not defensive, do not arise out of conflict, and are not understandable in terms of ego psychology. It urges analysts to limit their goals to those in the realm of character change and not to the expectation that successful analytic treatment will be reflected in the patient's ability to do away with medication or have a decreased number of affective episodes or hospitalizations.

More and more frequently, patients in analytic psychotherapy and psychoanalysis who have realized substantial gains from their treatment are being referred to psychopharmacologists for evaluations of subtle but clear-cut mood disturbances which have been unresponsive to psychological interventions (Kantor 1990). Whereas at one time they might have been viewed as having failed psychological treatments, such patients are increasingly seen as suffering from two disorders: one psychological, which has benefitted from analytic treatment, and one biological, which has not (Kantor 1989).

In undertaking the analysis of patients who suffer from affective disorders, the analyst's understanding of the relationship between the biological and the psychological will be crucial in determining which patients he or she elects to treat, to what extent formal analytic techniques must be modified for their treatment, to what extent medication will be relied upon, and what goals are realizable.

In the past, manic-depressive illness has been thought of as a single entity manifesting itself in alterations in mood states which shift between wild psychoses and suicidal depressions. In more recent years, manic-depressive illness has been viewed as a spectrum concept: patients have been characterized as Bipolar I or II based on the severity or intensity of their affective excursions and as Classical or Rapid Cycling based on the frequency of their oscillations in mood.

The patient I will present is a 20-year-old woman who has Rapid Cycling Bipolar Disorder. In addition, she has a severe character disorder, a central feature of which is the idea that, all things considered, she might just as well kill herself. The material to be presented includes 8 months of psychotherapeutic work, two hospitalizations prior to the adequate adjustment of her medications, and the initial 12 months of analysis.

My hope is that this material will illustrate the theoretical and practical questions which arise in working with patients who have both affective and character disorders and that a discussion of these problems will enable analysts to work more effectively with this type of patient.

Case Report

The patient is a 20-year-old woman whose parents separated when she was aged 11. She dates her earliest memory from age 5. Her mother was ill and reported that the doctor said the only way she could recover was if she went to France without her daughter. Her mother subsequently told the patient that she was only joking.

She recalls having been unhappy for much of her childhood, stating that she always felt herself to have been an "evil person." She felt like an outcast growing up, was picked on by class bullies, and felt she couldn't compete socially.

In junior high, she had a very low opinion of herself, felt her peers talked about her, and was eventually ignored by them. She often came home weeping. Fortunately, her superior intellect and ability to do schoolwork enabled her to become an honors student. Her life didn't improve until high school, where for the first time she was appreciated and liked by students as well as teachers.

Her mother vacillated between telling the patient that she was an evil child who didn't deserve to be loved, and telling her that she was the center of the mother's universe, the only thing that made her life worth living. The patient remembers verbal and sometimes physical battles, which at times would result in her mother throwing her out of the house and threatening not to allow her back.

This fighting went on throughout the patient's childhood and adolescence. She remembers scenes in which her mother would burst into her room, tear down curtain rods, throw books off the shelves, rip pages out of her books, and have frequent hysterical outbursts. Many times her mother would castigate the patient for ruining her own artistic career, saying she should never have had children in the first place.

To what extent her father, who had left home when she was 11 years old, was providing adequate financial support was a mystery to the patient and the subject of much acrimonious talk by her mother. While the patient was able to attend private high school financed by her father, every year there was great anxiety about whether or not her mother would pay the tuition. This was a matter of desperation for the patient, in that private school was the first time that she felt adequate, competent, and less of an outsider than she had felt throughout her earlier life.

Despite the verbal and physical outbursts, her mother held herself out to be the best possible, most perfect mother there ever was. The patient was uncertain about whether or not this was so. She felt that her mother often denied the truth of situations, fabricated responses, and completely reversed herself without acknowledging her former positions. This left the patient bewildered as to where the truth actually lay.

Despite these difficulties, the patient ultimately believed herself to have had a good relationship with her mother. She discounted the more serious and frightening aspects of her mother's behavior, including the mother's hysterical rages, in part by regarding her mother as somewhat "looney."

Recently her mother had a fight with the man she was dating. In the course of this fight, the mother took out a real gun, which her boyfriend didn't know was neither loaded nor functional. She held it to her boyfriend's head. Her mother found his terror hilarious and related this story to the patient. The patient reported this as yet another example of the "looney" things her mother does.

The patient's father is a highly regarded attorney. She remembers him with great fright and described a number of episodes in which he hit her or threatened to do so. When her mother would throw her out of the house and say she wouldn't let her return, she would call her father, who would tell her that this was her problem to work out with her mother and that she couldn't come to live with him.

In recent years he seems to have mellowed and become more emotionally available to her. They have developed a much better relationship and frequently talk and have dinner together.

Affective Disorder

The patient's father has a history of depression treated with antidepressants. His own father had a history of depression treated with electroshock therapy. The patient's cousin is manic-depressive.

The patient's journals, which she began in adolescence, reveal several periods of severe depression and suicidal thinking. It is not possible to determine at precisely what point these mood states (which may have represented some mixture of situational reaction, character disorder, and early bipolar mood disturbances) crystallized into the first manifestation of her affective disorder.

However, she does recall that on and off during adolescence she had a number of 1- to 2-week periods when she would become more severely depressed, sleep 14 hours a day, become withdrawn and unsociable, and have poor concentration.

At age 15–16 she believes she started having her first hypomanic episodes. The first one lasted about a week, during which she was "incredibly productive, ebullient, and sociable" and needed only 6 hours' sleep a night. She thinks she had four or five similar episodes during late adolescence, although they tended to last days and not weeks.

Six months prior to beginning treatment with me, she was referred to a psychiatrist because of severe depression. She was having some cycling during this time, and when she was started on an antidepressant, her cycling became exaggerated and her moods more volatile. She had multiple mood changes within a few days or even within 24 hours and was soon hospitalized in a full-blown manic state manifested by excessive talking, diminished need for sleep, and a sense of elation. She was hospitalized for 3 weeks and placed on lithium carbonate, which stabilized her mood.

She saw me in consultation shortly after her hospital discharge. At that time she was continuing to have mild cycles. They seemed manageable on lithium and there was the expectation that because lithium has increasing effectiveness as a person has been on it longer, her mood would level out entirely.

In addition to needing someone to follow her medication, the patient had a number of problems for which she wanted psychological help. These included:

1. Feelings that she wasn't genuine, as if she were "a constructed facsimile of a human being. I spend my whole life imitating others."

2. She wanted to write fiction and couldn't because her creative thinking was interrupted by intrusive thoughts. For instance, when attempting to write a humorous portrait of family life, her thoughts would lead to matricide.

3. She had "always" wanted to cut herself with razors but began actually doing so only in the past year.

4. She had been incapable of sustaining a good relationship with a man and repeatedly became involved with men who treated her badly.

At the time of my initial consultation, I felt the patient had two different types of illness for which she needed different and concurrent treatments. She had a yet-to-be-fully-stabilized Rapid Cycling Bipolar Disorder as well as character pathology, possibly of a borderline dimension, which needed intensive psychotherapeutic work. She was obviously very bright and suffering a great deal but was quite fearful of psychotherapy and somewhat reluctant to engage in treatment.

Twice-weekly psychotherapy was begun. However, she immediately began slipping into a depression of increasing severity. After 2 weeks, small doses of an antidepressant were added to her lithium. Over the next several days her depression began to lift, but she started to get high. The antidepressant was discontinued and the lithium increased, which stabilized her mood.

As she had begun to talk more openly about herself and was beginning to feel that treatment might be of benefit to her, therapy was increased to three times a week. However, she again became severely depressed. An antidepressant was added, but again she began to cycle into highs, lows, and mixed states in which she was simultaneously high and low.

During this period of great mood instability and when she was actually somewhat hypomanic, for the first time in her life, she began to have vivid images of having been molested by her grandfather, who died when she was 11.

These images were frequent, vivid, and detailed. She was quite bewildered by having them at all, and whereas they had an air of reality about them, she could not decide whether they were real or had been made up.

No psychotherapeutic work could be done with this because her mood instability increased, her hypomanic behavior accelerated, and she had to be hospitalized in a manic state 6 months after beginning treatment with me.

She spent the next 6 weeks in two different hospitals with her course complicated by drug toxicity, side effects, allergic reactions to medication, lithium-induced organicity, and self-mutilation. She was eventually stabilized on a combination of lithium carbonate and valproic acid, an antiseizure compound that has demonstrated considerable effectiveness in the stabilization of rapid cycling bipolar patients (see below, Rapid Cycling).

At the point of hospital discharge, her parents told her and me that they felt I was incompetent, that I had bungled their daughter's care, and that they did not want her to be treated by me any longer. After discussing this with the patient and agreeing that we wished to continue working together, I met with both parents together who ultimately agreed to let her continue working with me.

Three-times-weekly therapy thus resumed a week after her hospital discharge. With some minor medication adjustments her mood remained stable. She began to reveal that for the preceding 18 months she had increasingly felt that life held out no prospects for her and that she might just as well be dead. Three months before beginning treatment with me, at a time when she was euthymic, she was visiting a friend who happened to have a gun in the house. The patient put the barrel of this gun in her mouth. She said she was not suicidal but just "wanted to see what it felt like."

She discussed this material in a completely dispassionate way with no evidence of any biologic mood disturbance. She went on to tell me that she had set a date for her suicide and a method, neither of which she would reveal. She saw no reason to continue treatment because she didn't feel it would do any more than get her to accept some happy accommodation to life. She refused to be rehospitalized and stated that she would never speak to me again if I told her family of her suicidal plans.

Feeling I had no choice, I informed her father of her desperate condition and told him she needed immediate and long-term hospitalization. There was then a meeting between the patient and her family in which she convinced them that despite my alarm, her threat wasn't to be taken seriously.

Her father told his daughter and me that he had been suicidal at times in his life and knew what his daughter was experiencing. Although they certainly hoped that she wouldn't do anything to herself, they would not under any circumstances hospitalize their daughter against her will.

At her next appointment, she expressed her fury at me for the betrayal of having told her parents.

Over the next 2 weeks we discussed whether she was willing to continue seeing me and whether I was willing to continue working with her. She said that despite her anger at me she wanted to continue working together. She accepted my terms: she would increase the frequency of sessions to four times a week, she would dispose of whatever she had planned to kill herself with, she would remain in treatment for at least another 10 months, and she would guarantee not to attempt suicide during that period (Kernberg et al. 1989).

During the preceding months, as the extent of her character pathology had become increasingly evident, I had been thinking that if her mood disorder could be stabilized, she should be analyzed. Her mood disorder had now been stabilized for over 2 months, and I felt reasonably optimistic that the combination of lithium and valproic acid would continue to keep her affective disorder under control.

Although she represented a high risk for suicide, I felt I could rely on her to keep to her end of our contract. I did not think her suicidal potential would be increased by analysis more than by intensive psychotherapy, and that whereas there was a real potential for acting out, I felt it would remain within manageable limits.

Above all, I felt that only if she could develop an analyzable transference neurosis would I be able to understand fully the sources of her problems and have enough leverage to enable her to make some lasting change in her life.

Of course there were a number of factors that might complicate or even mitigate against a successful analysis.

1. Her bipolar disorder might again become uncontrollable. This would preclude analytic work, in that "real" interventions I would have to make might be so extensive that the analysis would lose its "as-if" character. Though this represents a real possibility for any bipolar patient, I did not feel it should deprive this patient of an opportunity to be psychoanalyzed when her character pathology warranted it.

2. Psychoanalysis might make her bipolar disorder worse. I did not think this possible any more than I thought it might make her bipolar disorder better. Of course, were she to appear to be becoming psychotic, I could not leave her on the couch and would have to make whatever interventions might be necessary to deal with and control the psychosis.

3. I had already developed a "real relationship" with her and her parents: I had treated her successfully with medication where a previous psychiatrist had failed; I had treated her during a very complicated hospitalization; I had "betrayed her" in telling her parents she should be rehospitalized; I had been roundly criticized by her parents but had gotten them to allow her to continue treatment with me. The transference implications of these actions were unknown.

4. In my explanations to her and through the direct action of recommending psychoanalysis, I had made it clear to her that I thought she had two completely separate disorders: one biologic, for which she needed medication, and one psychological, for which she needed psychoanalysis. I told her that I did not expect medication to help her feelings of alienation, her inability to establish a satisfactory relationship with a man, her episodes of cutting herself, or the suicidal thinking that was independent of her affective disorder; and that I did not expect psychoanalysis to influence the course of her Rapid Cycling Bipolar Disorder.

I did not know if these factors would preclude the development of a workable transference relationship. However, the ability to predict which patients will develop a satisfactory analytic process and which will not is notoriously difficult. I felt the only way to assess whether or not a workable transference would develop was with a trial of analysis. This was begun at the point she had been in therapy with me for 10 months.

The Analysis

Starting in the first session, and lasting throughout the period I am reporting, the patient would frequently look back over her shoulder at me. At times she would do this in a joking way, at time coyly, at times to ask a serious question. It was many months before she was willing to see this as something that had some meaning worth understanding.

Initially she felt it was difficult to talk, and complained that the analysis just made her more aware of the emptiness of her inner self: "This is like putting a mirror in an empty room." She was aware of feeling frustrated and angry much of the time.

The complaining soon gave way to thoughts about her grandfather that she'd had the previous day, and which had led to another episode of cutting herself. She expressed her fears of telling me the thoughts about him lest they take on a reality she couldn't control or, alternatively, lest I would think she was poisonous for having invented such thoughts. Had all this happened with her grandfather or not?

More memories surfaced: where she slept on sleep-overs at his house, him sitting next to her on the couch on which she slept, her fright of what he was doing to her, his threats that she remain silent about it. "Each time I speak of this it comes more into focus . . . like a Polaroid developing." "If this all really happened, I feel soiled, unclean. You will lose respect for me." She began to wonder whether this explained her feelings of debasement as a child, what she was afraid couldn't be concealed from her peers.

She complained of how empty she felt at times, how vulnerable she felt on the couch, "like a crab on its back." She had felt separated from me since the analysis started. On occasion she said that looking back made her feel less separate.

Cutting herself continued with no apparent pattern: "I was just in the mood. I liked dragging the razor across my skin." She continued to feel suicidal but stated that when she felt so, she reminded herself of our contract.

Three weeks after the start of the analysis, she had a 48-hour hypo-manic episode which occurred over a weekend and was self-limited. She reported this as one event among many over the weekend.

The analysis proceeded with her beginning to talk of her mother's possessiveness. Even as a child she felt smothered by her mother's adora-tion and would hide in a closet and read to avoid her. Her looking back persisted. "I want to make sure you're not being judgmental or hostile when I talk of her."

She spoke of tremendous fights between her and her mother (de-scribed above) and reported the development of childhood fears that prevented her from going into certain parts of the house at night lest she be attacked. She recalled calling her father during these fights and his telling her she had to work them out herself.

I pointed out the good humor with which she described some of these fights and the defensive nature of her need to see these frightening battles as humorous. She said, "When I was little and grew up, I felt I'd developed the ability to close everything out . . . some inner part of me had to be untouched by any of the violence, the noise, the anger, until I no longer needed shields."

I told her that she still used many shields to ward off the emotional impact on her of her mother's behavior. "I'd love to believe she was horrifying. It would exonerate me. But you are just trying to make me feel better. I can't believe you are sincere."

During these conversations she would frequently look back, joking that she wanted to make sure I was still there. I told her that her mother seemed like a character in a fairy tale, that she was either the good witch or the bad witch and she didn't know when one would disappear and be replaced by the other. She might have similar ideas about me disappearing and was just looking back to check. She thought this was ridiculous.

She went on to say that growing up, she thought her father was the problem, not her mother. It was always difficult, if not impossible, to refute her mother's refrain, that she was the most perfect mother in the world. She added, "My view of her is in flux since we started treatment. My overall opinion is that my mother was very damaging. But even now when she says weird things, I have trouble seeing she's being weird."

But she then complained, "I feel that overall you hear me with an ear toward helping me exonerate my self."

I told her that overall I heard her with an ear tuned to the notion that her ideas of killing herself were based on a set of erroneous conclusions and that we had to understand how she'd drawn them. She said that she still thought of killing herself several times a week but, "I'm glad I don't do it. I feel my comfort with being alive is getting stronger."

She thought of cutting frequently throughout the day and continued to feel bouts of overwhelming self-hatred that would culminate in her actually cutting herself.

"I experience self-inflicted pain as a clarifying, freeing sensation. . . . Sometimes I can't justify staying alive . . . I'd rather kill myself."

During the third month of analysis I observed that I seemed to be hearing little of her daily life, that the analysis seemed to exist in a vacuum. She said that she had been aware of this as well. She didn't want to become the kind of person who depended on her analyst to run her daily life.

In the next session she reported having dreamed of a boyfriend whose father actually is a psychiatrist. In the dream the father is secretly a Mafia boss.

In the next session, she said she'd not known what made her so anxious when reporting the Mafia dream. Her associations led me to say that I thought it had to do with the subject of telling me about her daily life. She responded, "I don't want to feel I use analysis to get me through life. I'd feel too ordinary, too helpless, and too dependent on you." She went on to say that she had initially trusted me but hadn't since I'd told her father that she should be rehospitalized (a month before the start of the analysis).

She subsequently reported the recurrence of dreams of being chased by vampires. Her associations were to vampires as sexual seducers. She thought the dream has to do with me, how she just couldn't trust me since I called her parents. I did it once and might do it again. "Maybe I should have dropped out of treatment after that happened."

I said that her father had already told me that her life was her responsibility. I didn't think he'd respond any differently in the future and therefore I didn't feel there would be any point going to him under similar circumstances. I also said that although I appreciated that this was a real concern, I thought it must be coming up now for some particular reason. She spoke of her worry that my role was to make her "well adjusted" and that this would diminish her and take away her creativity and uniqueness.

At the end of the fourth month of analysis, her father was notified by his insurance company that the patient had exhausted her benefits. This provoked a major crisis in the analysis; the insurance coverage was a crucial element in the financing of her care and had been carefully evaluated prior to the start of treatment.

After several telephone conversations with her parents and a meeting between her mother and me, her parents agreed to share the cost of three-times-a-week treatment with the hope that the misunderstanding with the insurance company would be clarified. The analysis proceeded at three times weekly.

She reported that she felt it cowardly to try to suppress thoughts relating to her grandfather and went on to talk of the detailed images she had: of his house; his bedroom; where she slept when she stayed over; sexual experiences she thought they'd had. She had a jumble of images, some pleasant such as being pushed on the swings, others terrifying such as his putting his hand on her mouth so she wouldn't call out to her grandmother.

She went on to talk of her own current sexual difficulties, of how during sex she sometimes feels a tremendous pressure inside her head, as if she'll lose her mind or become hysterical. Sometimes when involved sexually with men she actually did become hysterical.

Over the next week or so there were more episodes of cutting herself, including once after a nightmare in which she went to work and there were a thousand people following her, taking notes, commenting and criticizing everything she did. They said it was important to collect information. Another dream that night was of someone disemboweling her.

Her associations were to the analysis making her weaker as a person. She went on to describe that with her friends she is now much more self-revealing than she'd been in the past. She likes this but it makes her feel exposed. She feels this especially in analysis, where she is left open to betrayal.

I then received an unexpected telephone call from her mother who said that everyone had misunderstood her. She had said she would only contribute toward treatment for another month until my summer vacation began and not in an ongoing way. The patient said this made her feel like she did in high school when there was the constant threat that she wouldn't be able to return in the fall. Maybe she should just stop treatment to avoid this whole situation with her mother. Her mother subsequently gave some reassurance that the money for treatment would be there and we should continue.

Analysis resumed with the patient continuing to complain of the difficulty she had not knowing about me and not knowing my thoughts. She said that she felt vulnerable in general, not only in the analysis. She then reported a dream in which she was having boring, mechanical sex with the man who had been her boyfriend on and off for 3 years. What was significant, she said, was that in the dream she hadn't been tied up.

She explained that being tied up, which she referred to as "light bondage," was an almost obligatory part of their sexual life though it was at his insistence, not hers. She protested when I suggested that this type of sexual practice had some meaning. She complained, "That is another horrible thing I don't want to believe. It makes sex so complicated. A single kiss can remind you of your whole childhood."

She said this boyfriend treated her badly in a number of situations, not just sexually. "What is wrong with me that I am never involved with someone in a normal way?"

Three weeks after her insurance company's cutting off benefits, they informed her that they had made an error and that her benefits would continue. We agreed to resume four sessions a week in the fall.

She then reported that she had discontinued her medications 2 weeks before but had just resumed them. She thought maybe this had to do with the recent financial discussions between her parents and me owing to the insurance discontinuation.

I pointed out that stopping the medication was like playing Russian roulette and that it must have had some meaning just as her having put the gun in her mouth some months prior to beginning treatment with me had some meaning.

She was quite angry when I suggested that her friend's idea, that the way for her to get her parents to pay for continued treatment was to stop her medication and go crazy, might also be her own. "I manipulate my parents, but would never do anything like that." I told her that the motivation for many of her self-destructive thoughts was not in her awareness and that something must lie behind her impulses and actions.

She then reported that for the past 2 months she'd become aware that no matter what we talked about, she has been getting increasingly angry at me. "Is this legitimate or is this transference?" she jokingly inquired. She thought the anger might be because she wants me to be more responsive or perhaps because she feels she's not making progress. Or maybe she is angry because I haven't told her I was certain that her experiences with her grandfather had been real or perhaps her anger is a response to feeling trapped. She feels she has to submit to whatever I say. I told her that I didn't think her anger was attributable to anything as specific as the complaints she'd mentioned. Rather, I thought the anger she was beginning to experience toward me, as well as her persistent need to look back at me, must be related to experiences and feelings the origins of which lay in her childhood. She responded, "My vulnerability to you is a big thing in this analysis."

I said I thought she was frightened at what might come up in the treatment and angry with me because she felt so frightened and vulnerable. I told her it was important to find out what lay behind the anger and not just feel she was angry and that was that. Just as she had begun evaluate her actual feelings towards her family, she had to try and find out what was behind the anger towards me.

She then went on to talk of her increasing ability to see her mother's problems. After giving me some examples, she reported a dream in which she and I were chatting. She was annoyed to have a dream about me. "It means that analysis is getting to me. You must be pleased to have people all over the city dreaming of you," she joked.

A week before my vacation (a month after she had resumed the medication she had interrupted for 2 weeks) she had a 2-day hypomanic episode. In the session she was bubbly, giggly, couldn't lie on the couch, paced around the office, and couldn't follow her own thoughts.

This state persisted into the next night when, after a call to me, she took 20 mg of Thorazine. She slept well and the next day was euthymic.

She returned to the couch after sitting up for one session. She asked in passing about my vacation coverage, which I'd already explained to her. She then went on to talk about a number of unrelated subjects. I asked for her thoughts about the manic episode. "It's just another day, it comes and it goes." She then went on to talk of her manic-depressive cousin, who denied many aspects of her own illness.

I again asked her about her own recent episode and she said how worried she was that it wouldn't go away. I asked why she thought she'd again asked about my vacation coverage. "When you have rockets going off in your head, you want to know who is going to be around." She'd not had an episode in 4 months and was worried that if it happened now, it could happen again. She was upset when I told her that having a new episode meant she'd need to be on medication at least 6 more months.

I remarked on how if I hadn't asked, she wouldn't have said anything about her reaction to having gotten high. I said she was trying to deal with this as she'd dealt with other upsetting experiences in her life: to act as if they hadn't happened, that it was business as usual.

She wanted to know what I made of the fact that she cut herself when she was high as well as when she wasn't. I told her I didn't know. She said she hoped it didn't mean that getting high was psychological, because she wanted to keep the getting high separated from her character. If her manic-depression and her character were part of the same thing, it meant she was more severely disturbed, that her manic-depressive episodes were signs of a serious weakness in her character. I told her that I didn't think getting high was psychological but that when high she might do or say things that had psychological significance.

She ended the session with the hope that she wouldn't get high while I was on vacation and the thought that she was looking forward to the resumption of four-times-a-week treatment on my return: "It is very intense, it comes to rule your existence, but I think it is a good thing and I have hope."

When the analysis resumed, she began discussing her difficulties with creative work, which was impeded by intrusive, sometimes violent thoughts. She was also frightened that her creative work went off in unintended directions, sometimes leading to frightening material but more often frightening her because she didn't feel in control of where her thoughts would lead.

During the first month back it became evident that she was still cycling, although in a much milder fashion than before medication. This sometimes led to an exacerbation in suicidal thinking or to somewhat impaired concentration for a day or two. It sometimes led to analytic sessions in which she had little to say, or to depressive affect that seemed incongruous with either the mood or material that had been evident over immediately preceding days.

I elected to continue with her current medications in the hopes that these mood shifts would be further muted with more time at these dosages.

During the next several months the patient developed an increasing conviction that she had in fact been molested by her grandfather. This came as a consequence of readings she had done, of work in the treatment, and because increasingly coherent memories of the experiences had begun to emerge.

At the same time, she became involved with a man in whom she was interested, who respected and admired her, and who treated her well. However, she became preoccupied with the obsessional concern that he would harm or kill her. She knew this was absurd but couldn't get the thoughts out of her mind.

During the tenth month of analysis, these fantasies and obsessional concerns that he might harm her escalated into a delusional conviction that she was in actual physical danger.

This delusion was accompanied by visual hallucinations, gross tremors, and a pronounced facial tic. Whereas all her blood levels, including serum ammonia, were normal, and her lithium and valproate blood levels were within their therapeutic ranges, it seemed that she was experiencing a drug-induced delirium and not any type of schizophrenic episode. Lithium was discontinued, valproate was decreased, and these symptoms cleared within 72 hours. She was subsequently maintained on valproate alone with no return of delusional thinking, hallucinations, or myoclonic activity.

However, her obsessional concerns about being endangered by her boyfriend persisted. She was reminded that she had had similar concerns during childhood when she imagined she would be attacked in her house. She was told that these concerns must have been a consequence of worries and fantasies about her mother, which she did not allow into her awareness. I told her how these same frights have been expressed in the analysis through her fears of attack by me and how they must be arising in her current relationship and in the analysis because they recreated the intimacies and fears of her childhood.

This seemed true to her, and as a consequence of these interpretations her obsessions about attack by her boyfriend receded. In addition, while she continued to have self-mutilative fantasies, she stopped cutting herself and refrained from doing so throughout the next 4 months of analysis.

During the next several months, she reported herself as being intermittently moody, although much less intensely than before she was begun on medication, and she also reported an intermittent sleep disturbance. Whether these expressed an underlying mood disorder was unclear.

She then entered a period in which silence became a significant factor in the analysis. She said she felt she had to screen and censor what she reported: "I'm unwilling to expose anything but an elaborately filtered version of myself. I do that with you and I do it with the rest of my life. I worry that if I spoke without screening, I'd open myself to interpretations I don't want to make available to you. You'll end up thinking I'm evil."

The first year of analysis ended with her understanding that the period of silence would end only when she could take a chance of further exposing herself in the analysis.

Rapid Cycling Bipolar Disorder

Whereas most manic-depressives have one or two episodes of mania or depression a year or may go for years between affective episodes, some patients have a much greater frequency of highs and lows. Fieve and Dunner (1974) first described a group of patients who had more than four affective cycles in a year and coined the term Rapid Cycling Bipolar Disorder to describe them. Their observation that these patients represent a discrete subgroup has been substantiated and refined over the years.

However a recent collaborative project done by the National Institute of Mental Health came to the opposite conclusion: the findings of this group were that rapid cycling is not a distinct condition but simply represents one end of a cycle frequency spectrum. They also reported that rapid cycling was not a permanent feature of a patient's illness: in almost all cases it was only seen transiently during a 5-year period of observation (Coryell et al. 1992).

Other investigators suggest that rapid cycling is not only becoming increasingly reported but may actually be demonstrating an increased incidence in patients suffering from bipolar disorders (Wolpert et al. 1990).

The purely endogenous nature of rapid cycling has been of particular interest to investigators exploring the biologic underpinnings of psychological states. Patients have been shown to have fixed cycle length regardless of their environment and have been shown to continue to cycle even under conditions of sensory deprivation where there are no cues given with respect to time of day (Sack 1986).

Patients with this disorder may switch from one affective state to the other within a several-hour period. An example of such an abrupt mood change occurred in a rapid cycling woman I treated, who described herself as switching from depression to hypomania while having her nails done at a beauty parlor. Researchers have focused on this "switch process" in attempts to determine what biologic processes are responsible for the change from one affective state to another (Carney et al. 1989).

Some have looked at dopamine metabolism with respect to this switch process (Carney et al. 1989), whereas others have focused on disorders of the thyroid axis. Here (Bauer and Whybrow 1990 and Bauer et al. 1990), work suggests that the site of the biologic defect may be in the hypothalamus and that relative hypothyroidism within the central nervous system may lead to rapid cycling. Patients whose rapid cycling responds poorly to more traditional treatments are sometimes given high-dose thyroid medication, a therapy consistent with the theory that central nervous system hypothyroidism may play a role in rapid cycling.

In addition to having a different clinical picture and sex distribution from classic manic-depressives, rapid cyclers demonstrate a different treatment response: as a group, they tend to be less responsive to lithium carbonate and more likely to be provoked into manic states by antidepressants. (Haykal 1990, Prien and Gelenberg 1989, Roy-Byrne et al. 1984, Sack 1986).

Because of their relative unresponsivity to treatment with lithium, rapid cyclers are often concurrently treated with the antiseizure medications carbamazapine and valproic acid (McElroy et al. 1989, Prien and Gelenberg 1989).

Serendipitously discovered to have anti–manic-depressive properties approximately 10 years ago, these compounds have become the mainstay of treatment for rapid cyclers as well as for more typical manic-depressives who fail to benefit from, or cannot tolerate, lithium carbonate.

Psychoanalysis of Patients with Affective Disorder

A number of studies have been reported in which attempts have been made to work analytically with affectively disordered patients. The work of Fromm-Reichman's group (Cohen et al. 1954) offers perhaps the best summary of thinking during the prepsychopharmacologic era.

Whereas they appreciated the fact that manic-depression probably had a number of etiologic factors, they were particularly interested in pursuing the role that psychodynamic factors played in bringing about this illness.

They state, "We agree with Freud, Lewin, and others that dynamically the manic behavior can best be understood as a defensive structure utilized by the patient to avoid recognizing and experiencing his feelings of depression" (p. 122).

Loeb and Loeb (1987), on the other hand, discuss psychoanalytic observations on the effect of lithium on manic attacks. They cite the work of Kraepelin, Fenichel, and Jacobson, who felt that purely biologic determinants accounted for outbreaks of mania.

Rather than agreeing with Lewin who felt mania was a defense against depression, they viewed mania as the manifestation of an instinctual drive which needed to be defended against.

They state, "between manic attacks, the manic's ego seems to function like a neurotic's, and he uses neurotic defense mechanisms to resolve conflicts between his id and reality" (p. xx).

David Kahn (1990), in his *Psychotherapy of Mania* discusses the possibility that beyond its effect of enhancing medication compliance, psychological treatment may have an additive and independent impact on the course of properly medicated bipolar illness.

Kahn focuses his psychotherapeutic work on the traumatic experience of the illness itself and the effect this illness has on the patients' real and intrapsychic life. These include (1) interrupted developmental tasks, especially when the illness begins in adolescence; (2) problems in discriminating normal from abnormal moods; (3) fears of recurrence; (4) concerns about genetic transmission; (5) realistic losses, such as the sometimes diminished creativity and productivity owing to treatment; (6) symbolic losses such as feelings of defectiveness related to the illness and its treatment.

He advocates an eclectic psychotherapy that balances the needs between expressive/psychodynamic, cognitive, and behavioral approaches. Neither Kahn nor Loeb and Loeb seem to feel that early childhood issues have much to do with the development of manic-depressive illness.

Wylie and Wylie (1987) described an analytic case who could not be analyzed until her hysteroid dysphoria (Liebowitz and Klein 1979) was treated with medication. They felt "the character container for her neurotic conflicts was essentially sound" (p. 490). They reasoned that she suffered from a disorder of neurotransmitter regulation, the correction of which would enable her to benefit more broadly from psychoanalysis. With reference to the combination of medication and psychoanalysis, they concluded that "an adherence to psychoanalytic orthodoxy should not be cause for overlooking pertinent advances in understanding neurochemistry" (p. 492).

Of course, analyzing patients who have concurrent affective disorders creates certain technical difficulties not present in other cases. Cohen (1991) describes this dilemma in trying to determine whether her analytic patient's plummeting mood was the consequence of an anniversary reaction, a transference reaction, or an expression of the patient's endogenous depressive disorder, which had been unmasked because her antidepressant dosage had been decreased.

The idea as expressed by Loeb and Loeb (1987), that "between manic attacks, the manic's ego seems to function like a neurotic's" or as expressed by Wylie and Wylie (1987), that "the character container for the neurotic conflicts is essentially sound," is central to working analytically with patients who suffer from character pathology as well as concurrent affective disorders.

Clinical Case Discussion

The first question about analyzing a bipolar patient is whether or not treatment is making the affective disorder worse. Prior to stabilization with medicine this young woman had two hospitalizations and dramatic mood oscillations, sometimes daily, sometimes every 2 to 3 weeks. Since the start of intensive therapy and psychoanalysis, and while remaining on medication, she has had only two severe affective episodes lasting 48 to 72 hours each, which occurred 4 months apart. It would thus seem that, to date, the improvement in her rapid cycling brought about by medication has not been diminished by intensive treatment. Although she continues to cycle, her mood shifts are much less frequent and much milder than before having begun medication. Hopefully, with time or with further medication adjustments, these will become an even smaller factor in her life and in the analysis.

The next question concerns whether or not an insight-oriented treatment is developing.

The traumas that have organized this patient's life have been those of the emotional and actual abandonment by both parents, her mother's constant denial of the patient's own perceptions and reality, and her incestuous experiences.

Her childhood memories were replete with instances of extreme conflict, sometimes leading to physical violence with a mother who vacillated between smothering her daughter with love and affection and telling her that she had ruined her life, destroyed her career, was not deserving of a mother's love.

She had no help from her father with this, as he was a frightening, at times violent man who had little to do with his children after he left home and who constantly told his daughter to deal with her mother without his help.

Recollections of some kind of incestuous experience with her grandfather came into her awareness during the first several months of psychotherapy and have continued to be an important part of the analysis. In my experience it is not unusual for long-repressed incestuous material to spontaneously erupt into the awareness of incest victims. To what extent these memories emerged into my patient's awareness as a consequence of the treatment itself, the hypomanic state she was in when they first appeared, or some unrelated factors is uncertain.

During the course of the analysis these memories have continued to emerge and have been worked with therapeutically. The material has been related to her childhood perceptions of herself as damaged or soiled and to her current feelings of alienation and self-destructiveness.

Her relationship with her mother has been explored, and she has begun to see how she uses intense denial and a sardonic humor to deal with experiences that have been both infuriating and frightening. As a consequence, for the first time she has begun to distance herself from entanglements with her mother and to recognize and better cope with her mother's often irrational behavior.

She has not yet recognized the depths of her anger or the extent to which she turns it against herself. She rejects the possibility that such anger could have led her to have temporarily discontinued medication.

She has begun to examine some of her feelings of worthlessness and to see that they have something to do with her difficulty with romantic attachments.

All of these developments are signs that she has begun to benefit from and become engaged in the early stages of an insight-oriented treatment. But what of the transference? Is it developing? How has it been influenced by my active interventions, which included the prescribing of medication, hospital treatment, and family meetings, as well as frank discussions with her about her affective disorder?

If the transference were to have been shaped by my interventions in the treatment of her bipolar disorder, I would have expected this to have been in the direction of positive and trusting feelings towards me. After all, over a period of many months I had finally gotten her bipolar illness under control, had several frank discussions with her about her illness and its management, and had numerous meetings with her parents.

Furthermore, with the exception of my once telling her parents she needed to be hospitalized against her will, she knew that I had uniformly supported her position with respect to her continuing need for treatment, and that in a direct confrontation with them I had gotten them to back down when they wanted to stop her treatment with me because they had felt I was incompetent. Finally, their concern about her illness and my meetings with them had resulted in her parents speaking with each other and working together in a civil fashion for the first time in 10 years.

Despite all of these "real" interventions with the patient, her view of me in the transference was not of a caring and concerned physician who could be safely relied upon and who would protect her. To the contrary. The patient's uneasiness was evident from the first session in which she began looking back at me. After the first 2 months of analysis, she said that the reason that she wasn't reporting many details of her daily life was because she didn't want to depend on me and, as a subsequent dream in which I was represented as a Mafia don revealed, she couldn't trust me.

Another dream, one in which her friends turned into vampires whom she views as dangerous seducers, she also relates to me. How can she trust me after I betrayed her trust by telling her parents to rehospitalize her? Would I actually harm her by taking away her creativity and uniqueness?

Several weeks later she had dreams of being followed by an army of note takers and of being disemboweled. She associated to me and the recurrent theme of whether analysis will weaken or harm her. The more she comes to depend on me, the more she is worried about betrayal by me.

During the sixth month of the analysis, she observed that the mounting anger she felt toward me didn't seem to make sense. She went on to say that she thought it had something to do with the vulnerability she felt toward me. A partial interpretation of the transference fantasy that I might harm her has been used to show how fantasies that persist from her childhood interfere with her current romantic life, and has resulted in the dispelling of her obsessional concerns that her boyfriend might want to kill her.

After 12 months, the experience of me as dangerous and possibly malevolent figure, a consequence of internal fantasies that have remained unaltered despite my active interventions on her behalf, continues to play a dominant role in the analysis.

Conclusions

During the first 12 months of analysis, the "real" relationship that was necessitated by the management of this patient's affective disorder has not stood in the way of her developing a set of transferential attitudes stemming from lifelong feelings of distrust, fear, and vulnerability. Assuming that her bipolar disorder does not get out of control, there is no reason to feel that she cannot develop a workable transference relationship. In answer to the question posed by the title of this chapter, I would respond, "Yes, the transference is keeping up."

However, I would like to say more. The concept of signal-to-noise ratio, which is used in the study of many physical and biologic systems, may also be applied to psychoanalysis. In our work with patients we are constantly trying to discriminate the signals of unconscious communication from a confusing cacophony of background noises: reports of daily activity, dreams, acting out, historical information, screen memories, and transference as well as counter-transference reactions.

In working analytically with affectively disordered patients, we must be alert to the presence of a second set of signals: those emanating from biologically generated mood states. We must be prepared to observe and track them and determine how the patient and the analysis are being affected by them. We must evaluate the ways in which our patients' various ego strengths and weaknesses come into play in their attempts to cope with mood states that are not within their conscious or unconscious control.

We must accept the notion that although they may be an episodic or constant presence during the analysis, these mood states may be unaffected by analytic treatment. Even more important, we must have a place in our psycho-analytic thinking for the concept that biologically generated mood states may exist that are devoid of dynamic significance, are not defensive, do not arise out of conflict, and are not understandable in terms of ego psychology.

Although there are some theoretical notions to the contrary (Post et al. 1982, Post 1992) in fairness to him- or herself, the analyst must limit the goals of analysis to those in the realm of character change and not to the expectation that successful analytic treatment will be reflected in the patient's ability to do away with medication or have a decreased number of affective episodes or hospital-izations.

As I hope can be seen from this presentation, working with patients who have character pathology as well as concurrent affective disorders provides analysts with new challenges, enables us to reevaluate the ever-changing interface between psychology and biology, and provides new opportunities to patients who in the past might have been deprived of the potential benefits offered by psychoanalysis.

References

Bauer, M. S., and Whybrow, P. C. (1990). Rapid cycling bipolar affective disorder: treatment of refractory rapid cycling with high-dose levothyroxine. *Archives of General Psychiatry* 47:435–440.

Bauer, M. S., Whybrow, P. C., and Winokur, A. (1990). Rapid cycling bipolar affective disorder: association with grade 1 hypothyroidism. *Archives of General Psychiatry* 47:427–432.

Carney, M. W. P., Chary, T. K. N., Bottiglieri, T., and Reynolds, E. H. (1989). The switch mechanism and the bipolar/unipolar dichotomy. *British Journal of Psychology* 154:48–51.

Cohen, M. B., Baker, G., Cohen, R. A., et al. (1954). An intensive study of twelve cases of manic-depressive psychosis. *Psychiatry* 17:103–137.

Cohen, S. K. (1991). The use of medication with patients in analysis. *Journal of Clinical Psychoanalysis* 1:26–35.

Coryell, W., Endicott, J., and Keller, M. (1992). Rapidly cycling affective disorder. *Archives of General Psychiatry* 49:126–131.

Fieve, R., and Dunner, D. (1974). Clinical factors in lithium carbonate prophylaxis failure. *Archives of General Psychiatry* 30:229–233.

Haykal, R. F., and Akiskal, H. S. (1990). Bupropion as a promising approach to rapid cycling bipolar II patients. *Journal of Clinical Psychiatry* 51:450–455.

Kahn, D. (1990). The psychotherapy of mania. *Psychiatric Clinics of North America* 13:229–239.

Kantor, S. J. (1989). Transference and the beta adrenergic receptor. *Psychiatry* 52:107–115.

_____ (1990). Depression: when is psychotherapy not enough? *Psychiatric Clinics of North America* 13:241–254.

Kernberg, O. F., Selzer, M. A., Koenigsberg, H. W., et al. (1989). *Psychodynamic Psychotherapy of Borderline Patients*. New York: Basic Books.

Liebowitz, M. D., and Klein, D. F. (1979). Hysteroid dysphoria. *Psychiatric Clinics of North America* 2:555–575.

Loeb, F. F., and Loeb, L. R. (1987). Psychoanalytic observations on the effect of lithium on manic attacks. *Journal of the American Psychoanalytic Association* 35:877–901.

McElroy, S. L., Keck, P. E., Pope, H. G., and Hudson, J. I. (1989). Valproate in psychiatric disorders: literature review and clinical guidelines. *Journal of Clinical Psychoanalysis* 50(Suppl.):23–29.

Prien, R. F., and Gelenberg, A. J. (1989). Alternatives to lithium for preventive treatment of bipolar disorder. *American Journal of Psychiatry* 146:840–848.

Post, R. M. (1992). Transduction of psychosocial stress into the neurobiology of recurrent affective disorder. *American Journal of Psychiatry* 149:999–1010.

Post, R. M., Uhde, T. W., Putnam, F. W., et al. (1982). Kindling and carbamazapine in affective illness. *Journal of Nervous and Mental Disease* 170:717–731.

Roy-Byrne, P. P., Joffe, R. T., Uhde, T. W., and Post, R. M. (1984). Approaches to the evaluation and treatment of rapid-cycling affective illness. *British Journal of Psychiatry* 145:543–550.

Sack, D. A. (1986). An approach to the patient with rapid-cycling bipolar disorder. *Currents in Affective Illness* 5:5–12.

Wolpert, E. A., Goldberg, J. F., and Harrow, M. (1990). Rapid cycling in unipolar and bipolar affective disorders. *American Journal of Psychiatry* 147:725–728.

Wylie, H. W., and Wylie, M. L. (1987). An effect of pharmacotherapy on the psychoanalytic process: case report of a modified analysis. *American Journal of Psychiatry* 144:489–492.

Credits

Chapter 1: "The Psychology of Psychopharmacology," by Thomas G. Gutheil. Originally printed in *Bulletin of the Menninger Clinic* 1982, vol. 46, pp. 321–330. Copyright © 1982 The Menninger Foundation. Reprinted by permission of the *Bulletin of the Menninger Clinic* and the author.

Chapter 2: "Psychotherapy and Pharmacotherapy: Toward an Integrative Model," by Toksoz B. Karasu. Originally printed in the *American Journal of Psychiatry*, 1982, vol. 139, pp. 1102–1113. Copyright © 1982 by the American Psychiatric Association. Reprinted by permission of the American Psychiatric Association and the author.

Chapter 3: "Will Neurobiology Influence Psychoanalysis?" by Arnold M. Cooper. Originally printed in the *American Journal of Psychiatry*, 1985, vol. 142, pp. 1395–1402. Copyright © 1985 by the American Psychiatric Association. Reprinted by permission of the American Psychiatric Association and the author.

Chapter 4: "Adverse Response to Neuroleptics in Schizophrenia," by Donald B. Nevins. Originally printed in the *International Journal of Psychoanalytic Psychotherapy*, 1977, vol. 6, pp. 227–241. Copyright © 1977 by Jason Aronson Inc. Reprinted by permission of Jason Aronson Inc. and the author.

Chapter 5: "Psychoanalytic Observations on the Effect of Lithium on Manic Attacks," by Felix F. Loeb, Jr. and Loretta R. Loeb. Originally printed in the *Journal of the American Psychoanalytic Association*, 1987, vol. 35, pp. 877–902. Copyright © 1987 by International Universities Press. Reprinted by permission of International Universities Press and the authors.

Chapter 6: "Medication and Transitional Phenomena," by Robert Hausner. Originally printed in the *International Journal of Psychoanalytic Psycho-*

therapy, 1985–1986, vol. 11, pp. 375–398. Copyright © 1985–1986 by Jason Aronson Inc. Reprinted by permission of Jason Aronson Inc. and the author.

Chapter 7: "Pills as Transitional Objects: A Dynamic Understanding of the Use of Medication in Psychotherapy," by Steven A. Adelman. Originally published in *Psychiatry,* 1985, vol. 48, pp. 246–253. Copyright © 1985 by the Washington School of Psychiatry. Reprinted by permission of the Washington School of Psychiatry and the author.

Chapter 8: "How Does Psychiatric Drug Therapy Work?" by Mortimer Ostow. Originally published in the *Israel Journal of Psychiatry,* 1987, vol. 24, pp. 265–279. Copyright © 1987 by the *Israel Journal of Psychiatry* and Gefen Press. Reprinted by permission of the *Israel Journal of Psychiatry,* Gefen Press, and the author.

Chapter 9: "Comments on the Pathogenesis of the Borderline Disorder," by Mortimer Ostow. Originally published in *The Borderline Patient,* 1987, edited by J. Grotstein, M. Solomon, and J. Lang, vol. 1, pp. 137–162. Copyright © 1987 by The Analytic Press. Reprinted by permission of The Analytic Press and the author.

Chapter 10: "On Beginning with Patients Who Require Medication," by Mortimer Ostow. Originally published in *On Beginning an Analysis,* edited by Theodore J. Jacobs and Arnold Rothstein, 1990, pp. 201–227. Copyright© 1990 by International Universities Press. Reprinted by permission of International Universities Press and the author.

Chapter 11: "Combining Drugs and Psychotherapy in the Treatment of Depression," by Gerald L. Klerman. Originally published in *Drugs in Combination with Other Therapies,* edited by Milton Greenblatt, 1975, pp. 67–81. Copyright © 1975 by Psychological Corporation. Reprinted by permission of Myrna Weissman, Psychological Corporation, and the Group for the Advancement of Psychiatry (GAP).

Chapter 12: "Countertransference Aspects of Pharmacotherapy in the Treatment of Schizophrenia," by Steven T. Levy. Originally published in the *International Journal of Psychoanalytic Psychotherapy,* 1977, vol. 6, pp. 15–30. Copyright © 1977 by Jason Aronson Inc. Reprinted by permission of Jason Aronson Inc. and the author.

Chapter 13: "Psychotherapy and Pharmacotherapy: The Challenge of Integration," by Paul M. Goldhamer. Originally published in the *Canadian Journal of Psychiatry,* 1983, vol. 28, pp. 173–177. Copyright © 1983 by the *Canadian Journal of Psychiatry.* Reprinted by permission of the *Canadian Journal of Psychiatry* and the author.

Chapter 14: "Medication Consultation and Split Treatment during Psychotherapy," by David A. Kahn. Originally published in *Journal of the American*

Index